A Core Curriculum for Diabetes Education

SECOND EDITION

Published by the
**AMERICAN ASSOCIATION OF
DIABETES EDUCATORS AND THE
AADE EDUCATION AND RESEARCH FOUNDATION**

Virginia Peragallo-Dittko, RN, MA, CDE, Editor
Kathryn Godley, RN, MS, CDE, Associate Editor
Julie Meyer, RN, MSN, FAAN, CDE, Associate Editor

Managing Editor: Janet Schwarz
Medical Editors: Karen Moline
Martha Urban
Proofreader: Candace Kurinsky
Compositor: Sherry Meyer
Printer: Port City Press

A Core Curriculum for Diabetes Education, 2nd Edition
Published by the American Association of Diabetes Educators and the AADE Education and Research Foundation.

© 1993, American Association of Diabetes Educators, Chicago, Illinois.

First edition published under the title *Diabetes Education: A Core Curriculum for Health Professionals*
© 1988, American Association of Diabetes Educators.

Printed and bound in the United States of America.

TABLE OF CONTENTS

MANAGEMENT

SPECIAL POPULATIONS

COMPLICATIONS

RESEARCH

ACKNOWLEDGEMENTS

This book is greater than the sum of its parts because of the multidisciplinary professionals who are passionate about the education and care of people with diabetes.

Many experts have contributed to the success of *A Core Curriculum for Diabetes Education - Second Edition*. The chapter authors offered both their content expertise and their commitment to revisions, queries and schedules. For some, this is their first appearance as an author or co-author of a chapter. Many others were contributors to the first edition and greeted the task of modifying their original work with professionalism. We are indebted to each of the reviewers who took the role seriously and challenged to editors and authors through comments and literature searches.

We thank the readers of the first edition whose observations and suggestions were incorporated into the second edition. We remain grateful to the editorial team, advisory board and contributors of the first edition who were pioneers in presenting diabetes educators with a core curriculum for our specialty practice.

We would also like to recognize the work and support of those behind the scenes. We are grateful to the Board of Directors of the American Association of Diabetes Educators, and the AADE Education and Research Foundation for their trust and support, to our Advisors for their role in assuring multidisciplinary representation and input, to Kate Doyle for her encouragement and dedication to excellence, to Jan Schwarz for her skill in publishing and cheerful understanding that all of us involved in this project have "day jobs," to Martha Urban, Karen Moline and Candace Kurinsky for their skillful editing, to Sherry Meyer for her meticulous attention to detail in typesetting, to Marina Moore for her secretarial skill and dependability, to the Medical Librarians at Winthrop-University Hospital and all libraries for helping us prepare a scholarly, well documented text and to our spouses, families, friends and colleagues at work who faithfully encouraged us and are proud of our endeavors.

This book is dedicated to the people we serve who together with the health professionals involved in this project have taught us so much about diabetes, ourselves and the future of diabetes education.

INTRODUCTION

The first edition of *Diabetes Education: A Core Curriculum for Health Professionals* was published in 1988. It stands as the first publication documenting the core knowledge required by diabetes educators. The second edition has emerged as more than a revision because the challenge of caring for the patient with diabetes has continued to be stimulated by a rapidly expanding knowledge base. Since the publication of the first edition, issues that were accepted as dogma have been revisited, controversies have emerged and outdated approaches have been eliminated. The challenges that guided the development of the second edition were:

- to revise and update the content;
- to identify and present the diversified knowledge required as core for diabetes educators;
- to highlight the multidisciplinary nature of diabetes management;
- to identify that knowledge of learning theory plus diabetes management distinguishes the specialty practice of diabetes education.

Readers of both editions will find similarities and changes. Similarities include the narrative outline format and highly regarded case studies. The most notable differences are the revision of the content of the text and the chapters' order of appearance. To underscore the importance of learning theory as core knowledge for diabetes educators, the first chapter of the book is Educational Principles and Strategies. These principles are woven into each chapter and are given prominence at the end of the chapters under the heading Key Educational Considerations. This unique format was designed to highlight the anecdotal, often undocumented information that answers the question, "How would you teach this content?"

The section on Psychosocial Issues follows Education as these issues help us understand the experience of diabetes and how it impacts effective educational strategies. Nutrition, a cornerstone of diabetes management, is integrated throughout, just as nutrition related issues are found in practice. Nutrition is also covered in a separate chapter reflecting its importance.

New chapters have been added to focus on the educational needs of special populations such as children and adolescents, elderly people and visually impaired persons. Chapters devoted to cultural sensitivity and teaching patients with low literacy skills reinforce the diversity of practice of diabetes educators.

The last chapter brings the reader forward to examine research, the basis of our practice. Critical appraisal of published research is considered core knowledge for diabetes educators. The chapter deviates to a colloquial style inviting the reader to study the research process.

Because this book represents the *core* curriculum, not advanced practice, every important reference or fact could not be captured in this edition. Careful documentation and lists of suggested readings are included to guide the reader toward further study. The reviewers were invaluable in preventing regionalization of information. Many times the reader will be introduced to the diversity of approaches to the same topic. Lay literature is often included in the suggested readings as many educators have found the style useful in translating scientific information to a lay audience. The content of this book was written to be consistent with the Scope of Practice for Diabetes Educators,[1] the Standards of Practice for Diabetes Educators,[1] and the National Standards for Diabetes Patient Education Programs.[2] We have attempted to maintain a consistent format throughout the text to provide a framework for teaching and studying. Topics have been cross referenced to decrease repetition and tables have been used to more concisely present important material.

The intended use of this book is to provide a reference for diabetes educators in both novice and advanced practice.

Health professionals working in the inpatient setting on general patient care units, in specialized diabetes units, or in outpatient settings may use the text as a reference for developing individualized plans of care for patients with diabetes. Specialists in diabetes education may use the text for educational programming with different audiences such as health professionals, patients and families or community groups. The case examples can be particularly helpful in inviting active participation with staff education. *A Core Curriculum for Diabetes Education* can be used by faculty as a basis for curriculum development, for quality improvement indices, and for justification of personnel and policy changes.

This book may also be used as one of many study guides for the certification examination for diabetes educators. *However, examination questions are not necessarily written from the content in this book. Consequently, use of this book alone will not ensure success in passing the examination.* In conjunction with the AADE video series, "Diabetes Education: A Video Course Review," the core curriculum can reinforce the content that you know and identify areas that require further study.

Your feedback will ensure that subsequent editions exceed the former in promoting state of the art diabetes education. Please share your suggestions for the next edition.

We owe the profession the best and most valid information we can provide. To offer less is to undermine the very purpose that publication is supposed to serve. Ultimately, that purpose is tied to better care for the people for whom we care.[3]

Thank you for the privilege of serving as editor of the second edition.

Virginia Peragallo-Dittko, RN, MA, CDE

REFERENCES

1.   The scope of practice and standards of practice for diabetes educators. Diab Educ 1992;18:52-56.

2.   National standards for diabetes patient education and American Diabetes Association review criteria. Diabetes Care 1986;9:XXXVI-XL.

3.   Down FS. Accuracy counts too. Nur Res 1990;39(3):131.

ADVISORS

Special Advisor: Diana W. Guthrie, RN, PhD, FAAN, CDE

Dee A. Deakins, RN, MS, CDE
Allan L. Drash, MD
Gary M. Ingersoll, PhD
Karmeen Kulkarni, RN, MS, CDE
Hope S. Warshaw, MMSc, RD, CDE
Peggy Yarborough, RPh, MS, CDE, FAPP

EDITORS

Virginia Peragallo-Dittko, RN, MA, CDE, Editor
Winthrop-University Hospital
Diabetes Education Center
Mineola, New York

Kathryn Godley, RN, MS, CDE, Associate Editor
Diabetes Control Program
New York State Department of Health
Albany, New York

Julie Meyer, RN, MSN, FAAN, CDE, Associate Editor
University of Texas
Health Science Center
School of Nursing
San Antonio, Texas

The Scope of Practice for Diabetes Educators and the Standards of Practice for Diabetes Educators

Developed under the aegis of a multidisciplinary task force of the American Association of Diabetes Educators

---

The American Association of Diabetes Educators (AADE) was established in 1974 as a multidisciplinary organization of health professionals who teach people with diabetes. Since then the Association has achieved many milestones in the professional specialty, including the development of a Certification Program for Diabetes Educators, a Core Curriculum for Diabetes Education, and accreditation as a provider and approver of continuing education in nursing.

Mission of the Association

As a professional organization, AADE has a responsibility to foster high professional standards of diabetes education and practice, and to identify for the consumer competencies and excellence in practice. The Association's purpose is embodied in the following mission statement adopted by the AADE Board of Directors:

> *The American Association of Diabetes Educators is dedicated to advancing the role of the diabetes educator and improving the quality of diabetes education and care.*

In keeping with this mission, the AADE has developed the Scope of Practice for Diabetes Educators and the Standards of Practice for Diabetes Educators to provide guidelines for achieving excellence and improving the quality of diabetes patient education and care.

These documents represent the combined expertise and experience of a multidisciplinary task force of health professionals involved in diabetes education and an extensive review process embracing a broad spectrum of practice areas. Together the Scope of Practice and the Standards of

Practice provide a framework for health professionals who teach people with diabetes.

By also providing a consistent point of reference, the Standards of Practice may be used as the basis for the development of evaluation tools, quality assurance programs, orientation procedures, and performance appraisal systems.

Additionally they support the specialty by:

- Stimulating the process of peer review;
- Promoting documentation of the benefits and outcomes of the diabetes education experience;
- Encouraging research to validate practice and lead toward improved quality of patient education.

The Scope of Practice for Diabetes Educators and the Standards of Practice for Diabetes Educators are designed to complement the National Standards and Recognition for Diabetes Patient Education Programs, the Core Curriculum for Diabetes Patient Education, and the Certification Program for Diabetes Educators. Thus these documents will further enhance and promote quality diabetes education for people with diabetes.

SCOPE OF PRACTICE FOR DIABETES EDUCATORS

Purpose

The American Association of Diabetes Educators developed this Scope of Practice to delineate: (1) selected beliefs and definitions related to the practice of diabetes education, and (2) the dimensions of this practice in relation to other components of care for persons with diabetes, their families, and appropriate support systems. This Scope of Practice describes the present practice of diabetes education by multidisciplinary health care professionals.

Beliefs and Definitions

Living well with diabetes requires a positive psychosocial adaptation to, and the effective self-management of, the disease. To achieve effective self-management of diabetes mellitus, a patient must learn the body of knowledge, attitudes, and self-management skills related to the control of this chronic disease. *Diabetes education* is defined as the teaching and the learning of this body of knowledge and skills, with the ultimate goal being to promote the behavior changes necessary for optimal health outcomes, psychosocial adaptation, and quality of life. This planned educational experience is most effectively provided by qualified diabetes educators. Diabetes education is considered a therapeutic modality, and it is integral to the care of these patients.

A *diabetes educator* is defined as a health care professional who has mastered the core of knowledge and skill in the biological and social sciences, communication and counseling, and education, and who has experience in the care of patients with diabetes. The role of the diabetes educator can be assumed by various health care professionals, including but not limited to : registered dietitians, registered nurses, physicians, pharmacists, social workers, podiatrists, and exercise physiologists. A goal for all diabetes educators should be to meet the academic, professional, and experiential requirements to become a certified diabetes educator (CDE).

Dimensions of Practice

The role of the diabetes educator is multidimensional, with boundaries for accountability that interface with other members of the health care team. This role involves the education of patients, their families, and appropriate support systems, as well as other health care professionals who do not specialize in diabetes management, and the public. While a multidisciplinary team approach is the preferred delivery system for diabetes education, this specialty practice can occur successfully in a wide variety of settings and formats.

The primary area of responsibility for diabetes educators is the education of patients, their families, and appropriate support systems about diabetes self-management and related issues. The content of this educational experience should include, but not be limited to, the following topics:

- Pathophysiology of diabetes mellitus
- Nutrition management and diet
- Pharmacologic interventions
- Exercise and activity
- Self-monitoring for glycemic control
- Prevention and management of acute and chronic complications
- Psychosocial adjustment
- Problem-solving skills
- Stress management
- Use of the health care delivery system

The diabetes educator should present the necessary information, using established principles of teaching-learning theory and life-style counseling. The instruction is individualized for persons of all ages, incorporating their cultural preferences, health beliefs, and preferred learning styles, when feasible. The diabetes educator should perform the following:

- Assessment of educational needs
- Planning of the teaching-learning process
- Implementation of the educational plan

- Documentation of the process
- Evaluation based on outcome criteria

The Scope of Practice of a diabetes educator *should intersect* with the practice of other members of the health care team. The diabetes educator should appreciate the impact of acute or chronic problems on patients' health behaviors and on the teaching-learning process. Such appreciation is essential for the development of a comprehensive plan for continuing education and cost-effective, managed care.

Members of the various health care professions who practice diabetes education bring their particular focus to the educational process. This phenomenon widens or narrows the Scope of Practice for individual educators, as is appropriate within the boundaries of each health profession which may be regulated by national or state agencies or accrediting bodies. Other roles for the diabetes educator may involve consultation with other health care providers or agencies and research in diabetes management and education.

Diabetes education occurs in a variety of settings, depending on the needs of the patient, the practice of the educator, and the local environment. Inpatient and outpatient settings, as well as home settings, are used effectively for both individual and group education. Diabetes education should be a planned, individualized, and evaluated activity wherever it occurs.

Summary

This Scope of Practice incorporates definitions of *diabetes educator* and *diabetes education*, while providing statements of beliefs regarding the educational process inherent in this practice. The scope of practice of a diabetes educator has changing dimensions because of the multidisciplinary nature of the health care professionals who provide it. The primary role of a diabetes educator is to provide an educational experience for patients, their families, and appropriate support systems to learn the effective management of diabetes. Thus, the Scope of Practice delineates the multifaceted role and responsibilities of the health care professional who engages in this teaching-learning process. This Scope of Practice does not constitute an exhaustive description of diabetes education as a specialty practice because there are various interpretations of the role of the diabetes educator in a health care team.

STANDARDS OF PRACTICE FOR DIABETES EDUCATORS

Purpose

This document has been developed by the American Association of Diabetes Educators to: (1) provide standards for a nationally acceptable level of practice for diabetes educators; and (2) assure quality in the professional practice of diabetes education. The individual diabetes educator is responsible for adhering to these Standards.

The Standards of Practice will provide:

1. Diabetes educators with:
   - Direction to assess and improve the quality of their practice;
   - a framework within which to practice.

2. Patients with:
   - a means of assessing the quality of diabetes education services provided;
   - a basis for forming expectations of the diabetes education experience.

3. Health care professionals who do not specialize in diabetes management with a means of:
   - understanding the role of the diabetes educator;
   - assessing the quality of diabetes education services provided;
   - understanding diabetes education as an integral component of diabetes patient care.

4. Insurers, government agencies, industry, and the general public with:
   - a description of the specialized educational services provided by a diabetes educator;
   - information about the benefits of diabetes education in developing self-management skills;

- an awareness of the importance of diabetes education in improving the quality of life for persons with diabetes.

Standards of Education

Standard I. Assessment

The diabetes educator should conduct a thorough, individualized needs assessment with the participation of the patient, family, or support systems, when appropriate, prior to the development of the education plan and intervention.

Practice Guidelines

The needs assessment should include information from the patient on the following:

1. Health history;
2. Medical history;
3. Previous use of medication;
4. Diet history;
5. Current mental health status;
6. Use of health care delivery systems;
7. Life-style practices such as occupation, vocation, education, financial status, social, cultural, and religious practices;
8. Physical and psychological factors including age, mobility, visual acuity, hearing, manual dexterity, alertness, attention span, and ability to concentrate;
9. Barriers to learning such as education, literacy levels, perceived learning needs, motivation to learn, and attitudes;
10. Family and social supports;
11. Previous diabetes education, actual knowledge, and skills.

Standard II. Use of Resources

The diabetes educator should strive to create an educational setting conducive to learning, with adequate resources to facilitate the learning process.

Practice Guidelines

Appropriate resources for effective teaching should include:

1. A teaching environment that:
    a) provides privacy, safety, and accessibility;
    b) includes ample teaching and storage space, adequate furniture, lighting, and ventilation.
2. A variety of teaching materials and audiovisual teaching aids to meet the individual patient's needs.
3. Adequate staffing for the needs of the patient population.

Standard III. Planning

The written educational plan should be developed from information obtained from the needs assessment and based on the components of the educational process: assessment, planning, implementation, and evaluation. The plan is coordinated among diabetes health team members, including the patient with diabetes, family, and support system.

Practice Guidelines

The written educational plan should include the following:

1. Goals of the educational intervention;
2. Measurable, behaviorally stated learner objectives;
3. Content outline;
4. Instructional methods, including discussion, demonstration, role playing, simulations;
5. Learner outcomes based on the evaluation process.

Standard IV. Implementation

The diabetes educator should provide individualized education based on a progression from basic survival skills to advanced information for daily self-management.

Practice Guidelines

Considerations in developing the individualized education plan should include:

1. The need for diabetes education to be lifelong because of the chronicity of the condition;
2. The need for a dynamic education plan that will reflect the inevitable changes in life-style;
3. Survival skills that include safe practices of medication administration, meal planning, self-monitoring for glycemic control, and recognition of when to access professional assistance for emergencies;
4. Advanced information for daily self-management practices that may include prevention and management of chronic complications, problem-solving skills, exercise, psychosocial adjustment, stress management, and travel situations.

Standard V. Documentation

The diabetes educator should completely and accurately document the educational experience.

Practice Guidelines

Accurate documentation:

1. Establishes a record to substantiate the provision of education;
2. Contributes information for retrospective, concurrent, and prospective reviews;
3. Provides data for scientific and economic analysis;
4. Serves as a resource for continuity of care;
5. Aids in planning subsequent diabetes education.

Standard VI. Evaluation and Outcome

The diabetes educator should participate in at least an annual review of the quality and outcome of the education process.

Practice Guidelines

Evaluation of the diabetes education process should:

1. Occur periodically and as part of a comprehensive quality assurance program;
2. Be consistent with the National Standards for Diabetes Patient Education Programs as established by the National Diabetes Advisory Board;
3. Determine the impact of education on patients, institutions, and the community;
4. Use outcome measures such as:
    a) cost-effectiveness;
    b) changes in use of health care delivery systems, eg, emergency room visits, hospital length of stay;
    c) changes in knowledge and attitudes;
    d) changes in physiological measures, eg, glycosylated hemoglobin values, weight.

Standards of Professional Practice

Standard VII. Multidisciplinary Collaboration

The diabetes educator should collaborate with the multidisciplinary team of health care professionals and integrate their knowledge and skills to provide a comprehensive educational experience.

Practice Guidelines

The multidisciplinary education team should:

1. Include, but not be limited to, the registered nurse, registered dietitian, physician, pharmacist, social worker, psychologist, exercise physiologist, and podiatrist;
2. Observe professional practice boundaries in light of each member's discipline;
3. Have a responsibility to:

a)   share with team members information from individual patient assessments;

b)   prioritize learning needs;

c)   make education relevant to medical management;

d)   promote delivery of consistent information from various team members to patients;

e)   hold patient management conferences on a regular basis;

f)   provide referrals for appropriate follow-up.

Standard VIII. Professional Development

The diabetes educator should assume responsibility for professional development and pursue continuing education to acquire current knowledge and skills.

Practice Guidelines

The diabetes educator should:

1.   Incorporate into practice the generally accepted new techniques and knowledge acquired through continuing education;
2.   Deliver education based on a continuous process of review and evaluation of scientific theory, clinical and educational research;
3.   Pursue professional education based on progression from basic through advanced curriculum;
4.   Strive to meet the academic, professional, and experiential requirements to become a certified diabetes educator (CDE).

Standard IX. Professional Accountability

The diabetes educator should accept responsibility for self-assessment of performance and peer review to assure the delivery of high quality diabetes education.

Practice Guidelines

The diabetes educator should:

1. Participate in an annual systematic review and evaluation of practice;
2. Incorporate into practice the appropriate changes based on the results of self-evaluation, peer review, and patients' evaluations.

Standard X. Ethics

The diabetes educator should respect and uphold the basic human rights of all persons.

Practice Guidelines

The diabetes educator should:

1. Maintain confidentiality of appropriate information, and allow freedom of expression, decision making, and action;
2. Demonstrate concern for personal dignity;
3. Consider that a person with diabetes balances many daily tasks for management which may require a gradual incorporation into life-style;
4. Appreciate the impact of diabetes management on daily living so that reasonable expectations are established with the patient;
5. Display honesty, warmth, and openness to reinforce positive behavior change.

AUTHORS

Robert M. Anderson, EdD
The University of Michigan, DRTC
Ann Arbor, Michigan
Educational Principles and Strategies

Jean Betschart, RN, MN, CDE
Children's Hospital of Pittsburgh
Pittsburgh, Pennsylvania
Childhood and Adolescence

Elaine J. Boswell, MSN
Vanderbilt DRTC
Nashville, Tennessee
Managing Diabetes During Intercurrent Illness

R. Keith Campbell, RPH, FAPP, MBA, CDE
Washington State University
College of Pharmacy
Spokane, Washington
Pharmacologic Therapies

Belinda P. Childs, RN, CDE
Mid-American Diabetes Association
Wichita, Kansas
Perioperative Issues

Linda Cohen, RN, CDE
State University Hospital of New York
Health Science Center
Brooklyn, New York
Nephropathy

Mayer B. Davidson, MD
Cedars-Sinai Medical Center
Division of Endocrinology
Los Angeles, California
Hyperglycemia

James Fain, RN, PhD, FAAN
Yale University School of Nursing
New Haven, Connecticut
Teaching Patients with Low Literacy Skills

Marion J. Franz, MS, RD, CDE
International Diabetes Center
Minneapolis, Minnesota
Nutrition

Martha Mitchell Funnel, MS, RN, CDE
University of Michigan
Ann Arbor, Michigan
Neuropathy

Claudia Graham, PhD, MPH, CDE
Long Beach, California
Exercise

Douglas Greene, MD
University of Michigan
Ann Arbor, Michigan
Neuropathy

Diana Guthrie, PhD, RN, CDE
University of Kansas School of Medicine
Wichita, Kansas
Stress Management

Debra Haire-Joshu, PhD, RN
Diabetes Education Center
St. Louis, Missouri
Cultural Sensitivity in Diabetes Education

Deborah Hinnen Hentzen, RN, MN, CDE
Saint Joseph Medical Center
Wichita, Kansas
Monitoring and Management
Special Issues in Management

Lucy A. Levandoski, PAC
Washington University
St. Louis, Missouri
Hypoglycemia

Marvel Logan, RN, MSN, CDE, CST
Saint Joseph Medical Center
Wichita, Kansas
Lower Extremity Problems

Nelda Martinez, PhD, RN, CDE
San Antonio, Texas
Research: Continuing Education

Anne T. Nettles, RN, MS, CDE
University of Minnesota Hospital
Minneapolis, Minnesota
Diabetes in the Elderly

Virginia Peragallo-Dittko, RN, MA, CDE
Winthrop-University Hospital
Diabetes Education Center
Mineola, New York
*Adaptive Diabetes Education for Visually
Impaired Persons*

William W. Quick, MD, CDE
Midwest Diabetes Care Center
Kansas City, Missouri
Pathophysiology

Richard R. Rubin, PhD, CDE
Baltimore, Maryland
Behavioral Change

Stephanie Schwartz, MPh, RN, CDE
Kansas City, Missouri
Hyperglycemia

Catherine Stewart Sackett, RN
Glen Arm, Maryland
Eye Disease

Julio V. Santiago, MD
Washington University
St. Louis, Missouri
Hypoglycemia

Diana Speelman-Rhiley, MA, CDE
Saint Joseph Medical Center DRTC
Wichita, Kansas
Psychological Assessment and Support

Condit F. Steil, PharmD
Ashland, Kentucky
Pharmacologic Therapies

Frank Vinicor, MD
Center for Disease Control
Division of Diabetes Study
Atlanta, Georgia
Macrovascular Disease

Candace J. Wason, BSN, MS
Birmingham, Alabama
Pregnancy: Preconception to Postpartum

John R. White, PharmD
Washington State University
College of Pharmacy
Spokane, Washington
Pharmacologic Therapies

Neil H. White, MD, CDE
Washington University
St. Louis, Missouri
Hypoglycemia

Contributor
Teresa Scarpulla, RN
Birmingham, Alabama

REVIEWERS

Jo Ann Ahern, RN, BSN, CDE
Trial Coordinator of
the Diabetes Control
& Complications Trial
Yale-New Haven Hospital
New Haven, CT

Gary Arsham, MD, PhD
California Pacific
Medical Center
San Francisco, CA

Paul J. Beisswenger, MD
Associate Professor
of Medicine — Dartmouth
Medical School
Dartmouth Hitchcock
Medical Center
Lebanon, NH

George E. Bennett,
LCSW, ACSW, BCD
Founder/Director
Life Educators
Lexington, KY

Barbara H. Bodnar,
RN, BSN, CDE
Diabetes Nurse Consultant
Pennsylvania Department
of Health
Pittsburgh, PA

Peggy Bourgeois,
RN, MN, CNS, CDE
Director, Diabetes Center
Baton Rouge General
Medical Center
Baton Rouge, LA

Jeanne Bubb, MSW, ACSW
Diabetes Research
Social Worker
St. Louis Children's
Hospital
Washington University
St. Louis, MO

Madonna Carlson, RN, MEd
Program Coordinator
California Diabetes and
Pregnancy Program
San Diego, CA

Jerry D. Cavallerano,
OD, PhD
Staff Optometrist
Joslin Diabetes Center
W.P. Beetham Eye Institute
Boston, MA

Stephen Clement, MD, CDE
Chief, Diabetes Clinic,
Endocrinology Service
Walter Reed Army
Medical Center
Washington, DC

Sara E. Crawford,
RN, MSN, CDE
Diabetes Nurse Specialist
Alliant Health
System-Diabetes
Care Center
Louisville, KY

Ellen D. Davis, MS, RN, CDE
Diabetes Clinical
Nurse Specialist
Duke University
Medical Center
Chapel Hill, NC

Judy Davis, RN, BA, CDE
Director, Idaho Diabetes
Management Center
St. Alphonsus Regional
Medical Center
Boise, ID

Dee A. Deakins, RN, MS, CDE
Diabetes Specialist
Department of Veterans Affairs
Medical Center
Lexington, KY

Carolyn Dennis, MS, RD, CDE
Nutritionist
Lexington/Fayette County
Health Department
Lexington, KY

Elizabeth A. DeShetler,
MS, RD, CDE
Nutritionist
Diabetes Care Center
Riverside Methodist Hospitals
Columbus, OH

Allan Lee Drash, MD
Professor of Pediatrics
University of Pittsburgh
Children's Hospital
Pittsburgh, PA

Jacqueline D. Dudley, RN, CDE
Coordinator of Diabetes
Education Programs
Kilo Diabetes & Vascular
Research Foundation
St. Louis, MO

Samuel Engel, MD
Clinical Assistant Professor
 of Medicine
Albert Einstein College
 of Medicine
Bronx, NY

Ruth Farkas-Hirsch,
MS, RN, CDE
Diabetes Clinical Specialist
University of Washington
Diabetes Care Center
Seattle, WA

Janine Freeman, RD, CDE
Diabetes Nutrition Specialist
Georgia Center for Diabetes
Atlanta, GA

Martha M. Funnell,
MS, RN, CDE
Associate Director
Michigan Diabetes Research
 & Training Center
Ann Arbor, MI

James R. Gavin, III, MD, PhD
Senior Scientific Officer
Howard Hughes Medical Institute
Bethesda, MD

Beverly P. Giordano, RN, MS
Editor; former Pediatric
 Diabetes Clinical Specialist
Denver, CO

Frederick C. Goetz, MD
Professor of Medicine Emeritus
University of Minnesota
Medical School
Minneapolis, MN

Liz Grabowski,
MSN, CDE, ARNP
Diabetes Clinical
 Specialist/Owner
Diabetes Resource Center, Inc.
Louisville, KY

Diana W. Guthrie,
RN, PhD, FAAN, CDE
Professor
University of Kansas School
 of Medicine
Wichita, KS

Linda B. Haas, PhC, RN, CDE
Endocrinology Clinical
 Nurse Specialist
Veterans Affairs Medical Center
Seattle, WA

Broatch Haig, RD, CDE
Director Minnesota Diabetes
 in Youth Program
International Diabetes Center
Minneapolis, MN

Robert J. Hanisch, MA, CDE
Exercise Specialist
Diabetes Treatment Center
 at Columbia Hospital
Milwaukee, WI

Joyce L. Hayman,
RN, PhD, CDE
Program Manager, Diabetes
 Education Program
St. Joseph's Hospital
Tampa, FL

Marcia Hegstad,
RN, MN, CS, CDE
Clinical Nurse
 Specialist/Diabetes
Catherine McAuley
 Health System
Ann Arbor, MI

Joan M. Heins, MA, RD, CDE
Project Director
Center for Health
 Behavior Research
Washington University
St. Louis, MO

Joan Hill, RD, CDE
Director of Nutrition Services
Joslin Diabetes Center
Boston, MA

Irl B. Hirsch, MD
Assistant Professor of Medicine
University of Washington
Seattle, WA

Priscilla Hollandar, PhD, MD
International Diabetes Center
St. Louis Park, MN

Edward S. Horton, MD
Medical Director
Joslin Diabetes Center
Boston, MA

Cheryl C. Hunt,
MSEd, RN, CDE
Diabetes Nurse Specialist
The Diabetes Treatment
 Center at the Washington
 Hospital Center
Washington, DC

James B. Huy, BS, PHA
Supervisory Public
 Health Advisor
CDC/NIOSH
Morgantown, WV

Gary M, Ingersoll, PhD
Executive Associate Dean
 of Education
Professor of Counseling and
 Educational Psychology
Indiana University
Bloomington, IN

Donna L. Jornsay,
RN, BSN, CPNP, CDE
Clinical Coordinator
Diabetes and
 Pregnancy Program
Maternal-Fetal Medicine
North Shore University
 Hospital
Manhasset, NY

Aaron Kassoff, MD
Clinical Professor
 of Ophthalmology
Albany Medical College
Albany, NY

Karmeen Kulkarni,
RD, MS, CDE
Clinical Dietitian
Diabetes Health Center
Salt Lake City, UT

Steven Kurtz, PhD
Director of Child and
 Adolescent Services
Counseling Associates
 of Rockland
New City, NY

Matthew Leinung, MD
Assistant Professor
 of Medicine, Division
 of Endocrinology
Albany Medical College
Albany, NY

Marvin E. Levin, MD
Clinical Professor of Medicine
Washington University
 School of Medicine
St. Louis, MO

Deborah K. Lloyd, MSW
Clinical Social Worker
Children's Hospital of Pittsburgh
Pittsburgh, PA

Daniel Lorber, MD, FACP
Medical Director
Diabetes Control Foundation
Flushing, NY

Rachel B. Lyon, MS, RD, CDE
Consulting Nutritionist
Diabetes Control
 & Complications Trial
Massachusetts General Hospital
Diabetes Research Center
Boston, MA

Linda Marcuz, RN, CDE
Pilot Director - Rural Outreach
General Hospital
California Diabetes
 and Pregnancy Program
UCSF Medical Center
Eureka, CA

Margaret C. Marinelli,
MS, RD, CDE
Diabetes Nutritionist
Diabetes Education Center
Winthrop University Hospital
Mineola, NY

David G. Marrero, PhD
Director of Training
Diabetes Research
 & Training Center
Indiana University School
 of Medicine
Regerstriet Institute
Indianapolis, IN

Melinda Maryniuk, MEd, RD
Administrative Director
Joslin Diabetes Clinic
St. Barnabas Medical Center
West Orange, NJ

Barbara J. Maschak-Carey,
RNCS, MSN, CDE
Diabetes Clinical Nurse Specialist
Hospital of the University
 of Pennsylvania
Philadelphia, PA

Wylie L. McNabb, EdD
Assistant Professor of Medicine
The University of Chicago
Chicago, IL

Susan Rush Michael,
RN, MS, CDE
Assistant Professor of Nursing
University of Nevada-Las Vegas
Las Vegas, NV

Anne T. Nettles, MS, RN
Clinical Nurse Specialist, Diabetes
University of Minnesota Hospital
Minneapolis, MN

Cynthia A. Pasquarello,
RN, BS, CDE
Pediatric & Adolesent Diabetes
 Nurse Specialist
Joslin Diabetes Center
Boston, MA

Ruth Ann Petzinger,
MS, RN, CDE
Patient Education Coordinator
St. Peter's Medical Center
New Brunswick, NJ

James W. Pichert, PhD
Associate Professor of
 Medicine (Education)
Vanderbilt University School
 of Medicine
Nashville, TN

Margaret A. Powers,
 MS, RD
President
Powers and Associates
St. Paul, MN

Sandra Puczynski,
RN, MS, CDE
Project Director
Center for Nursing Research
Childrens Hospital
 of Pittsburgh
University of Pittsburgh
Pittsburgh, PA

Robert E. Ratner, MD, CDE
Director of Endocrinology
Washington Hospital Center
Washington, DC

Diane M. Reader, RD, CDE
Diabetes Nutrition Specialist
International Diabetes
 Center & Park Nicollet
 Medical Center
Minneapolis, MN

Linda S. Reyle,
RN, BSN, CDE
Diabetes Educator
Germantown, TN

Janice L. Roth,
RN, BSN, CDE
Manager, Diabetes
 Nurse Educator
Allenmore Hospital
 Diabetes Center
Tacoma, WA

Marita M. Sension,
RN, MS, CDE
Coordinator of Patient
 Education
Joslin Diabetes Center
Berwyn, IL

Connie Shella, RN, CDE
Pediatric Diabetes Educator
Joslin Diabetes Clinic
 at Methodist Hospital
Indianapolis, IN

Patricia D. Stenger, RN, CDE
Diabetes Coordinator
Diabetes and Nutrition Centers
Eastern Maine Medical Center
Bangor, ME

Cathie J. Stepien, MPH, RN
Community Health Educator
Michigan Diabetes Research
 and Training Center
Ann Arbor, MI

Frances Stracqualursi,
BSN, CDE
Nurse Educator Consultant
Indian Health Services
 Diabetes Program
Albuquerque, NM

Susan L. Thom, RD, LD, CDE
Partner and Clinical Specialist
Diabetes Associates
Cleveland, OH

Elizabeth A. Walker,
RN, DNSc, CDE
Assistant Professor,
 Department of Epidemiology and
 Social Medicine
Albert Einstein College
 of Medicine
Bronx, NY

Joseph A. Ward, MA, LPC
Medical Psychotherapist
San Antonio, TX

Elizabeth Warren-Boulton, RN
President
Diabetes Education
 Consulting Associates
Washington, DC

Hope S. Warshaw,
MMSc, RD, CDE
Nutrition Consultant
 /Freelance Writer
Hope Warshaw Associates
Atlanta, GA

Madelyn L. Wheeler,
MS, RD, CDE
Coordinator, Research Dietetics
Diabetes Research
 and Training Center
Indiana University Medical Center
Indianapolis, IN

Ann S. Williams, MSN, RN, CDE
Senior Diabetes Educator
Cleveland Sight Center
Cleveland, OH

Mary E. Wood, RN, MS, CDE
Diabetes Clinical Nurse Specialist
Dartmouth-Hitchcock
 Medical Center
Lebanon, NH

Peggy Yarborough,
RPh, MS, CDE, FAPP
Clinical Consultant
Pharmacy Department
Wilson Memorial Hospital
Wilson, NC

Education

I   EDUCATIONAL PRINCIPLES
    AND STRATEGIES   1

EDUCATION

I. EDUCATIONAL PRINCIPLES AND STRATEGIES

Some of the material in this chapter is also contained in Anderson RM, Funnell MM. Strategies for diabetes patient education: a review of fundamentals. In: Home PD, Marshall SM, Alberti KGMM, Krall LP, eds. The diabetes annual/7. Amsterdam, The Netherlands: Elsevier Science Publishing, 1993.

INTRODUCTION

Most of the sections in this core curriculum are concerned with the content of diabetes patient education programs, that is, the knowledge and skills to be acquired by patients. This section is concerned with the process of diabetes patient education. It focuses on the program design and the educational methods used to help patients learn about diabetes. How diabetes knowledge and skills are taught can have as much impact on patient outcomes as what is taught. The instructional design of a diabetes patient education program can affect patients' acquisition of knowledge and skills, their attitudes about diabetes, their motivation to practice appropriate diabetes self-care, their willingness and ability to change behavior, and their degree of psychosocial adjustment to diabetes. To be effective, diabetes educators need to be both knowledgeable about diabetes and skilled in teaching. This chapter will outline educational process issues relevant to diabetes patient education.

OBJECTIVES

On completion of this chapter, the learner will be able to:
- compare and contrast the compliance and empowerment approaches to diabetes patient education;
- discuss nine issues to consider when designing a diabetes patient education program;
- compare and contrast formative and summative evaluation;
- explain the rationale for employing a multidisciplinary team in diabetes education;
- list eight areas to consider when assessing an individual patient's needs and readiness to learn;
- describe four characteristics of adult learners;
- list 10 teaching and learning strategies used in diabetes patient education;
- describe seven techniques that can be used to enhance learning and decision making;
- explain the importance of follow-up diabetes patient education.

A. Approaches to Education

1. The compliance-based approach[1,2] to diabetes patient education is intended to improve patient adherence to the treatment recommendations of health care professionals. It is based on the assumption that health care professionals are diabetes care experts and that patients should, in most cases, comply with their recommendations regarding diabetes self-care. Patient education is seen as a means of influencing patients to follow treatment recommendations in order to improve their glucose control and prevent the short- and long-term complications of diabetes.

2. In the empowerment approach,[3,4] the primary purpose of diabetes patient education is to prepare patients to make informed decisions about their own diabetes care. This approach assumes that most patients with diabetes are responsible for making important and complex decisions while carrying out the daily treatment of their diabetes. The empowerment approach also assumes that because patients are the ones who experience the consequences of both having and treating diabetes, they have both the right and the responsibility to be the primary decision makers regarding their own daily diabetes care.

3. Very few educators will use one approach all the time to the exclusion of the other. Most educators will use some combination of the two approaches based on their own values and understanding of the purposes and methods of patient education as well as the needs of their patients. Patients will have varying needs and tolerance for autonomous decision making in their diabetes self-care based on a number of factors. For example, a newly diagnosed patient with diabetes may wish to have the majority of decisions made by the health care team until he or she becomes more familiar with the cost and benefits of various options in diabetes self-care.

B. Considerations in the Design of Patient Education Programs

1. Design an education program that fits your setting and your patients. The program and educational materials should be geared to the disease type, age, education, experience, needs, abilities, and cultural background of your patients.

2. Program philosophy is an important consideration. The program's educators should agree on whether they are comfortable with the compliance approach, the empowerment approach, or some other educational philosophy that expresses the values and sense of purpose shared among the program's educators. A written philosophy statement can be a very useful tool in helping develop and express the program's philosophy.

3. Designing a diabetes patient education program requires first selecting appropriate goals and objectives, and then determining the program's level(s) of comprehensiveness, ie, deciding what material to cover and in what depth.

    a) Diabetes patient education programs should have clear and realistic goals. These goals can be somewhat general in nature, such as "the program will prepare patients to make informed choices about their diabetes care goals and methods." Well-written goals will guide the formulation of the program's objectives.[5]

    b) The specific changes in patient behavior that will contribute to goal achievement should be expressed as behavioral objectives. For example, "using their own meter, patients will demonstrate the ability to assess their own blood glucose level with no errors." Objectives should be written in terms of observable and measurable behavior, and contain a criterion for acceptable performance.[6]

    c) Diabetes education programs should offer courses of study with different levels of comprehensiveness. Patients cannot, and should not, learn everything there is to know about diabetes in one course of study.

(1) The basic course should focus on the initial skills that a newly diagnosed patient must learn immediately to care for diabetes.

(2) Next, for patients who have had time to adapt to having diabetes, a more comprehensive course in the self-management of diabetes should be available.

(3) Finally, diabetes education for review, for lifestyle flexibility, and for special situations should be available (eg, instruction in insulin adjustment when traveling across time zones, and use of adaptive devices should visual changes occur).

4. Issues related to educational format are also an important design consideration. One-on-one teaching and group teaching both have costs and benefits that should be considered. Also, consider issues of when and where classes will be held and whether classes will be given for one type of patient (eg, insulin-dependent patients) only. Flexibility and adaptability are the keys to developing appropriate educational formats.

5. The design of a patient education program should reflect the needs and values of those groups of people (stakeholders) who have an investment in the program and its outcomes. Patients, referring physicians, hospital or clinical administrators, the patient's family, and the program's educators are all examples of program stakeholders. A program benefits from an advisory committee with representatives from each stakeholder group.

6. Availability of resources is an important design consideration. The availability of financial resources will have a significant impact on the design of the program. The availability of people to teach in the program is an equally important resource. It is also helpful to consider physical resources such as space, equipment, education materials, and so forth.

7. The makeup of the educational team (eg, nurse, dietitian, physician, psychologist, pharmacist, exercise physiologist) is

crucial to the design of a program and should be identified early in the planning process. Team teaching in a program has significant benefits, such as providing patients with multidisciplinary expertise. However, effective team teaching also requires a significant investment of time for planning and team meetings.

8. Another important issue is documentation and record keeping. Diabetes education programs should develop a system that allows for the most complete documentation possible of educational assessment, education, and follow-up. Such documentation may be required to meet standards, such as the National Standards for Diabetes Patient Education developed by the National Diabetes Advisory Board[7] and promulgated by the American Diabetes Association.

9. The design of diabetes patient education should take into account the National Standards for Diabetes Patient Education programs developed by the National Diabetes Advisory Board. These standards address important issues such as needs assessment, program planning and management, communication and coordination, patient access to teaching, the content of the educational curriculum, the qualifications of the instructor, the importance of follow-up education and program evaluation, and record keeping and documentation.

C. Program Evaluation

1. Formative evaluation,[8-10] also called process evaluation, involves collecting information about how well the program is functioning. Formative evaluation provides information that can be applied almost immediately to change the program and increase its effectiveness. Formative evaluation data are often gathered by having patients complete questionnaires about their reaction to the course content, physical and social environment, teaching, audio visual aids, and so forth.

2. Summative evaluation,[8-10] also called outcome evaluation, involves gathering and analyzing information to determine if the program achieved the outcomes that it intended to produce. Summative evaluation domains include knowledge, attitudes, self-care practices, and psychosocial adaptation. Some metabolic indices, such as blood glucose control and weight, are sometimes considered outcome measures by education programs. Educators should choose outcome measures that occur shortly after the end of the program, and outcomes that can be attributed to the program with a high degree of confidence.

D. Multidisciplinary Teams in Diabetes Education

1. A coordinated team approach is recommended in diabetes care because of the multidisciplinary nature of the treatment.[11] This recommendation is especially true for patient education in which learners must acquire knowledge and skills from a variety of disciplines.

2. Additional benefits of multidisciplinary teams include improved coordination of care and education, multiple reinforcement of the same educational objectives, and consistency of approach to treatment. For example, although a physician may not spend much time teaching, he or she can reinforce the importance of diabetes patient education and transmit other core messages to the patient, such as "diabetes is a serious disease."[12]

3. A program coordinator should be chosen to plan and coordinate the efforts of the educational team. This person should be responsible for scheduling team meetings and producing the agenda.

4. Team membership is crucial and should, whenever possible, include a registered dietitian, a physician, and a registered nurse as core team members. Other team members will vary, depending on need and availability. These could include a

psychologist, social worker, pharmacist, exercise physiologist, or podiatrist.

5. Team meetings can be used to share information gained from individual patient assessments (eg, nursing, nutrition, medical); to identify and assign priority to patients' learning needs; to plan, implement, and evaluate a patient education program; and to provide for patient referrals, follow-up care, and education.

E. Assessing Individual Patient Educational Needs and Readiness to Learn

1. The process of teaching and learning is generally divided into three domains — knowledge, psychomotor skills, and affective (or attitudinal) learning. Assessment should focus on these three domains as well. It is useful to assess a patient's attitudes[13] and health beliefs[14] about diabetes and its care.[15,16] Patients who think they have mild diabetes or are immune from complications are not very likely to be motivated to learn. It is also important to assess the patient's attitude about participating in the education program. For example, the educator could discuss the patient's learning goals by asking questions about what the patient hopes to get out of the education program and the patient's goals related to daily self-care.[3,17] The educator should also assess the patient's metabolic goals regarding blood glucose control, weight, and lipid levels.

   a) Patients' experience with diabetes, and/or other health problems, can shape their attitudes and affect their readiness to learn and apply diabetes self-care skills. For example, a patient who is admitted to the hospital for gallbladder surgery, or a patient who is newly diagnosed with an acute illness is likely to have a diminished readiness to learn about diabetes. Acutely ill (including hypoglycemic) patients should learn only basic survival skills until they feel well enough to be more active learners.

b) Families can have a significant impact on a patient's attitudes and readiness to learn by providing or withholding social support. Patients are more likely to have a positive attitude about learning about diabetes when family members are supportive and enthusiastic about diabetes education.[18]

2. Current level of self-care is another important area to assess.[17,19] An educator can glean important information about a patient's tolerance for complexity in the regimen and/or which self-care behaviors will be most difficult by assessing the patient's current self-care practices.

3. Patients' preferred style of learning can affect their willingness to participate in the education program and whether or not they will learn. Some patients prefer to read, others like to listen, and still others learn best in discussions. Ask patients how they prefer to acquire other (than diabetes) types of information, eg, from newspapers, TV, discussion with friends, and so forth. This information will provide clues about how to tailor the education to the patient's needs. Finally, everyone does not belong in a group; some patients require individualized instruction.

4. The psychological status of patients can affect their interest in learning about diabetes. Marked denial, depression, and anxiety can interfere with learning while low to moderate anxiety about diabetes can increase readiness to learn. Patients will also display various degrees of alertness and ability to concentrate on educational issues.

5. Severe stress can seriously impair a patient's ability and interest in learning about diabetes. Stress is a reaction to factors that force persons to adapt to situations that are perceived on some level as a threat to their well-being. For patients experiencing severe stress, patient education (with the possible exception of

basic survival skills) should be postponed (see Chapter III: Stress Management).

6.   Assess patients' sociocultural and religious milieus that can influence their interest and willingness to learn about and apply specific diabetes self-care recommendations. Diabetes patient education should be tailored to the cultural needs and perceptions of the patient.

7.   Literacy can be difficult to assess. Years of schooling completed only gives a clue to literacy. Educational and literacy levels can influence how patients learn, ie, reading versus listening or viewing illustrations, and the amount of complexity they can tolerate in an education program. Unfortunately, complexity is part of diabetes; the challenge lies in using this part of the assessment to direct learning and management issues (see Chapter XVIII: Teaching Patients with Low Literacy Skills).

8.   Other assessment areas include physical factors such as age, mobility, visual acuity, hearing loss, and dexterity. These factors can influence a patient's willingness and ability to learn and apply diabetes self-care skills.

F.   Characteristics of Adult Learners[20]

1.   Adults are usually self-directed and have to have a felt need to learn in order to participate fully in the educational process. It is not relevant that the educator feels the patient should learn something if the patient does not also perceive the need. Sometimes, however, the diabetes educator will have to help patients discover what they need to know. For example, if a patient is being started on insulin for the first time, there are certain safety issues that the educator must address. In this case, the educator may have to take a leadership role in pointing out to the patient certain crucial areas for diabetes education (eg, signs, symptoms, and treatment of hypoglycemia)

rather than wait for the patient to discover these educational needs on his or her own.

2. Adults tend to be problem-oriented learners rather than subject-oriented learners. Adults usually want to acquire information that will help them solve specific diabetes problems rather than complete a comprehensive study of the subject of diabetes.

3. Adults learn better when their own experience with diabetes is incorporated into diabetes education. This includes their past experiences and consideration of how they will apply their learning in the future.

4. Adults usually prefer to participate in the learning process actively rather than passively. Education programs should give patients an opportunity to ask questions, solve problems, share their own experiences, and otherwise be actively engaged in the educational process.

G. Teaching and Learning Strategies

1. A short lecture is useful for presenting information. Patients can participate in the learning process through listening and note taking. However, this kind of instruction provides a very passive learning experience for the patient. Because lectures are easy for teachers to plan and control, this method is sometimes overused.[21,22]

2. Discussion is a more participatory and active learning experience than a lecture. It allows patients to acquire information, to ask and answer questions, and to share feelings and personal experiences. Discussions cannot be planned and controlled as precisely as lectures; therefore, they require the educator to tolerate a certain amount of ambiguity. Furthermore, leading discussions effectively requires good interpersonal skills on the part of the educator.[19] For example,

a discussion leader must know how to gracefully interrupt a nonstop talker so that other members of the group will have a chance to speak.

3. Demonstration is useful for teaching psychomotor or social skills. After a skills demonstration, patients should be encouraged to practice skills they have seen demonstrated.[15] Finally, patients should be given the opportunity to demonstrate their skills to the educator and receive feedback. Teaching insulin injection and/or home blood glucose monitoring are the classic examples of when to use this teaching sequence.

4. Print material can provide information for individual study, reinforce previously presented information, and be a resource for reference and review. Print material should employ readable type (patients with vision loss may need large type) and be written at an appropriate reading level for the learner. Materials written at approximately the sixth- to eighth-grade level will meet the needs of most learners. The SMOG[23] formula and Fry[24] readability graph are two techniques that can be used to determine the reading level of written information. Clarity, nontechnical language, and good illustrations enhance the effectiveness of printed material. Printed material should not replace interaction with the educator (see Chapter XVIII: Teaching Patients with Low Literacy Skills).

5. Audiovisual (AV) aids such as slides, films, videotapes, food models, and overhead transparencies can enhance the presentation of information.[22,25] Varying the presentation by using audiovisual aids can help increase learner concentration and prevent boredom. Also, learning can be reinforced when the same concepts are presented through a variety of formats. Self-made audiovisual materials give the instructor the opportunity for flexibility and creativity. The use of AV media can be very helpful to patients who do not learn well by reading.

6. Role playing gives patients a chance to practice social skills, explore interpersonal (eg, family conflict) problems, discuss alternative solutions, and share feelings in a psychologically safe environment.[26,27] Role playing usually works best with a verbal group of learners who know and trust each other and the instructor. Effective role playing requires an instructor with good interpersonal and group process skills.

7. Games can make education more enjoyable and improve learner participation. Many board games (eg, Trivial Pursuit®) or television game shows (eg, Jeopardy®) can be adapted for diabetes patient education. Also, some games appropriate for diabetes education are produced commercially.

8. Computers are now being used in diabetes education. Patients who are amenable to using computers may find computerized clinical problems and simulations a useful mechanism for testing and increasing their knowledge and improving their problem-solving skills.[28]

9. Patient examples provide a psychologically safe and useful way for learners to explore problems related to having diabetes and to discuss solutions. Patient examples can be written to meet the needs of different types of learners and to address a variety of learning domains (eg, knowledge, self-care behavior or attitudes).[26,27]

10. Affective exercises[26,27] are techniques for helping patients express, explore, and change feelings and personal values related to having diabetes. Affective exercises can include some of the techniques described above, such as discussion and role playing, or they can employ activities designed specifically to elicit an affective response. Existing books on values clarification[28] and human relations training[29] provide many techniques that can be adapted for diabetes education.

H. Techniques to Enhance Learning and Decision Making

1. Most diabetes educators desire to have their patients be motivated, involved, responsible, and committed learners. Diabetes education is much more rewarding and enjoyable for both the educator and the patient when the patient is an active and committed learner. The techniques listed below can enhance the involvement and learning of most patients.

   a) Learning is enhanced when it is related to what the learner already knows. The educator should fit what is being taught into the patient's existing frame of reference.[26,27]

   b) Learning is improved when patients have confidence (self-efficacy) in their ability to actually perform the behavior being taught. Educators should continually reinforce the idea that the patient is a person who can master diabetes self-care skills. This process is enhanced when diabetes patient education is structured as a series of carefully planned "success" experiences.

   c) Practice and rehearsal increase the retention of knowledge and skills. Patients should be given opportunities to practice both psychomotor and social skills (eg, asking family members for their support when following a diet).

   d) Learning is enhanced by feedback. Patients should be given feedback on how well they are acquiring knowledge and skills. Continued learning can be encouraged by making patients aware of their incremental progress.

   e) Learning is reinforced and retained when it can be applied immediately and repeatedly. Patients will retain knowledge and skills longer if they have opportunities for frequent application. For example, having non-insulin-requiring patients sit through a class on insulin injection because they "might have to go on insulin someday" is unlikely to produce any important or lasting learning.

   f) Educators will occasionally need to adjust the pace at which they teach to accommodate variations in the patient's ability to absorb and retain information. Patients do not always learn at a constant rate. Periodic plateaus in learning can result from changes in mood, stress level, or health status.

g) Knowledge and skills need to be reviewed. People forget much of what they have learned as time passes. Core diabetes knowledge and skills should be reviewed and updated on a regular basis.

I. Follow-Up Learning Opportunities

1. Learning should be ongoing. One of the most serious impediments to effective diabetes education is the notion that diabetes patient education is a one-time event. Patients change, their situations change, their diabetes changes; therefore, new learning needs arise. Also, patient education can provide the emotional support and behavioral reinforcement necessary for good diabetes self-care. To be most effective, patient education should be thought of as an ongoing process (similar to medical care) that plays a role in diabetes care for as long as the patient lives.

2. Educators should look for opportunities to provide continuing education to their patients. These opportunities include interactions with patients during ongoing diabetes care, such as a return visit to the physician's office or clinic. Educators can also offer courses that are promoted as diabetes updates or refresher courses for patients who have already been through basic education. Support groups, periodic health appraisals and screenings, and annual meetings of affiliates and chapters of the American Diabetes Association also provide opportunities for follow-up diabetes education.

REFERENCES

1. Raymond MW. Teaching toward compliance. Diabetes Educ 1984;10:42-44.

2. Resler MM. Teaching strategies that promote adherence. Nurs Clin North Am 1983;18:799-811.

3. Funnell MM, Anderson RM, Arnold MS, et al. Empowerment: an idea whose time has come in diabetes education. Diabetes Educ 1991;17:37-41.

4. Strowig S. Patient education: a model for autonomous decision-making and deliberate action in diabetes self-management. Med Clin North Am 1982;66:1293-1307.

5. Goals for diabetes education. Alexandria, Va: American Diabetes Association, 1986.

6. Mager RF. Preparing instructional objectives. Belmont, Calif: Fearon Publishers, 1975.

7. American Diabetes Association. National standards for diabetes patient education and American Diabetes Association Review Criteria. Diabetes Care 1986;9(4):36-50.

8. Haire-Joshu D. The process of evaluation in diabetes education. In: Haire-Joshu D, ed. Management of diabetes mellitus. St. Louis: CV Mosby, 1992:593-612.

9. Gronlund NE. Measurement and evaluation in teaching. 6th ed. New York: Macmillan, 1990.

10. Mehrens WA, Lehmann IJ. Measurement and evaluation in education and psychology. 3rd ed. New York: Holt, Rinehart & Winston, 1984.

11. Anderson RM. The team approach to diabetes: an idea whose time has come. Occupa Health Nurs, 1982;30:13-14.

12. Anderson RM, Funnell MM. The role of the physician in patient education. Practical Diabetol 1990;9:10-12.

13. Anderson RM, Donnelly MB, Dedrick RF. Measuring the attitudes of patients towards diabetes and its treatment. Patient Educ Couns 1990;16:231-45.

14. Becker MH, Janz NK. The health belief model applied to understanding diabetes regimen adherence. Diabetes Educ 1985;11:41-47.

15. Beeney LJ, Dunn SM. Knowledge improvement and metabolic control in diabetes education: approaching the limits? Patient Educ Couns 1990;16:217-29.

16. Funnell MM, Merritt JH. Diabetes mellitus and the older adult. In: Haire-Joshu D, ed. Management of diabetes mellitus. St. Louis: CV Mosby, 1992:505-59.

17. Haire-Joshu D. Promoting behavior change: teaching/learning strategies. In: Haire-Joshu D, ed. Management of diabetes mellitus. St. Louis: CV Mosby, 1992:556-90.

18. Fain JA, D'Eramo-Melkus G. Diabetes mellitus in young and middle adulthood. In: Haire-Joshu D, ed. Management of diabetes mellitus. St. Louis: CV Mosby, 1992:480-502.

19. Davis WK, Hull AL, Boutaugh ML. Factors affecting the educational diagnosis of diabetic patients. Diabetes Care 1981;4:275-78.

20. Knowles M. The modern practice of adult education. Chicago: Follett, 1980.

21. Padgett D, Mumford E, Hynes M, Carter R. Meta-analysis of the effects of educational and psychosocial interventions in the management of diabetes mellitus. J Clin Epidemiol 1988;41:1007-30.

22. Funnell MM, Donnelly MB, Anderson RM, Johnson PD, Oh MS. Perceived effectiveness, cost, and availability of patient education methods and materials. Diabetes Educ 1992;18:139-45.

23. McLaughlin G. SMOG grading — a new readability formula. J Reading, 1969;12:639-46.

24. Fry E. Fry's readability graph: clarification, validity and extension to level 17. J Reading, 1977; 21:242-52.

25. Bowbeer MM, Hiss RG. Use of educational resources in diabetes patient education [Letter]. Diabetes Educ 1990;16:15.

26. Anderson RM. The personal meaning of diabetes: implications for behavior and education, or kicking the bucket theory. Diabetic Med 1986;3:85-89.

27. Anderson RM, Nowacek GW, Richards F. Influencing the personal meaning of diabetes: research and practice. Diabetes Educ 1988;14:297-302.

28. Simon S, Howe L, Kirschenbaum H: Values clarification. New York: Hart Publishing Co, 1972.

29. Pfeiffer JW, ed. Developing human resources. Annuals 1-22. San Diego: University Associates, 1971-1993. (Pfeiffer JW, ed. Series in human resources development).

SELF-REVIEW QUESTIONS

If you are unsure of the answers to the following questions, please review the materials.

1. Compare and contrast the two educational philosophies (compliance and empowerment approaches) described in the beginning of the chapter.

2. If you had time to ask a patient only three or four questions when assessing educational needs and readiness to learn, which questions would you ask and why?

3. If you were asked to design a patient education program, what would you do first and why?

4. When designing a patient education program, whose input would you seek and why?

5. How would you decide what to evaluate in your patient education program?

6. Which characteristics of adult learners appear most relevant for diabetes patient education?

7. Describe the teaching/learning strategies that you think are most useful in diabetes patient education.

8. Describe the teaching/learning strategies that you think are least useful in diabetes patient education.

9. Describe four techniques that you believe could enhance the learning of patients.

10. If you had to justify the team approach in diabetes education to your supervisors, what would you say?

11. What would you say to a patient to reinforce the idea that diabetes patient education needs to be ongoing?

CASE EXAMPLE 1

JL is a dietitian who has recently finished her master's degree and a 1-year internship. She has been hired to be a diabetes educator at an 800-bed urban hospital in Texas. She will overlap for 6 months with the experienced dietitian who is currently teaching the nutrition component of the diabetes education program. JL is confident that she will know enough about diabetes and nutrition to teach the classes when she takes over in 6 months but she is concerned because currently the two 1-hour classes are given entirely as lectures by the dietitian. JL has been told that lecturing to patients for 2 hours is not the best educational technique, but she is unsure about what teaching method she should substitute for the lecture.

QUESTIONS

1. If JL has 2 hours' worth of material on nutrition and diabetes to teach, which part of the class should be lecture and which part should be changed to another educational method?
2. How can JL decide which alternative methods to use instead of a lecture?

SUGGESTED SOLUTIONS

JL could start by using the simple rule of thumb that most people have an attention span of about 15 to 20 minutes for a lecture. Using that rough guideline, she could decide that she wants to use two to three different teaching/learning activities for each hour of class. Another rule of thumb could help JL choose methods; it is that after 15 to 20 minutes of listening to information, patients should be able to interact with that information. For example, JL could give a 15- to 20-minute presentation on diabetes and nutrition, followed by a discussion session among the patients about the application of this information to their own lives. This session could be followed by an opportunity to do some problem solving, such as calculating ideal body weight or practice reading the new nutrition information labels on food. JL's choices should be guided by the introduction of two or three new methods per hour; the opportunity to give patients a chance to participate actively in the learning process; activities that will move the patients closer to the application of the knowledge in their own lives; and activities that will give patients the opportunity to share their own experiences and express their own needs to insure that the education is relevant.

CASE EXAMPLE 2

MW is a patient with non-insulin-dependent diabetes mellitus (NIDDM) who has been treated with diet only for the past five years. MW's physician has referred him for patient education because his diabetes control has been worsening for the past 18 months, and the doctor has prescribed oral agents. MW informed the teaching nurse that he doesn't see why he needs diabetes education. He said, "Do they think I'm an idiot, that I can't take a couple of pills without going to an education program? Besides I feel fine, I don't know why I have to take these pills anyway." The physician is convinced that MW is denying the seriousness of his diabetes and expects the nurse educator to change MW's attitude. MW seems resentful that he has been referred to the program. It is not at all clear to the nurse educator that MW will actually show up for classes.

QUESTIONS

1.   How should the nurse educator deal with this patient?

SUGGESTED SOLUTIONS

The answer to this question involves judgment, and judgment is always debatable. However, it is unlikely that the nurse educator can (or should) persuade MW to value and attend the education program, the reason being that when we try to persuade people that they are wrong in their point of view, they are likely to defend that point of view with increasing vigor. It is psychologically threatening to one's self-image to be told that one's point of view is wrong or inappropriate, and most people resist such threatening messages. The approach that would probably be most useful with MW would be to ask him a series of questions about his diabetes and his feelings about it and listen to his responses. Question him about how long he has had diabetes, how he feels, and what he knows about the progression of the disease; and give him an opportunity to express and explore his point of view and perceptions. Such exploration may allow him to work through some of his thoughts and feelings. It will also help him to perceive the teaching nurse as an ally rather than as someone who is judging him. If at the end of such a discussion MW is still unconvinced that he needs to attend the education program, the nurse could acknowledge the validity of his point of view but suggest that he may wish to consider attendance at some future time, since the nurse and the program are available to him if and when he should desire to use them. The nurse could also suggest that MW try at least one class or meet for one-on-one education. The nurse educator should communicate to the referring physician that MW is not open to attending a patient education program at this time and that pushing him to do so may increase rather than decrease his resistance to patient education. If MW feels safe, accepted, and valued by the nurse educator, he is more likely to return at some point and participate in the education program.

CASE EXAMPLE 3

JR is a nurse educator in a 200-bed hospital in a rural town in Wisconsin. The hospital has had both outpatient diabetes education classes and one-on-one education by nurses and dietitians for the past 15 years. However, the hospital has never evaluated its education program. The nurse in charge of patient education informs JR that it is time to develop an evaluation for their education program because the hospital may want to apply for Recognition for meeting the National Standards for Diabetes Patient Education in the near future. She asks JR to be in charge of developing a program evaluation.

QUESTIONS

1. How should JR begin to develop an evaluation?
2. What aspect of the program should be evaluated?

SUGGESTED SOLUTIONS

JR could begin by putting an together an advisory committee if one does not already exist. The advisory committee should be composed of program stakeholders such as teaching nurses and dietitians, a patient, a referring physician, an administrator, and anyone else who has an investment in the education program. The committee can help JR develop an evaluation plan. Furthermore, having such a committee moves the program one step closer to meeting the national standards.

The committee could make a series of recommendations about which things to measure for a program evaluation. Those decisions should be based on the answers to the following questions: What is the purpose of the evaluation? Whom are we collecting data for? For example, if the major purpose of the evaluation is Program Recognition, then the committee should examine the guidelines and information provided by the recognizing body (eg, the American Diabetes Association) to determine its requirements for program evaluation.

Evaluation should also be linked to the staff's desire to improve the quality of the education program. The advisory committee should design an evaluation that will help the hospital answer meaningful questions about the program. For example, does the hospital know how the program is perceived by patients? Do patients find the program helpful? Do they recommend it to their friends with diabetes? Does the program produce changes in diabetes knowledge, attitudes, or self-care behaviors? What kinds of changes do physicians who refer patients to the program expect? What is the cost of the program? Does it generate revenue?

The important first step in developing a program evaluation is to set priorities among the questions to be answered. Measures can then be either developed or selected to obtain answers to those questions. Valid and reliable measures of knowledge, attitudes, psychosocial adaptation, and self-care behavior exist and can be employed or adapted if these are the areas that the advisory committee decides to focus on during the evaluation. The most important question that the advisory committee should answer is, How are we planning to use the information that we gather during the evaluation? It is important to have a well-thought-out and agreed upon answer to this question before proceeding.

OTHER SUGGESTED READINGS

Brown SA. Effects of educational interventions in diabetes care: a meta-analysis of findings. Nurs Res 1988;37:223.

————. Studies of educational interventions and outcomes in diabetic adults: meta-analysis revisited. Patient Educ Couns 1990;16:189-215.

Dunn SM, Turtle JR. Education: new definitions, new directions. In: Alberti KGMM, Krall LP, eds. The diabetes annual/5. New York: Elsevier Science Publishing, 1990:186-201.

Falvo DR. Effective patient education. Rockville, Md: Aspen Publishers, 1985.

Heins JM, Nord WR, Cameron M. Establishing and sustaining state-of-the-art diabetes patient education programs: research and recommendations. Diabetes Educ 1992; 18:501-9.

Knowles M. Self-directed learning: a guide for learners and teachers. Chicago: Follett Publishing Co, 1975.

————. The modern practice of adult education. Chicago: Follett, 1980.

Lorenz RA, Pichert JW. Evaluation of education program development: illustration of the research and development cycle. Diabetes Educ 1989;15:253-56.

Mager RF. Preparing instructional objectives. Belmont, Calif: Fearon Publishers, 1975.

Maggard A. Handbook of patient education. Rockville, Md: Aspen Publishers, 1989.

Pichert JW. Teaching strategies for effective nutrition instruction. In: Powers MA, ed. Handbook of diabetes nutrition management. Rockville, Md: Aspen Publishers, 1987.

Redman BK. The process of patient teaching in nursing. 6th ed. St Louis: CV Mosby, 1988.

Smith C, ed. Patient education: nurses in partnership with other health professionals. Orlando, Fla: Grune & Stratton, 1987.

Strowig S. Patient education: a model for autonomous decision-making and deliberate action in diabetes self-management. Med Clin North Am 1982;66:1293-1307.

Woldum K, ed. Patient education: foundations of practice. Rockville, Md: Aspen Systems Corp, 1985.

————. Patient education: tools for practice. Rockville, Md: Aspen Systems Corp, 1985.

Psychosocial Issues

PSYCHOSOCIAL ISSUES

II. PSYCHOSOCIAL ASSESSMENT AND SUPPORT

INTRODUCTION

The emotional adjustment to diabetes by the patient and the family can be a crucial element in the long-term success of living with this disease. This chapter focuses on some of the psychological hurdles faced by patients with diabetes and provides guidelines that the health care professional can utilize to help patients and families process their feelings and create a healthy lifestyle conducive to good diabetes management. Helping patients process their feelings and assess their behavior can be therapeutic and can lead to a stronger commitment to health care. Also discussed in this chapter are barriers to adherence, considerations of the impact of living with diabetes, and potential resources available to patients and to the diabetes educator.

OBJECTIVES

Upon completion of this chapter, the learner will be able to:

- discuss the potential adjustment process that patients may experience upon receiving a diagnosis of diabetes;
- compare the differences in adaptive and maladaptive coping behaviors for patients and family members;
- explain how diabetes may affect the family;
- list and discuss potential barriers to adherence to the diabetes regimen;
- describe the impact of living with diabetes;
- discuss some of the research related to psychosocial adjustment;
- list and discuss various psychological resources available to the patient or the health professional.

A.   Coping With the Diagnosis

1.   It is quite common for a grief process to occur after the diagnosis of diabetes. Research indicates that most persons will resolve their psychological distress within the first year.

   a)   Kovacs et al[1] evaluated the psychosocial adjustment of children after diagnosis and found that the majority of children showed no significant distress. Of those who did show signs that were clinically diagnostic of psychiatric disorders, 50% had recovered within 3 months and 93% had recovered by 9 months.

b)   Holmes[2] reported that adults with non-insulin-dependent diabetes mellitus (NIDDM), also called type II diabetes, may experience psychological distress after diagnosis, but typically have adjusted within one year. The adjustment process is easier for adults who have experienced a good quality of life prior to diagnosis, who have social and emotional support, and who are able to resume their usual level of activity. Even after the onset of complications, Holmes[2] reported that patients were able to adjust to simpler lifestyles.

2.   Feelings of loss typically trigger the grief process. Patients may sense a loss of functioning, loss of freedom, or loss of control.

3.   Various models of grieving can help the educator understand the process. Kubler-Ross described a stage theory for the terminally ill in her book, *On Death and Dying.*[3] Parallels may be drawn to a population with chronic illness. Kalish[4] described affective expressions of grief and normalized grief as an appropriate response to loss. The following reactions or stages may be observed when working with patients who are grieving.

a)   Shock may be the initial response. The individual and the family may be at a loss for how to proceed. At this time, the diabetes educator should offer calm encouragement.

b)   Fear and anxiety may be quite overwhelming for a patient. Many of the short-term anxieties (Whom to tell that I have diabetes? Can I give myself a shot? Will I be able to do all this?) are resolved with education and the experience of living with the diabetes regimen. Other fears (Will I go blind? lose a leg? be on dialysis? Will I die from hypoglycemia?) are more persistent. While fear may provide a certain amount of motivation, if the patient becomes overwhelmed, denial can develop and become debilitating. Diabetes educators should not threaten patients with complications, but educate them as to the risks and help them identify and process their fears.

c) Denial is a common defense mechanism that can interfere with one's care. At first it may be helpful in easing the pain associated with the reality of having diabetes. Many persons with diabetes use a partial denial, in which they refuse to acknowledge the seriousness of the disease. For example, they may follow only certain parts of the regimen, such as taking an oral hypoglycemic agent or insulin, but eat an unrestricted diet.

d) Anger and guilt are common reactions during the adjustment process. Anger may be directed outward toward medical professionals or family members. Some anger may be directed inward in the form of guilt (Why didn't I lose weight? Why didn't I listen to my doctor?). Many patients who live with diabetes for a period of time before receiving extensive education wrestle with anger toward the physician who failed to tell them they should be actively involved in preserving their future health. Anger frequently is a clue that deeper feelings exist (eg, fear of rejection, guilt, embarrassment, frustration, and feelings of inadequacy).

e) Bargaining is a stage from Kubler-Ross' theory[3] that educators may observe in persons with diabetes. For example, the patient may bargain by saying, "If I lose 10 pounds, will I be able to go off insulin?" or "Can I have a hot fudge sundae if I exercise an extra half hour?" A bargain also may be silent, even subconscious, made with God or the physician. Here the patient mentally promises to follow a self-care regimen, often to perfection, in return for a cure. When the requested outcome does not happen, the patient may become discouraged and depressed. An attitude of adherence may be replaced with the attitude, "Why bother?"

f) Depression, sadness, and sorrow are among the most common reactions to loss. Depression that does not lift, however, is of concern (see the discussion of depression in this chapter, section F. Psychopathology).

g) Relief is an emotional response that may be mingled with other initial reactions. One might experience relief at finally knowing what is wrong. Relief often is present for patients who may have suspected something they consider to be worse, usually cancer. The diabetes educator should remain alert to the possibility of other reactions that might follow the patient's sense of relief.

h) Acceptance (adjustment, adaptation) is marked by the patient's acknowledgment of personal self-care responsibility for diabetes management in conjunction with the medical team. Acceptance is a fragile condition that frequently is challenged by other life stressors.

4. Some patients may experience other reactions to loss.

a) Somatization, with symptoms such as diarrhea, headaches, and loss of appetite, may occur when people are not resolving the underlying problem.

b) Patients may experience confusion, disorientation, or difficulty comprehending information.

B. Long-Term Coping

1. The adjustment process continues with each new stage of life. The challenges and responsibilities of diabetes care are different in childhood than in adolescence. In adulthood, the goals and challenges differ between young adults, adults at mid-life, and senior citizens. Each of these transitions may involve a reworking of the adjustment process and questions concerning how diabetes fits into the particular stage of life. The diabetes educator should keep in mind that having had diabetes for several years does not preclude a reemergence of adjustment issues later.

2. The Health Belief Model identifies specific attitudes and beliefs that influence people to choose preventive health behaviors

and to comply with medical regimens. The following factors are examined in determining compliance.

a) The health and willingness of the patient to accept medical recommendations.

b) The patient's subjective estimate of susceptibility, vulnerability, and extent of negative consequences.

c) The degree to which the regimen interferes with the patient's lifestyle.

d) The patient's perception of his or her ability to perform the regimen.[5]

3. Coping styles vary among individuals depending on their previous experiences and current level of stress. The patient's perceptions of the situation, available resources, and social support also influence coping ability.

4. An adaptive style of coping includes the following behaviors.

a) Patient responsibilities for health care are identified, and a commitment is made by the patient to carry out these responsibilities. Mutual goal setting with the educator or diabetes team may lead to the following actions.

   (1) The patient agrees to wear medical identification.

   (2) The patient uses glucose monitoring as a source of information from which self-management decisions can be made.

b) The patient is able to make lifestyle changes appropriate to the diabetes regimen.

c) The patient establishes a pattern of continuing education to stay abreast of new information and to help maintain a commitment to self-care, including regular contact with health care providers.

5. Some of the research on adjustment and glycemic control is summarized in the following descriptions.

a) Adolescents with poor metabolic control reported more problematic symptoms of diabetes such as slow healing, thirst, frequent urination, fatigue, vision problems, and leg pain. They also reported higher anxiety, decreased regard for physical appearance, less personal happiness, and lower self-esteem.[6]

b) In a comparison of youth with diabetes in good control and youth with diabetes in poor control, and a matched nondiabetic control group, Simonds[7] found very little difference between the nondiabetic group and the group in poor control. The group with diabetes in good control appeared to have better mental health.

c) Many researchers have looked for factors that influence metabolic control. Hanson, Henggeler, and Burghen[8] studied adolescents and found that adherence behaviors and stress had a direct effect on control. Adherence was affected by three areas: diabetes knowledge, family relationships, and adolescent age. Further research evaluating factors that influence adult adherence behaviors might be enlightening.

d) Cox and Gonder-Frederick[9] reviewed the research on factors affecting glycemic control and the psychosocial impact of diabetes.

C. Diabetes and the Family

1. The family's adjustment to the diagnosis of diabetes is extremely important. Family members need education, just like the patient, to help them make necessary lifestyle changes and support the patient. It is especially important that all family members living with the patient have an understanding of the demands of the diabetes self-care regimen.

a) The diabetes educator needs to make sure that both parents receive education in the case of a child with diabetes. It is important to involve the father and to avoid establishing the mother as the diabetes "expert," especially if it is a traditional family in which she does the cooking.

b) Other family members should be included in education and support (eg, children, siblings, and grandparents) whenever possible. In some cultures and situations, other extended family members may be in primary care roles with a patient. These persons also have to make emotional adjustments and lifestyle changes and will benefit from education.

2. The diabetes educator can gain insight into the interactive nature of the disease and the family dynamics by utilizing family systems theory.[10] Family characteristics such as family conflict are predictive of adherence difficulties. Other characteristics such as family support, cohesion, and organization are associated with better adherence and metabolic control.[9,11,12]

3. A patient in a dysfunctional family system may use illness-maintaining behaviors (poor management of the regimen, noncompliance behaviors, or dependency on the sick role) as a way to organize the family.[13]
    a) An adolescent may use illness-maintaining behaviors to regulate marital distance or parental conflict.
    b) A couple may avoid dealing with long-standing issues by directing their energies toward health care issues.

4. An adaptive reaction to a diagnosis of diabetes in a family member is characterized by involvement with the diabetes regimen and having realistic expectations. Typically the family members become educated about the disease, offering encouragement and showing concern when warranted, but remain nonjudgmental.

5. A maladaptive reaction by a family member may be expressed in one of two ways.
    a) A family member may withdraw and be nonsupportive of the patient, sabotaging the patient's efforts or putting obstacles to good diabetes management in the patient's path. This approach often is characterized by fear, denial, and lack of education.

b) A family member may be overly protective and foster dependency. This approach denies natural opportunities for risk-taking that help promote a good self-image. Overprotectiveness and enmeshment also may halt the natural progression through the developmental stages of life.

D. Barriers to Adherence

1. Many obstacles interfere with adherence to the diabetes regimen. Estimates of noncompliance with long-term medical regimens range from 41% to 69%, depending upon illness, patient population, and complexity of regimen.[13] Therefore, the diabetes educator must assess those barriers. Some obstacles, such as grief, health beliefs, and family dynamics, have already been discussed; other potential barriers are described in this section.

2. A limited support system may hinder adherence to the diabetes regimen. A person living alone or separated from loved ones may lack the support and encouragement often necessary to follow the regimen.

3. A poor self-image and a sense of powerlessness can be devastating to adherence behaviors. Subconscious thoughts such as "I'm not worth the effort" or "What's the use?" can sabotage the regimen.

4. Other stressors in a person's life may push the diabetes regimen lower on the list of priorities. These other stressors may consume so much time and energy that the patient has very little of either to direct toward personal health care.

5. Insufficient financial resources often interfere with adherence. The treatment of diabetes is expensive, and many patients do not have insurance or qualify for assistance programs. Many do not have funds for proper food. Some patients have insurance;

but if insurance does not cover the cost of supplies and prescription items, many patients will find it difficult to afford the items necessary for diabetes care (see Section G, Resources).

6. A lack of diabetes education can be a barrier to adherence. For example, if the patient and family do not receive an explanation as to why a particular regimen is important, the motivation for adherence may disappear over time.

7. Multicultural issues and concerns need to be addressed by the diabetes educator (see Chapter XIX: Cultural Sensitivity in Diabetes Education).

    a) Because some cultural practices may create barriers to adherence, the diabetes educator should determine how customs, traditions, values, and ethnic foods may present obstacles to a traditional diabetes regimen.

        (1) In some cultures, being overweight is considered desirable, and the eating and sharing of rich foods often is valued.

        (2) Some European cultures and American Indians consider it impolite to refuse food that is offered when visiting another person's home. The gifts that are exchanged often are sweet foods. Holidays are celebrated with special foods that are high in calories and simple sugars.

        (3) Fasting may be a cultural or religious practice, and must be done very carefully with supervision and adequate understanding of the impact on the person with diabetes.

        (4) Other cultural factors may relate to acceptance. A parent or spouse may feel that the person with the diagnosis of diabetes now is contaminated, or imperfect. Macho images also may be affected.

    b) The diabetes educator may need to work with an interpreter. The following recommendations should be followed.

(1) Use a nonrelative, ideally someone fluent in the language with an understanding of diabetes or medical terms.

(2) Look at and speak to the patient, not the interpreter.

(3) Use simple explanations and avoid analogies.

(4) Allow sufficient time.

(5) Determine whether the patient reads or writes in the native language.

8. If diabetes interferes with one's lifestyle, the associated frustration may greatly diminish adherence.

E. The Impact of Living With Diabetes

1. The impact of living with diabetes varies with individuals. Some experience few difficulties, while others feel diabetes is a threat to their lifestyle.

2. The demands of the diabetes regimen can be considerable and overwhelming. It may be difficult for friends and family members to fully appreciate these demands (eg, insulin injections, blood glucose monitoring, dietary restrictions, scheduling concerns, treatment of hypoglycemia, and the need to make routine decisions regarding these concerns.)

3. The fear of hypoglycemia frequently is expressed as one of the greatest worries of persons with diabetes. Severe hypoglycemia reduces independence, and even mild reactions can create a feeling of loss of control. Persons who have had diabetes for a number of years often find that the epinephrine response decreases over time, thus minimizing warning signals that the blood glucose level has dropped. As a result, the patient may fail to treat hypoglycemia in the early stages. The fear of hypoglycemia is magnified for those who live alone, especially the elderly who may be trying to maintain independent living.

4. Persons with diabetes should be able to perform most jobs. The Americans with Disabilities Act of 1990 states that a person cannot be discriminated against because of a "handicapping condition," which is how diabetes mellitus is identified.

    a) Persons with diabetes are prohibited from working in certain vocations, however. A person with diabetes requiring insulin cannot join the US military, hold a pilot's license, or drive an interstate truck. (Legislation is pending in the United States Congress to have such cases decided on an individual basis.) The Occupational Safety and Health Administration guidelines also limit the machinery in construction and factory work that a person with diabetes can operate.

    b) In all career fields, an employer who has had a negative experience with an employee with diabetes may be reluctant to hire another person with diabetes.

    c) Many jobs present scheduling obstacles for ideal diabetes self-care. Third shifts and swing shifts can make it challenging to schedule meals and injections. Many jobs do not recognize break or snack times. (see Chapter X: Special Issues in Management).

    d) Persons with diabetes need to know their legal rights. Other than the exceptions already listed, it is against the law to discriminate against a person with diabetes who is applying for a job.

5. Personal relationships can be affected by diabetes. Difficulties that already exist in a relationship may become more intense.

    a) Diabetes may prove a source of frustration, sadness, and occasional embarrassment to family members or friends.

    b) There is a tendency for others to assume that changes in mood are related to blood glucose levels and to sometimes discount legitimate feelings. When patients are irritable during periods of low or high blood sugars, family and friends may misinterpret these actions and take them personally.

c) Diabetes can become a tool for manipulation, especially if others are not educated about the disease.

d) Marriages may be strained when a spouse or child is diagnosed with diabetes. Underlying issues may get ignored because of the energy focused on the disease.

e) Persons with diabetes may become reluctant to enter into new relationships for fear of rejection. Often a fear of abandonment is associated with already existing relationships.

6. Sexual functioning may be affected by diabetes and further strain a significant personal relationship. Sexual health is a product of the integration of many components. The biological effect of diabetes on erection in men has been well documented. Less is known about the possible biological effects on female sexual adaptation. The psychological and social consequences associated with sexual dysfunction and diabetes in both men and women also are less well known. Assessment of sexual health and guidance with sexual problems are important aspects of diabetes care.

7. Recreation and leisure activities may be affected by diabetes.

a) Getting and keeping a driver's license is an issue for many persons. Many states now require a doctor's statement indicating that the person's diabetes is well controlled in order to obtain a driver's license.

b) Patients frequently complain that diabetes limits the flexibility and spontaneity in their lives. Persons with diabetes need to plan ahead and think about when and where they will eat their next meal or snack. They need to make decisions about whether they can expend physical energy at a given time and how to prevent hypoglycemia or hyperglycemia from such exertion.

c) People with diabetes need to be aware of personal safety. Solitary expeditions, especially ones that include intense physical activity, are not for the person uneducated or inexperienced in diabetes self-care skills.

d) There is no vacation from diabetes. Supplies must be packed and taken with the patient, and the disease must be taken into account with every activity.

F.   Psychopathology

1.   Depression, even though expected, should not be taken lightly. The health care professional should know the symptoms of clinical depression: feeling down; sleep disturbances; change in eating patterns; loss of interest in activity; withdrawal from others; feelings of helplessness and hopelessness; suicidal ideation or attempt; and feeling alone, worthless, tired, lethargic, or irritable. The health care professional should assess the duration and severity of these symptoms and make referrals for treatment as appropriate. Leahy[14] reported research showing that depression is significantly higher in the diabetes population than in the general population. Because health professionals may think it normal for a person with chronic illness to be depressed, they may be less likely to refer the patient for counseling, thus denying the patient the help that is needed.

2.   Recurrent diabetic ketoacidosis may be a sign that further psychiatric and psychological assessment is warranted, especially if the diabetes is relatively easy to control within the hospital setting.

3.   Diabetes may create or increase a tendency towards eating disorders.
     a)   Stancin, Link, and Reuter[15] studied 59 women with IDDM, age 18 to 30 years, and reported that over half of the subjects had eating binges, and nearly 40% admitted to using glycosuria as a means of weight control. Many (12%) met the criteria for a diagnosis of bulimia. Birk and Spencer[16] studied 550 women with diabetes, age 13 to 45 years, and reported no greater prevalence of anorexia or bulimia in this group of females with diabetes than in the

general population. Both of these studies[15,16] describe the seriousness of eating disorders in persons with diabetes.

   b)   Wing, et al[17] described the high incidence of subclinical eating disorders with frequent binge eating and reduced insulin dosage. LaGreca, Schwarz, and Satin[18] found that 70% of young women in poor control used a reduced insulin dosage as a means of weight reduction or control, compared with 0% of females in good control.

   c)   Overeating has been reported as more common in persons on a restrictive meal plan once their restrictions already have been exceeded.[19]

G.   Resources Available to the Family and Health Care Provider

1.   The health care team serves as a lifeline for many patients. It consists of a physician, diabetes nurse educator, dietitian, psychosocial professional (psychologist, social worker, counselor), pharmacist, and exercise physiologist. This group provides education, support, and motivation (see Chapter I: Educational Principles and Strategies).

2.   Third-party insurance coverage is ideal, but not always affordable.

   a)   The most economical situation is group coverage by the employer. Still, group policies vary considerably in coverage, especially concerning outpatient supplies.

   b)   Individual coverage for a person with diabetes can be very costly.

   c)   Many states have pooled-risk insurance. Qualifications and coverage differ from state to state.

   d)   Third-party reimbursement for diabetes education is available in many states.

   e)   Patients who qualify for Medicaid typically can access diabetes supplies. Other state programs sometimes assist with medical expenses.

   f)   Medicare coverage seems to change frequently. It is advisable to develop a working relationship with someone in the local office who can provide regular updates about relevant changes.

3. Community and financial resources may be available for short- and long-term counseling, and consultations with specialists.

    a) Government assistance for those who qualify can be beneficial. Medicaid or Medicare needs can be assessed and initiated by a social worker through Social and Rehabilitation Services.

    b) Counseling needs may include a need for a psychiatrist, psychologist, social worker, marriage and family therapist, sex therapist, mental health counselor, and/or vocational counselor. County mental health departments may be a good resource. Peer support groups for patients and family members also are available in many areas.

    c) Vocational rehabilitation through the state government can be a resource for vocational counseling, job placement, and financial assistance for job training and education.

    d) Community food banks may have some appropriate choices of foods for person with diabetes and may assist in providing staples on a monthly basis. Meals on Wheels is another food resource for those who qualify.

    e) Some communities have agencies or medical supply businesses that offer short-term leases or lease-to-buy contracts for blood glucose meters. Such arrangements may be useful while waiting for authorization from third-party carriers. Because prior Medicaid authorization may take 4 to 6 weeks, a loaner or rental meter may be needed.

    f) The Salvation Army or American Red Cross often can help with emergency financial assistance.

    g) Housing for families of inpatients or outpatients from out of town sometimes is available through a local Ronald McDonald House.

    h) Local chapters and affiliates of the American Diabetes Association (ADA), the Juvenile Diabetes Foundation (JDF), the American Association of Diabetes Educators

(AADE), and other diabetes organizations have many services to offer.

i) Other educational resources include the National Diabetes Advisory Board, the Centers for Disease Control Division of Diabetes Control, and the National Diabetes Information Clearinghouse. Newsletters and journals may be available from these organizations and from companies that market diabetes supplies.

REFERENCES

1.   Kovacs M, Brent D, Steinberg F, Paulaukas S, Reid J. Children's self reports of psychologic adjustment and coping strategies during the first year of insulin-dependent diabetes mellitus. Diabetes Care 1986;9:472-79.

2.   Holmes DM. The person and diabetes in psychosocial context. Diabetes Care 1986;9:194-206.

3.   Kubler-Ross E. On death and dying. New York: Macmillan, 1970.

4.   Kalish R. Death, grief, and caring relationships. Monterey, Calif: Brooks/Cole Publishing Co, 1985.

5.   Ryan P. Strategies for motivating life-style change. J Cardiovasc Nurs 1987;1(4):54-66.

6.   Anderson B, Miller JP, Auslander W, Santiago J. Family characteristics of diabetic adolescents: relationship to metabolic control. Diabetes Care 1981;4:586-94.

7.   Simonds J. Psychiatric status of diabetic youth matched with a control group. Diabetes 1977;26:921-25.

8.   Hanson C, Henggeler S, Burghen G. Model of associations between psychosocial variables and health-outcome measures of adolescents with IDDM. Diabetes Care 1987;10:752-58.

9.   Cox D, Gonder-Frederick L. Major developments in behavioral diabetes research. J Consult Clin Psychol 1992;60:628-38.

10.   Anderson B, Auslander W. Research on diabetes management and the family: a critique. Diabetes Care 1980;3:696-702.

11.   Anderson B. Diabetes and adaptation in family systems. In: Holmes CS, ed. Neuropsychological and behavioral aspects of diabetes. New York: Springer-Verlag, 1990:85-101.

12. Schafer L, Glasgow R, McCaul K, Dreher M. Adherence to IDDM regimens: relationship to psychosocial variables and metabolic control. Diabetes Care 1983;6:493-98.

13. Frey J. A family/systems approach to illness-maintaining behaviors in chronically ill adolescents. Family Process 1984;23:251-60.

14. Leahy M. Depression in adult insulin dependent diabetes [Dissertation]. Wichita, Kan: University of Kansas School of Medicine, 1985.

15. Stancin T, Link D, Reuter J. Binge eating and purging in young women with IDDM. Diabetes Care 1989;12:601-3.

16. Birk R, Spencer M. The prevalence of anorexia nervosa, bulimia and induced glycosuria in IDDM females. Diabetes Educ 1989;15:336-41.

17. Wing R, Nowalk M, Marcus M, Koeske R, Finegold D. Subclinical eating disorders and glycemic control in adolescents with type I diabetes. Diabetes Care 1986;9:162-67.

18. LaGreca A, Schwarz L, Satin W. Eating patterns in young women with IDDM: another look. Diabetes Care 1987;19:659-60.

19. Herman CP, Mack D. Restrained and unrestrained eating. J Pers 1975;43:647-60.

KEY EDUCATIONAL CONSIDERATIONS

1. To assist the patient in the therapeutic process of dealing with feelings, help the patient identify trigger events that prompt negative feelings. For example, some social events may trigger such feelings because in planning for the event, the patient is confronted with certain losses and demands in life because of having diabetes. Have the patient and family generate a list of the losses and demands they have experienced or that they anticipate experiencing if diabetes is newly diagnosed. This list will open several areas for discussion and education.

2. Role play "What if?" situations. Describe a situation that requires decision making and ask the patient to explain what he/she would do in those circumstances. For example, friends call and invite you to a late evening dinner. Or you decide to go play tennis this afternoon, knowing that your NPH insulin will peak while you are away. What would you do? These kinds of questions get the patient involved in diabetes management, decision making, and problem solving, and provide reassurance that an active lifestyle is possible with effective plans of action.

3. Have the patient list personal priorities. How close to the top is health care? Is this a surprise to the patient? Is the patient satisfied with his or her priorities or do they need to be revised?

4. Involve families whenever possible. Have family members discuss what impact diabetes will have on their lives and on the patient's life. Have patients share what they would like family members to do to support them. Ask family members what they are willing to do.

5. Help patients process and clarify feelings by giving them an opportunity for a cathartic experience. Ask them to imagine that you could set them up with a canvas, an easel, and a palette of paints. Their assignment is to paint a picture (or imagine a picture) that describes their experience of living with diabetes.

SELF-REVIEW QUESTIONS

If you are unsure of the answers to the following questions, please review the materials.

1. Discuss the possible adjustment process for the person newly diagnosed with diabetes or with newly developed complications of diabetes.
2. Describe behaviors that would indicate a person is adjusting to having diabetes.
3. Explain how a person with diabetes might use the disease to protect another family member.
4. Discuss the effect of cultural practices on adherence to the diabetes regimen.
5. What is the likelihood of an eating disorder in a young female with IDDM?
6. Discuss how diabetes may affect a chosen profession.
7. List and describe some community resources that patients with diabetes may find helpful.

CASE EXAMPLE 1

MD is a 77-year-old widow. She lives in a rural area of your state and has come to your diabetes center to be started on insulin. In visiting with her, you learn that MD's husband died 4 months ago. She is very stressed by trying to settle the estate and getting her finances in order. She is a little apprehensive about starting insulin, but willing to do that because her doctor says her blood sugar levels are too high. As you proceed with her instruction, you find that although MD does a good job of self-injecting, she cannot see well enough to fill the syringe. MD is proud of her independent nature and apologizes for her tearfulness during the teaching session.

QUESTIONS

1. How does MD's emotional adjustment affect her learning needs?
2. How can you help MD continue living independently?

SUGGESTED SOLUTIONS

During your interaction, you identify that MD is experiencing multiple losses (eg, loss of her husband, perceived loss of financial stability, and loss of her usual state of health). MD also is fearful of losing her independence.

When MD realizes that she cannot fill the syringe accurately, you validate her need to remain independent by offering the option of using an adaptive device for filling the syringe. Slowly, through the tears, you discover that MD has a decreased appetite and is skipping meals. After calling MD's physician to report your concern for her safety and the potential for hypoglycemia, the physician decides to postpone MD's transition to insulin.

MD is open to the need for emotional support during this crisis but refuses to attend a bereavement group. She is willing to meet with clergy and makes an appointment before she leaves your office. MD plans to return to the diabetes center when she is ready to make the transition to insulin therapy.

CASE EXAMPLE 2

The diabetes educator is requested to see a newly diagnosed 10-year-old and his family. The child came out of intensive care yesterday. He is bright and very verbal, and tells you about his school and activities. He enjoys sports. When you meet the parents, you can detect tension in the atmosphere. Dad has insulin-dependent diabetes mellitus (IDDM) with retinopathy and has just finished a series of laser treatments. Both parents work full time. There is a younger sister, age 7 years.

QUESTIONS

1. How will you proceed with education?
2. If you detect blaming behavior between the parents, how would you deal with this?
3. Sometimes when parents are caught up in their own schedules or have unresolved issues between them, much of the diabetes care may be delegated to the young child. This is especially true if the

child is very capable and responsible. How can you help this family avoid overburdening their child with such responsibility?

4.   What can you offer for the sibling?

SUGGESTED SOLUTIONS

Try to schedule both parents for education at the same time if possible. This arrangement will let both parents hear the same thing and you will not have to worry about whether you told them the same things. Invite anyone else who is involved with the child's care, such as grandparents or baby-sitters.

Sometimes parents experience guilt that their child has diabetes, especially when one parent has diabetes. The other parent may blame the one with diabetes, or the parent with diabetes may experience self-blame. Or both parents may feel guilty for not having identified the symptoms earlier. Try to assess for these reactions. Parents need to work through any feelings of blame or guilt. Occasionally a mental health professional may be needed for this purpose.

Praise the child's capabilities and maturity, but warn the parents about giving the child too much responsibility too early. This situation often occurs if either parent is very stressed by other issues, eg, making a living, dealing with an ex-spouse, or trying to start a new relationship.

Encourage parents to bring the sister to the hospital for visits. She needs to see that her brother is in good health. Involve her as appropriate in any education you provide for the child with diabetes.

OTHER SUGGESTED READINGS

Cox D, Gonder-Frederick L. Major developments in behavioral diabetes research. J Consult Clin Psychol 1992;60:628-38.

Feste C. The physician within. Minneapolis: Diabetes Center, Inc, 1987.

Holmes CS, ed. Neuropsychological and behavioral aspects of diabetes. New York: Springer-Verlag, 1990.

Fogel CI, ed. Sexuality and diabetes: an issue for both sexes. Diabetes Spectrum 1991;4:18-40.

Kurtz S. Adherence to diabetes regimens: empirical status and clinical applications. Diabetes Educ 1990;16:50-56.

Rubin R, Bierman J, Toohey B. Psyching out diabetes. Los Angeles: Lowell House, 1992.

PSYCHOSOCIAL ISSUES

III. STRESS MANAGEMENT

INTRODUCTION

Stress management is important for patients with diabetes to help them cope more effectively and manage their disease during difficult times. This chapter will describe the important role that stress and stress management play in diabetes.

Stress is defined as a feeling of tension, both physical and emotional, that occurs in certain situations. Managing stress is particularly important for people who have diabetes because stress can affect metabolic control in two different ways. First, stress tends to raise blood glucose levels in many people. Second, stress tends to have a debilitating effect that often leads to diminished self-care and, ultimately, poorer metabolic control.

Coping strategies are useful techniques for working through potentially difficult situations (stressors) that are a part of everyday life. Stress management refers to efforts to control and minimize the tension associated with situations that are perceived as difficult or unpleasant. The goal of stress management and coping strategies is improved metabolic and emotional control.

OBJECTIVES

Upon completion of this chapter, the learner will be able to:
- define the effects of stress on the body;
- identify four potential sources of stress for the person with diabetes;
- list three manifestations of stress;
- describe the six steps of the PARENT approach to stress management;
- describe six programs related to cognitive restructuring;
- list three methods of behavior modification;
- discuss the role of social support in a coping-strategy response.

A. Effects of Stress on the Body

1. Stress management is the ability of an individual to handle stress and may involve both physical and mental alterations. The intensity of the stressors and the internal physiologic

activity resulting from that stimulation will determine the degree of change and the stability of blood glucose levels. In some people, blood glucose levels may not become elevated despite tremendous stress. Blood glucose levels may rise and remain elevated if the person under stress is less active or if the stress becomes chronic. Blood glucose levels may drop sharply if the person becomes very active or agitated.[1]

a) The physiology of acute stress involves a sympathetic response of the autonomic nervous system and release of the counterregulatory hormones, epinephrine and norepinephrine.

(1) The sympathetic nervous system regulates the involuntary functions of the body, such as dilation of the pupils, dilation of the bronchioles, decreased peristalsis, increased closure of external sphincters, and increased heart rate. Blood pressure and pulse rate increase as the heart attempts to get the glucose-laden fuel in the blood to the cells in the muscles to enhance the person's abilities to fight or flee.

(2) Release of *epinephrine and norepinephrine* is indirectly stimulated by the hypothalamus, which biochemically signals the medulla of the adrenal gland to release these catecholamines.

(a) Epinephrine results in vasoconstriction of the superficial peripheral vessels and dilation of the blood vessels as they transverse the muscle fibers.

(b) Norepinephrine causes vasodilation of the peripheral vessels and diaphoresis. If stimulation lasts long enough, however, vasodilation will be followed by vasoconstriction of the same vessels.

(c) Both hormones will stimulate glycogenolysis.

(3) If the individual does not respond to acute stress with greatly increased activity, enhanced glycogenolysis in the face of insufficient insulin is likely to result in increased blood glucose levels.

(4) If activity is greatly increased, a greater sensitivity of the receptor sites allows glucose to enter cells more readily, lowering blood-brain glucose levels. Hypoglycemia could result, which could be reversed by the release of glucagon.

(5) Major dangers of the autonomic response are cardiac vasoconstriction with angina or heart attack. The symptoms of fright or excitement, which mimic hypoglycemia, are still of some concern. Without blood glucose monitoring, inappropriate treatment might occur.

b) Chronic stress is associated with a parasympathetic response that involves the release of cortisol and related hormones.

(1) The *parasympathetic nervous system* pertains to the craniosacral division of the autonomic nervous system and it consists of the oculomotor, facial, glossopharyngeal, vagus, and pelvic nerves. It is mediated by the release of acetylcholine and participates in the protection, conservation, and restoration of body resources. A few of these responses involve slowing the heart, stimulating peristalsis, constricting pupils, relaxing external sphincters, and constricting bronchioles.

(2) Cortisol and other associated hormones are secreted from the cortex of the adrenal gland through the reception of a biochemical message sent by the hypothalamus through the release of adrenocorticotropic hormone (ACTH) from the pituitary gland. Cortisol release results in a decrease in inflammatory reaction, a decrease in white blood cell count, and the promotion of gluconeogenesis.

2. The body's response to stress may most simply be described by Selye's theory of the general adaptation syndrome (GAS).[2]

a) The alarm reaction represents acute stress; at this point, the blood glucose levels may spike or hypoglycemia may occur.

b) The stage of resistance is marked by chronic stress. Cortisol secretion is elevated and the blood glucose levels may stay elevated during this stage or may become more labile and therefore harder to control.

c) The stage of exhaustion marks the end of life or the manifestation of the full disease process.[2]

3. Hobfoll[3] suggests that Selye's descriptors of stress are archaic in light of today's findings that stress responses in the body are very complex. We are looking not at just the physical, mental, and emotional components of stress, but at the person's genetic makeup and the perceptions that person has related to the stressors of life as reflected by the release of counterregulatory hormones.

4. One or more aspects of self-care may be diminished when chronic stress occurs. It may become more difficult to follow through with expected behaviors. As the person omits self-care activities related to monitoring, medication, dietary intake, and hygiene, a greater chance of elevated blood glucose levels occurs.

B. Potential Sources of Stress for the Person With Diabetes

1. Scheduling. Most people would rather do what they want to do when they want to do it. If the individual is an organized person who is used to eating correctly and exercising appropriately, the change in lifestyle when diabetes is diagnosed may not be that great. But if the person is less organized or enjoys an unpredictable lifestyle, adjusting to diabetes can be a major problem. Setting up a schedule to live by day after day not only gets boring for some but close to impossible for others. Work or school demands may be such

that a different schedule is needed every day, making scheduling more of a challenge.

2. Invasive procedures. Anything that brings about discomfort in any form becomes stressful. Some individuals may accept the fact that an invasive procedure, such as blood testing or injecting insulin, is needed and therefore useful. Others consider these procedures just a nuisance, while some may even fear the thought of the process.

3. Being different. We're all different in one way or another but problems may arise when differences are obvious (eg, having an insulin reaction or wearing a diabetes ID bracelet) and the individual feels uncomfortable being the center of attention. Consequently, some individuals may hide their diabetes. This delusion could be dangerous, especially if a person had an insulin reaction and people around him just assumed he was drunk.

4. Peer pressure. The wish to appear the same, not different, is an aspect of peer pressure. Even when people know that an individual has diabetes, they may still participate in unintentional sabotage by offering forbidden foods or encouraging just one taste.

5. Cost of care. The expense of diabetes supplies and medical care can be very stressful. If the individual with diabetes already has limited financial resources, the added strain of having to pay for supplies and medical care may lead to omitting tests and medication, and canceling appointments. The conflict of knowing the importance of adhering to a treatment regimen, but not being able to because of limited finances, also causes increased anxiety.

6. Time. Each action of care takes time. Whether it is waiting in a doctor's office or taking the time to do a blood glucose test, time becomes an enemy for many people. Participating in

activities that take time may be thought to interfere with more important or routine activities. Anything that "borrows" time can too often be considered a negative.

C. Assessment and Manifestations of Stress

1. A variety of methods exist for assessing stress levels.

    a) Holmes and Rahe's Social Readjustment Rating Scale predicts the chance of developing a stress-related illness.[4] The test takes about 10 minutes to administer.

    b) The Stress Map[5] identifies a state of stress level at the time the test is completed, and includes the interventions that work for the participant, as well as suggestions for correcting the stressful state. This test usually takes more than 30 minutes to complete.

    c) The Energy Director Assessment[6] categorizes an individual's stress responses according to the following groups: grounding energy, creative energy, relationship energy, and logic energy. This assessment provides guidelines for building skills to develop "weak energies" that have been identified.

    d) The Parenting Stress Index[7] is an assessment tool that utilizes multiple choice questions to determine the stressors associated with dysfunctional families. The responses can identify among others, the permissive parent and the abusive parent. At least 30 minutes are needed to complete this assessment.

    e) The Berkeley Stress and Coping Project's Daily Hassles Scale[8] reveals the extent to which daily irritants or hassles serve as stress indicators.[9] This assessment is available in a combined form (including an uplift scale and a hassles scale) and usually requires 20 to 30 minutes to complete.

2. Indicators of a person's attitude are measured in a generalized format or in relation to a specific emotion. A person's attitude can influence the perception of a stressor. For example, a

person with a negative attitude often sees a particular stressor as a greater threat than a person with a positive attitude.

   a)   A negative attitude can be a predictor of stress. Andreoli's Health Belief Scale[10] can be used to assess attitudes toward health care. Indirectly, an individual assessed to have a negative attitude is assumed to respond with a greater amount of stress than if that same person had a positive attitude.

   b)   Scheier and Carver's Levels of Optimism Test (LOT)[11] indirectly indicates an attitude by revealing greater or lesser levels of optimism. Higher levels of optimism appear to correspond with better attitudes.

3.   Poor nutritional status may be the result of a physically stressed state. Stressors could lead to inappropriate timing and choices of food or fluid intake and eating too much or too little of the needed nutrients. A 24-hour diet history, plus skinfold measurements, weight, and height, can help reveal the need for nutrition counseling.

4.   Lack of exercise or decreased activity may indicate a stressed state. A regular exercise program contributes to an increased feeling of well-being and a decreased sense of depression, as well as other improved physiologic factors. (see Chapter VII: Exercise).

5.   Lack of social support may indicate problems within the family structure or in social interaction. Social patterns can reflect physical or psychological problems with which the individual is unable to cope.

   a)   Olson and colleagues[12] developed a number of assessment scales (Family Inventories) to determine support systems.

   b)   Sarason and colleagues[13] developed the Social Support Questionnaire to identify external support systems.

6.   Lack of relaxation practices (eg, hobbies, physical activity) may indicate an inability to handle tension. Family history and

disclosure of interests in a hobby outside of work or school indicate a subconscious awareness of a need for varied activities. A baseline biofeedback reading obtained by monitoring temperature, electrical muscle activity, galvanic skin response, and/or an electroencephalogram can be used to assess the level of tension a person is experiencing.[14]

7. The professional can determine an individual's stressful state, without the use of paper and pencil tests, by measuring the blood pressure (systolic reading often elevated during stress), pulse rate (usually rapid), and respiration rate (also rapid). Questions should elicit responses that reflect the person's self-perceptions: "Are you feeling a little nervous? If you had three wishes, what would they be? How are you feeling? What are you thinking about? On a scale of 1 (least stressed) to 10 (most stressed), where do you rate yourself?"

D. Stress Management Programs

1. Program development for effective stress management should include methods to improve one's attitude and to help one think positively; appropriate training for assertiveness and relaxation practices; an exercise program; good nutrition guidelines; and a way to develop social interactions and a social support system (see Table III.1).

   a) Positive thinking can be achieved through behavioral conditioning, such as the daily use of positive affirmation statements (eg, "Each day I am doing better and better. I'm OK. I just happen to have diabetes. I can allow obstacles in my life, such as having a chronic illness, to become opportunities to learn"). The process of reframing[15] (turning a negative statement into a positive one) also can contribute to positive thinking[15] (eg, changing "I hate having diabetes" to "Having diabetes helps me learn how to take better care of myself").

   b) Assertiveness is needed at work, at school, and in social settings. If people are not assertive, they have a tendency

TABLE III.1:
A PARENT Approach to Stress Management

Focus/Concept	Strategies
Positive Thinking	Practice positive affirmation Reframe the negative into positive Use positive self-talk Stop negative thoughts Plan to have fun
Assertiveness	Alter stressors via assertive communications such as listening Give and receive feedback Effectively manage time Effectively negotiate
Relaxation	Listen to your body Use relaxation techniques Take a mini-retreat Plan time for hobbies Use SIT (Stop, Inhale, Think)
Exercise	Prepare for exercise the FITT way (Frequency, Intensity, Time, Type) Develop an individualized exercise program
Nutrition	Eat for optimal health and well-being Follow recommended dietary allowances (high-fiber, low-fat, low-sugar, low-salt) Eat fewer processed foods and more fresh fruits and vegetables Eat proper distribution and amounts of food
Touch	Seek social interaction that involves daily touching (eg, hugging) Utilize self-nurturing and spiritual nurturing Reach out to others

to feel neglected, hurt, angry, and pushed around, resulting in physiological stress responses. When assertiveness is used appropriately, the individual feels a sense of accomplishment, fairness, and improved self-esteem and self-confidence. Role playing is an effective technique for practicing new assertiveness skills.

c) Relaxation training develops a skill that is particularly helpful for persons with diabetes. Because blood glucose levels can become lower as the person becomes more relaxed, regular monitoring is essential. A change in medication may be necessary if the blood glucose levels decrease considerably. Learning relaxation skills can be enhanced by the use of biofeedback, an external process, that gives information about internal physiological activity. Some parameters that can be monitored include pulse, temperature, skin conductance (galvanic skin responses), blood pressure, muscle activity, blood glucose levels, and brain waves. An increase in peripheral temperature, a decrease in the muscle output of electrical activity, lower blood glucose levels, and lower blood pressure suggest a more relaxed state. As a number of studies have documented, the more the person is able to relax, the better the control of blood glucose levels.[1,16-19] A positive specific response with relaxation training has been reported in people with non-insulin-dependent diabetes mellitus (NIDDM), also called type II diabetes,[20] although this outcome has been controversial in people with insulin-dependent diabetes mellitus (IDDM), also called type I diabetes.[21]

(1) Progressive relaxation, developed originally by Jacobson,[22] is a process in which a person contracts muscle groups one at a time, concentrates on the feeling of the contracted muscles, then relaxes muscle groups one at a time, and again concentrates on how the muscles feel in this relaxed state. The training takes about 6 to 10 weeks of daily practice, monitoring peripheral temperature or muscle

response before and after contractions to develop an awareness of the feeling of relaxation.

(2) Autogenic therapy, developed originally by Luthe et al,[23] may be used in the more complex, six-step version, or the simplified version designed by Benson and colleagues.[24] This therapy involves concentrating on various parts of the body and imagining a feeling of heaviness followed by warmth. Feedback may involve electromyography (EMG), galvanic skin response (GSR), or measuring peripheral temperature. Six to 10 weeks are needed to develop this skill.

(3) Deep abdominal breathing increases the flow of oxygen to the brain, thus aiding the relaxation process. Usually only 2 to 3 breaths are needed to aid in the relaxing process. To increase relaxation further 9 or 10 deep breaths are followed by a short period of normal breathing then the deep breaths are repeated.

(4) Imagery may be used for relaxation purposes as well as for problem-solving. Pleasant imagery experiences help keep the person focused on positive ideas and feelings that facilitate relaxation.

(5) Meditation can promote relaxation by focusing one's thoughts away from daily stressors. This relaxation technique involves concentrating on a thought, verse, picture, or a spot on the wall, or making a repetitive sound, such as a mantra saying "ohm" or "one."

(6) Music therapy fosters relaxation through concentration on the tune and tempo of the music. As the music becomes calmer and the beat slower, the body attempts to mimic the musical response. As body activity slows, fewer counterregulatory hormones are released, and relaxation can begin.

(7) Color therapy enhances relaxation through the visualization of increasingly quieter tones.

d) Exercise can be a valuable means of releasing tension. Sessions should be at least 20 to 30 minutes long, 5 times per week to achieve a desired fitness level, or 3 to 4 times per week for maintenance (see Chapter VII: Exercise).

e) Nutrition guidelines provide information for following a well-balanced meal plan that is high-fiber, low-fat, and includes few concentrated sweets. Obesity may be a stressor and should be corrected within cultural and perceptual limits (see Chapter VI: Nutrition).

f) Social interaction in the form of touch involves hugging, plus self-nurturing, spiritual nurturing, and reaching out to others.

2. Biofeedback-supported relaxation training involves a method of enhancing or accelerating the learning process and may be used to determine the effectiveness of certain relaxation techniques (see Table III.2).

TABLE III.2: Techniques for Stress Reduction

Assertiveness Training	Increased Self-Awareness
Autogenic Therapy	Meditation
Biofeedback-Supported Relaxation Training	Nutritional Choices
	Personal Counseling
Communications Skills Development	Progressive Relaxation
	Refuting Irrational Ideas
Coping Skills Training	Self-Hypnosis
Deep Breathing Techniques	Self-Talk
Exercise	Thought Stopping
Imagery: Guided or Non-Guided	Time Management
	Transactional Analysis

E. Cognitive Restructuring

1. *Cognitive restructuring* is a purposeful attempt to reframe or take a new perspective on a troublesome problem in an effort to deal with the problem more effectively.

2. A number of cognitive restructuring approaches have been found to be successful.

   a) Relapse prevention is the process of determining cues or identifying high-risk situations that can direct one's thoughts and actions on a predetermined path toward effective self-care.[25,26] The Gorski and Miller[25] program helps people become aware of warning signs that indicate a probable decrease in self-care activities. These warning signs then are associated with action(s) that assist in maintaining or improving self-care activities. Marlatt[26] directs people to recognize high-risk situations in their lives and to plan what they would do to decrease the risk of getting off track.

   b) Problem solving is an active process in which a person assesses a troublesome situation, plans an intervention, implements the intervention, and then evaluates the outcome and refines the intervention to maximize its effectiveness.

   c) Assertiveness training uses education, role playing, and other techniques to teach how to state personal ideas and feelings in a nonaggressive manner. Many aspects of daily living with diabetes generate conflicts that can compromise good metabolic control. Learning to be assertive with peers and supervisory personnel, family and friends, and members of the health care team promotes good emotional and metabolic control.

   d) Time management skills enable the person to have sufficient time for planned activities and free time. Diabetes care takes time. Learning time management skills can be helpful in balancing the needs of life and good self-care.

   e) Self-talk involves saying positive affirmations to oneself or repeating general thoughts directed toward positive action. Some diabetes-related situations make a person feel overwhelmed. Learning to say specific things to oneself that facilitate resolving the actual problems can be very helpful and self-supporting.

f) Thought-stopping is the purposeful ceasing of negative mental thinking. Some thoughts can be overwhelming, especially when a person is faced with daily self-care activities or adjustment to a potentially life-threatening disease. Learning to say stop to such defeating thoughts can be a helpful stress reducer.

F.   Behavior Modification

1.   *Behavior modification* is a way of changing behavior that involves the use of reward or punishment, or informational impact to reach a desired goal.

2.   Three basic methods of behavior modification may be used alone or in combination.

a)   Positive behavior modification[27] involves the use of tokens, points, contracting, shaping (gradually changing behavior by steps), or modeling to reach an end point. This process has been helpful for people who wish to lose weight. Once a specified number of pounds has been lost, or a certain number of tokens has been obtained, or points accumulated, a preset reward may be obtained.

b)   Negative behavior modification involves the use of punishment, removal from the stressor (time-out), or removal of the stressor from the environment (extinction). The most common negative behavior modification recommended for a person who has diabetes is to remove all the tempting sweets from the house.

c)   Implosion (intensive information input) and desensitization (learning to relax in the proximity of the stressor) have been found useful for treating people who experience a variety of fears associated with having diabetes (eg, having an insulin reaction).

G. Coping Strategy Responses

1. Coping strategies work best when the support system is adequate. A social support system allows a person to know that someone else is there to help.

    a) A person may accept a distasteful regimen if a family member or friend shows concern and support.

    b) The interaction in a social support system helps a person feel accepted or acknowledged. Such a system reduces stress, improves adherence, aids in motivation, and reinforces positive behavior. Social support helps a person feel cared about and not alone in the human struggle.

2. Unless the person chooses to take responsibility for personal thoughts and actions, coping ability will not be enhanced and, therefore, little will be accomplished. Stress management is easier to practice if a support system is utilized or biofeedback is obtained. The result is a person better able to overcome both major and minor obstacles and to have a greater potential for stable blood glucose levels.

REFERENCES

1.   Cox DJ, Taylor AG, Nowacek G, Holley-Wilcox P, Pohl SL. The relationship between psychological stress and insulin-dependent diabetic blood glucose control: preliminary investigations. Health Psychol 1984;3:63-75.

2.   Selye H. The stress of life. London: Longmans, Green, 1957;36-38.

3.   Hobfoll SE. Conservation of resources: a new attempt to conceptualizing stress. Am Psychol 1989;44:513-24.

4.   Holmes TH, Rahe RH. The social readjustment rating scale. Psychosom Res 1967;11:213-18.

5.   Orioli EM, Jaffe EM, Scott CD. Stress map. New York: Newmarket Press, 1991.

6.   Tager MJ, Willard S. Transforming stress into power: the energy director system. 2nd ed. Beaverton, Ore: Great Performance Inc, 1991.

7.   Abidin, RR. Parenting stress index. 3rd ed. Charlottesville, Va: Pediatric Psychology Press, 1990.

8.   Delongis A, Coyne JC, Dakof G, Folkman S, Lazarus RS. Relationship of daily hassles, uplifts, and major life events to health states. Health Psychol 1982;1:119-36.

9.   Weinberger M, Hiner SL, Tierney WM. Support of hassles as a measure of stress in predicting health outcomes. J Behav Med 1987;10(1):19-31.

10. Andreoli KG. Self-concept and health beliefs in compliant and noncompliant hypertensive patients. Nurs Res 1981;30:323-27.

11. Scheier MF, Carver CS. Optimism, coping, and health: assessment and implications of generalized outcome expectancies. Health Psychol 1985;4:219-47.

12. Olson DH, McCubbin HI, Barnes H, Larsen A, Muxen A, Wilson M. Family inventories. St. Paul, Minn: University of Minnesota, 1986.

13. Sarason IG, Levine HM, Basham RB, Sarason BR. Assessing social support: the social support questionnaire. J Pers Soc Psychol 1983;44(1):127-39.

14. Fisher-Williams M, Nigl AG, Sovine DL. A textbook of biological feedback. New York: Human Sciences Press, 1986:470-86.

15. Rubin RR. Reframing: an approach to facilitating self-care. Changing Behav 1986;6:1,4,5.

16. Guthrie DW, Moeller T, Guthrie RA. Biofeedback and its applications to the stabilization and control of diabetes mellitus. Am J Clin Biofeedback 1983;6:82-87.

17. Lammers, CA, Naliboff BD, Straatmeyer AJ. The effects of progressive relaxation on stress and diabetic control. Behav Res Ther 1984;22:641-50.

18. Rosenbaum L. Biofeedback-assisted stress management for insulin-treated diabetes mellitus. Biofeedback Self Regul 1983;8:519-32.

19. McGrady A, Bailey BK, Good MP. Controlled study of biofeedback-assisted relaxation: type I diabetes. Diabetes Care 1991:14(5):360-65.

20. Surwit RS, Feinglos MN. The effects of relaxation on glucose tolerance in non-insulin dependent diabetes. Diabetes Care 1983;6:176-79.

21. Feinglos MN, Hastedt P, Surwit RS. Effects of relaxation therapy on patients with type I diabetes mellitus. Diabetes Care 1987;10:72-75.

22.   Jacobson E. Anxiety and tension control. Philadelphia: JB Lippincott, 1964.

23.   Luthe W, Jus A, Geissman P. Autogenic state and autogenic shift: psychophysiologic and neurophysiologic aspects. Acta Psychother Psychosom 1963;11:1-13.

24.   Benson H, Beary JF, Carol MP. The relaxation response. Psychiatry 1974;37:37-46.

25.   Gorski TT, Miller M. Counseling for relapse prevention. Independence, Mo: Herald House-Independence Press, 1982:17-26.

26.   Marlatt GA. Situational determinants of relapse and skill-training interventions: In: Marlatt GA, Gordon JR, eds. Relapse prevention. New York: The Guilford Press, 1985.

27.   Corey G. Theory and practice of counseling and psychotherapy. 3rd ed. Montgomery, Calif: Brooks/Cole Publishing Co, 1986:172-206.

KEY EDUCATIONAL CONSIDERATIONS

1. Stress management is an essential skill for people with diabetes and should be included as an important part of a total education program.

2. Approaches to stress management may be woven into consecutive individual sessions, incorporated within a group program, or taught as a separate class.

3. Create a list of resources for stress management, including helpful books, local workshops, counselors, biofeedback centers, behavioral therapists, etc. Referral is essential when the patient requires counseling with a specialist.

4. During the assessment, listen for and ask questions regarding possible sources of stress (scheduling, finances, family situations, etc). To encourage discussion, begin by saying, "Each one of us experiences stressful times and for some stress is continuous. Tell me about your daily stressors."

5. Using a pencil and blank piece of paper, ask the patient to identify personal signs of stress (binge eating, decreased exercise, withdrawal, etc) and the associated feelings. Using the PARENT approach to stress management, guide the patient in choosing methods of relaxation and stress reduction that suit personal interests, culture, and lifestyle.

6. Demonstrate some relaxation techniques, such as guided imagery, deep breathing, or progressive relaxation. Have audiotapes and videotapes available for loan. Some educators begin each teaching session with a short relaxation exercise to help the patient release outside concerns and focus on the teaching session.

7. Use blood glucose records to identify blood glucose levels as a marker for both the impact of stressors and the effectiveness of stress management.

8. Identify your own stressors and seek assistance for stress management to become a more effective educator and role model for your patients. A rushed, distracted and exhausted educator often delivers conflicting messages.

SELF-REVIEW QUESTIONS

If you are unsure of the answers to the following questions, please review the materials.

1. Describe how stress may affect the body.
2. Explain what should be included in an assessment of stress in preparation for developing a stress-management program.
3. List five methods for relaxation training.
4. Define cognitive restructuring.
5. Give two examples each of positive behavior modification and negative behavior modification.
6. What is the importance of the support system in relation to coping strategies?

CASE EXAMPLE

LL, who has insulin-treated NIDDM (type II diabetes), recently was admitted to the hospital for cystoscopy to evaluate the cause of recurring urinary tract infections. From the hospital's medical record you note that LL's glycosylated hemoglobin values have been close to the normal range for over 2 years. LL's latest hemoglobin A_{1c} value was 11.7% (normal <6.2%). During discharge planning rounds, the attending health professionals assumed that LL's elevated glycosylated hemoglobin level was secondary to the urinary tract infections. Your assessment reveals a different story. You discover that LL has been experiencing repeated crises, including sudden unemployment, financial difficulties, and family problems. LL stopped monitoring her blood glucose levels, skipped meals, overate in fear of developing hypoglycemia, stopped exercising, and reduced her usual dose of insulin but never missed an injection. LL is scheduled for discharge tomorrow and you have 20 minutes to consult with her today.

QUESTIONS

1. What was the value of your assessment?
2. In the limited time available to you, where would you begin?

SUGGESTED SOLUTIONS

Your assessment revealed a reason for LL's recurring urinary tract infections. Because of repeated crises, LL did not have the interest, time, or energy required to carry out the demands of diabetes self-management. To cope, LL tried to do what she thought was safe by reducing her insulin dose and eating to prevent hypoglycemia with resultant hyperglycemia. It is no surprise that LL became host to pathogens.

With 20 minutes for a consultation, you can accomplish a lot by listening to LL's story and validating her concerns. She may find relief in learning that it is common for people to neglect their health when experiencing stressors. This hospitalization gave LL an opportunity to stop and evaluate stress management. With this thought, you can begin to guide LL toward stress management using the positive thinking technique of the PARENT approach.

LL is tired and overwhelmed. You can use relaxation techniques and invite LL to participate in a brief guided imagery experience. Pull the curtain around the bed, ask LL to sit comfortably, and then guide her through the vision of a cool, rushing stream. Ask how she feels and if she found the imagery helpful. End the session by referring LL to some local resources, including a diabetes educator who works in the community.

OTHER SUGGESTED READINGS

Arnold LE, ed. Childhood stress. New York: John Wiley & Sons, 1990.

Benson H. Your maximum mind. New York: Avon Books, 1989.

Cooper CL, Cooper RD, Eaker LH. Living with stress. New York: Penguin Press, 1988.

Dossey B. Relaxation and imagery: awakening the inner healer. Temple, Tex: Bodymind Systems, 1989.

Faelten S, Diamond D. Take control of your life: a complete guide to stress relief. Emmaus, Pa: Rodale Press, 1988.

Goldstein DS. Neurotransmitters and stress. Biofeedback and Self-Regul 1990;15(3):243-71.

Guthrie DW, Sargent L, Speelman D, Parks L. Effects of parental relaxation training on glycosylated hemoglobin of children with diabetes. Patient Educ Couns 1990;16(3):247-53.

Lloyd CE, Robinson N, Stevens LK, Fuller JH. The relationship between stress and the development of diabetic complications. Diabetic Med 1991;8(2):146-50.

Ryan RS, Travis JW. Wellness: small changes you can use to make a big difference. Berkeley, Calif: Ten Speak Press, 1991.

Travis JW, Callander MG. Wellness for helping professionals. Mill Valley, Calif: Wellness Associates Publications, 1990.

Vranic M, Miles P, Rastogi K, et al. Effect of stress of glucoregulation in physiology and diabetes. Adv Exp Med Biol 1991; 291:161-83.

PSYCHOSOCIAL ISSUES

IV. BEHAVIORAL CHANGE

INTRODUCTION

Self-care behavior is critical to maintaining physical and emotional health for people who have diabetes. Technological advances in recent years offer the promise of better health, often at the cost of additional self-care demands. One key to helping patients with diabetes achieve good self-care is understanding the factors that determine diabetes-related behavior. These factors include health beliefs, locus-of-control orientation, self-efficacy, social support, self-care skills, coping skills, emotional well-being, cognitive maturity, health status, regimen complexity and aversiveness, and organizational factors related to health care delivery. To be effective, the diabetes educator must be able to assess these factors in individual patients. The educator and patient must then work together to develop an individualized treatment or education plan designed to foster and maintain mutually agreed upon patterns of self-care. This chapter will guide the reader through this process.

OBJECTIVES

Upon completion of this chapter, the learner will be able to:
- describe the role of behavior in diabetes;
- identify two models of behavior change in diabetes;
- discuss the determinants of diabetes-related behavior;
- assess these determinants in an individual patient, and use the results of this assessment to help the patient develop a healthy self-care plan.

A. The Role of Behavior in Diabetes

1. The relationship between self-care behavior and health outcomes (metabolic control and complications of diabetes) has not been formally established.

   a) The rationale for all our efforts to help patients change their behavior is the belief that good self-care will lead to improved metabolic control and, in turn, to a reduction in the long-term complications of diabetes and to enhanced quality of life.

b) While these assumptions are widely held, and find some support in the literature, the evidence is not clear-cut.

    (1) Self-care (sometimes described as adherence) is a multidimensional construct: adherence varies across areas of the regimen (highest for medical aspects such as taking medications; lowest for lifestyle aspects such as diet and exercise).[1] Adherence to different areas of the regimen are often uncorrelated,[2] thus it is difficult to formally establish relationships between self-care behaviors and metabolic control.

    (2) Evidence for the relationship between metabolic control and complications is somewhat more abundant, although still not unequivocal.[3]

    (3) New research findings, including those of the Diabetes Control and Complications Trial (DCCT), may clarify these relationships.

    (4) Despite the fact that we can draw only tentative conclusions about the benefits of behavior change in the service of more intensive self-care, there is substantial agreement that efforts in this direction are worthwhile.

2. Burgeoning technology affects diabetes self-care behavior.

a) Examples of such technological advances include: self--monitoring of blood glucose (SMBG); intensive conventional therapy (ICT) involving multiple daily insulin injections (MDII); and continuous subcutaneous insulin infusion (CSII).

b) The effects of this technological progress are greatest for those patients who take insulin.

c) Technological advances are a two-edged sword: they offer hope for better health on the one hand but often involve greater self-care demands on the other.

3. The diabetes self-care regimen requires substantial behavior change.

a) People who develop diabetes are asked to make major lifestyle changes (eg, practice SMBG; follow a sophisticated medications regimen; meet exercise requirements; carefully control nutritional composition and timing; manage hypo- and hyperglycemia and associated mood swings; stop smoking; maintain healthy body weight; and manage common illnesses).

b) Research and clinical experience suggest that the behavior change required to maintain good diabetes self-care is difficult for most people.

B. Models of Behavior Change in Diabetes

1. The *Compliance Model* is a traditional medical view of the relationship between health professionals and their patients.

   a) The Compliance Model assumes that the health care professional is responsible for the diagnosis, treatment, and outcome of diabetes care, while the patient is a recipient of this care.

   b) The Compliance Model assumes that change occurs as a result of the professional's efforts to get the patient to follow the prescribed treatment regimen.

2. The *Empowerment Model*[4] assumes that most of the responsibility for diabetes care rests with the person who has the disease, so final decisions regarding diabetes-related behavior are the right and responsibility of the individual.

   a) The Empowerment Model holds that the costs and benefits of diabetes care must be seen in the broader personal and social context of a person's life; and that patients must be seen as experts on their own lives, while professionals are experts on diabetes.

   b) According to the Empowerment Model, behavior change takes place as the professional helps patients prepare to make informed decisions about self-care through education, appropriate care recommendations, and support. The patient has the right and responsibility to operate as an informed, equal, active partner in the treatment program.

c) While empowerment is a desirable goal, not all patients may seek empowerment. Professionals must respect different styles.

(1) Some people are more comfortable in a less active role, preferring to follow the recommendations of their health care providers.

(2) Sometimes empowerment may be achieved by steps. For example, patients who present in very poor control may be first encouraged to closely follow a set treatment regimen. Once they have succeeded in this endeavor, they may choose to take a more active role in self-management.

C. Determinants of Diabetes-Related Behavior

Determinants of Diabetes-Related Behavior

1. Health beliefs
2. Locus of control
3. Self-efficacy
4. Self-care/Self-management
5. Coping skills
6. Emotional well-being
7. Cognitive maturity
8. Health status
9. Social support
10. Regimen complexity
11. Organizational factors related to health care delivery

---

1. According to the *Health Belief Model*,[5] behavior reflects a person's subjective interpretation of a situation.

a) In relation to diabetes self-care, the behavior of patients with diabetes is influenced by four perceptions: their susceptibility to the negative consequences of diabetes; the severity of their diabetes and its complications; the benefits of self-care activities; and the cost of self-care.

(1) Susceptibility: How vulnerable does the person feel to the negative consequences of the illness? People

with non-insulin-dependent diabetes mellitus (NIDDM), also called type II diabetes, may feel less susceptible, telling themselves that they are less vulnerable because they have a "milder form of the disease." On the other hand, people who have insulin-dependent diabetes mellitus (IDDM), also called type I diabetes, or people who are suffering from complications of diabetes may feel more vulnerable or susceptible. The more susceptible a person feels, according to this theory, the more likely it is that the person will practice good self-care.

(2) Severity of diabetes and its complications: Perceptions of issues such as impairment, disability, and job loss are relevant here. The more severe the perceived consequences of having diabetes, the more likely the person is to adhere to good self-care practices.

(3) Benefits of self-care activities: Questions such as, Will it work? Will it help me avoid complications? Will it help me do the things I want to do? are relevant here. An affirmative answer will reinforce good self-care behavior.

(4) Cost of self-care: Financial costs; personal costs, such as the extra time involved in efforts to achieve tight control, as well as the costs of tight control, such as weight gain and increased incidence of hypoglycemia, influence self-care behavior. To be open to behavior change, a person must believe that the benefits of these changes outweigh the costs. For example, the answer to questions such as, If I exercise and change my eating habits, will that help to control my diabetes? or, If I monitor my blood glucose levels and follow my regimen, will I be more likely to avoid eye problems? must be yes.

b) Research yields some confirmation for the predictions of the Health Belief Model. In particular, susceptibility and severity seem to predict self-care. These relationships may be curvilinear, however. For example, those who experience the lowest and highest levels of susceptibility may have the lowest levels of self-care. Those who feel very susceptible may not be motivated to change their behavior because they feel overwhelmed or fatalistic.

2. Beliefs concerning who or what controls health-related outcomes also influence behavior. The *Locus of Control Theory* suggests three such beliefs (often called orientations): internal orientation, powerful-other orientation, and chance orientation.

   a) Internal orientation: People who have an internal orientation tend to believe that diabetes-related health outcomes are controlled primarily by their own efforts. Research shows that internal orientation is associated with positive outcomes, particularly active, independent self-care management.[6]

   b) Powerful-other orientation: People who have a powerful-other orientation tend to believe that outcomes are controlled primarily by other people, generally by health care professionals. Research shows that powerful-other orientation is also associated with positive outcomes, particularly with close adherence to prescribed treatment regimens.[7]

   c) Chance orientation: People who have a chance orientation tend to believe that outcomes are primarily determined by fate or chance. Research shows that chance orientation is associated with a range of negative outcomes, including poor self-care, poor metabolic control, and low levels of emotional well-being.[7]

3. According to *Self-Efficacy Theory*,[8] a person's sense of self-efficacy affects behavior.

   a) The more confident a person feels about performing a set of behaviors, the more likely that person is to actually perform those behaviors.

   b) Some studies suggest that patients with diabetes who have a high degree of self-efficacy exhibit better self-care, emotional well-being, and metabolic control.

4. Behavior may also be influenced by the degree of actual *self-care and self-management skills* that a person has achieved in managing aspects of the diabetes self-care regimen.

    a) Skill may be defined as knowledge in action, because it is achieved through the acquisition of knowledge and through guided practice.

    b) Self-care skill involves the ability to accomplish specific tasks (eg, to accurately monitor blood glucose levels, to properly administer insulin, and to eat healthy meals), and the ability to coordinate a variety of specific tasks to promote physical and emotional well-being (eg, to coordinate the amount and timing of food, medication, and exercise when planning to attend a party).

    c) The foundation of self-care skill is the ability to solve problems, by coordinating activities, and using information and experience to make decisions. The ability to problem solve may be thought of as a self-management skill.

5. Self-care behavior can be affected by a patient's *skill in coping* with the emotional stresses of day-to-day life with diabetes.

    a) Emotional resourcefulness or hardiness can be a critical factor in determining a person's ability to change behavior and maintain good diabetes self-care.

        (1) Clinical experience reveals that major obstacles to self-care are often emotional (eg, denial and feeling overwhelmed).

        (2) Improving coping skills can lead to improved metabolic control by facilitating self-care.

        (3) Improving coping skills can also lead to improved metabolic control by reducing the direct effects of stress on glycemia.[9]

    b) Some evidence suggests that improved diabetes-specific coping skills may be associated with better self-care and glycemic control.[10]

6. *Emotional well-being* also influences patient self-care behavior.

a)   Causal relationships between emotional status and self-care are probably reciprocal (ie, high levels of emotional well-being tend to facilitate self-care, and high levels of self-care tend to facilitate emotional well-being).

b)   Self-esteem (feeling generally good about oneself) is positively related to diabetes self-care.[9]

c)   Depression is negatively related to self-care.[9]

d)   Anxiety is negatively related to self-care.[9]

7.   Behavior reflects the level of *cognitive maturity* that a person has achieved.

a)   Some young people (up to about 15 years of age) are not cognitively ready to assume responsibility for independent self-care.[11]

b)   To be considered cognitively mature, a young person must be able to reason about abstract concepts inherent in diabetes management (eg, balancing multiple unknowns).

c)   Parents, motivated by frustration or the advice of professionals, often withdraw from responsibility for their children's diabetes care. When young people aren't ready to assume the responsibility divested by their parents, gaps in care may develop. These gaps often go unrecognized and can lead to critical difficulties.

8.   A patient's *health status* influences self-care behavior. Acute and chronic complications of diabetes may either hamper or facilitate behavior change in the direction of improved self-care.

a)   Acute complications may adversely affect self-care behavior. For example, hypoglycemic episodes may discourage efforts to achieve tight control, while hyperglycemia may lead to exhaustion which, in turn, may sap energy required for self-care.

b)   Acute complications may encourage self-care. For example, blurry vision caused by hyperglycemia may be so frightening that the patient is motivated to improve self-care behaviors.

c) Chronic complications can also have an adverse effect on self-care. For example, neuropathy or cardiovascular complications may interfere with exercise, and poor vision may interfere with the patient's ability to self-monitor blood glucose (SMBG) levels.

d) Chronic complications may encourage better self-care. Patients often report that they were "scared straight" by the onset of complications.

9. Self-care behavior may also be affected by the amount of *social support* a patient receives.

  a) Potential sources of support include family, friends, and co-workers; medical staff; and other persons with diabetes.

  b) Some evidence suggests that peer group support facilitates self-care by providing practical help, increasing learning, and improving emotional well-being while decreasing the person's sense of isolation.[12]

10. *Regimen complexity and aversiveness* can have an effect on self-care behavior.

  a) Patient behavior may be influenced by the perception of the regimen as complicated and/or unpleasant.

    (1) The diabetes regimen is inherently complex.

      (a) The diabetes regimen involves many behaviors: meal planning, foot care, SMBG, exercise, and taking medication, to name a few.

      (b) Each behavior presents its own complexities: eg, following an exercise plan may require timing the activity to avoid the peak action time of injected insulin, testing blood glucose levels before and after exercise, establishing a habit of regular exercise, and remembering to carry food to avoid hypoglycemia.

    (2) The regimen must be taken into account during every aspect of daily living, thus complicating social situations, work activities, and personal life.

(3) The regimen must be followed for life or until a cure is developed.

b) Research on other medical conditions, and clinical experience in diabetes, suggests that regimen complexity may be a major obstacle to obtaining optimal patterns of self-care.

11. A person's self-care behavior is influenced by certain *organizational factors related to health care delivery*.

a) The quality of patient-provider interactions can affect self-care behaviors. A non-judgmental approach by the provider encourages behavior change by the patient. A cooperative/ consultative relationship between patient and provider also encourages change (eg, working together to develop a nutritional plan designed to meet a weight goal set by the patient rather than having the provider dictate a plan to produce a predetermined weight loss).

b) Financial resources affect behavior. Those with limited financial means are less likely to seek care and to activate the process of change.

c) Practices of the clinic or organization providing care can also have an effect on behavior.

(1) Long waits for appointments discourage people from seeking health care and from maintaining their own behavior change.

(2) Ready access to providers by means of on-call availability or follow-up phone contacts encourages self-care.

(3) Availability of a multidisciplinary care team including a nurse, nutritionist, mental health professional, and social worker, also facilitates self-care.

(4) Availability of high-quality diabetes education, conveniently timed and located, facilitates self-care.

D. Facilitating the Process of Behavior Change

1. The first step in facilitating behavior change is to assess the patient.

   a) Facilitating behavior change in a patient must begin with a thorough assessment of the factors currently influencing that person's diabetes-related behavior. Such an assessment allows the educator to identify strengths as well as areas of difficulty for the patient, and provides a structure for designing a plan for treatment and education.

   b) The following are some of the factors an educator may choose to assess, along with specific suggestions for assessment techniques where useful standardized techniques exist.

      (1) *Diabetes-related health beliefs* can be assessed by asking questions to determine the patient's beliefs concerning susceptibility to negative consequences of diabetes, the severity of these consequences, and costs and benefits of self-care. The patient's responses provide information about overall motivation to change as well as specific areas in which further education might increase motivation. Remember, people who feel highly susceptible might actually be less motivated than those who feel moderately susceptible, so interventions designed to temper fears about susceptibility may be required for these patients.

      (2) Diabetes-specific *locus-of-control* orientation may be assessed by means of standardized questionnaires such as those developed by Ferraro, Price, Desmond et al,[13] and Bradley, Brewin, Gamsu et al.[14] The patient's beliefs about what or who controls diabetes-related health outcomes can provide critical information about approaches likely to be effective for facilitating behavior change in that individual. Patients with a predominately chance orientation are at special risk for negative outcomes, and all efforts

must be taken to shift this orientation. The educator may find it impossible to shift patients from a chance orientation to an internal orientation in a single step, even though the latter orientation may be an ultimate goal. In many patients this process is best accomplished in stages. The first step might involve shifting from a chance locus-of-control orientation (belief that health outcomes are basically uncontrollable) to a powerful-other orientation (belief that health outcomes are controllable through reliance on the advice of health professionals). A second step might involve shifting from powerful-other to internal locus of control.

(3) A 30-item instrument originally developed for use with adolescents[15] provides an effective way to measure a patient's perceptions of diabetes *self-efficacy*, or the confidence that a person feels about performing diabetes-related behaviors. Because the degree of confidence is related to the individual's willingness to actually engage in healthy behaviors, diabetes self-efficacy responses provide useful data about the patient's overall confidence and about specific behaviors that need special attention during the education or treatment process.

(4) The patient's ability to carry out critical day-to-day *self-care skills* must be assessed as a guide to planning individual treatment or education. The level of these skills is best assessed by observation, when possible (eg, procedure of insulin administration or SMBG), or by having the patient describe in detail how the activity is performed (eg, meal planning or sick-day management). The patient's ability to coordinate activities to maintain physical well-being and quality of life should also be assessed, particularly because the level of these problem-solving or self-management skills seems to be a powerful predictor of health outcomes. Assessing

self-care and self-management skills can be an invaluable tool for targeting educational and treatment interventions.

(5) *Coping style, coping skills, and emotional well-being* may substantially affect a patient's self-care, glycemic control, and quality of life and should be assessed.

 (a) Coping style can be evaluated using structured instruments.[16]

 (b) Coping skills may be assessed by asking patients how they would respond to hypothetical diabetes-related emotional issues. Low self-esteem and high levels of anxiety or depression may severely hamper a patient's efforts to establish and maintain adequate patterns of self-care.

 (c) The presence of psychological disorders can be assessed through standardized questionnaires or by referral to a qualified mental health professional.

(6) Cognitive immaturity may preclude children and young adolescents from assuming substantial responsibility for their self-care. While the educator may not choose to assess *cognitive maturity* directly, this issue should be considered when working with young patients.

(7) A complete history of the patient's *health status* including acute and chronic complications of diabetes and other health issues and problems is essential for effective educational or treatment planning. These issues may critically influence a patient's motivation for self-care and ability to engage in important aspects of the self-care regimen.

(8) A patient's social environment may either support or undermine efforts to change behavior, so it is important to determine the *social supports* available, including involvement of family, friends, and co-

workers in the patient's life with diabetes. What practical help is provided? What emotional support? What (if any) barriers to self-care do other individuals represent? What changes would the patient like to see in these areas? The answers to these questions need to be determined.

(9) *Regimen Complexity* can have an effect on self-care behavior. Identifying aspects of the regimen that the patient considers particularly difficult can be critical to establishing positive patterns of self-care. Patients often report that they "give up" on self-care because one particular aspect of the regimen is impossible to manage. A direct question, What is the part of the regimen you find most difficult? will generally elicit invaluable information. Finding a more effective way to deal with such aggravating problems can have a major impact on overall motivation for self-care. Similarly, identifying aspects of the regimen that a patient finds particularly complex may also effectively focus educational efforts.

2. To facilitate behavior changes, patients must be taught self-management and coping skills.

   a) Developing and maintaining healthy patterns of self-care requires three basic skills: specific self-care skills, self-management skills, and coping skills.

   b) Educational interventions should be directed toward facilitating the development of each set of skills.

      (1) Specific self-care skills training: Meta-analyses (which statistically combine the results of many different studies) reveal that active diabetes education, involving demonstration of skills, practice, and direct practical feedback for efforts, is the most effective approach to improving self-care skills and metabolic control.[17] More didactic approaches are less effective, because they tend to increase knowledge without increasing skill or improving glycemia.

While these findings may seem obvious, their implications for the design of educational interventions are profound and often not adequately taken into account. The "bottom line" is clear: to facilitate behavior change, don't talk, teach behavior.

   (a) To make the inherently difficult process of behavior change as manageable as possible, educators must learn to help patients get the most "bang for their buck." If the goal is improved glycemic control, some studies show that one behavior — situational adjustment of insulin — can lead to significantly improved glycosylated hemoglobin levels even in the absence of changes in such basic aspects of lifestyle as meal planning and exercise.[18]

(2) Self-management skills training: Rigid adherence to a regimen prescription may be less effective than juggling components of treatment in response to daily events and SMBG results.[19]

   (a) Given the exigencies of life with diabetes, the patient's physical and emotional well-being is most enhanced by flexibility, or skill in problem solving.

   (b) To be effective, diabetes education must incorporate interventions designed to foster the development of these skills. One productive approach involves discussing in detail situations in which the patient finds his or her diabetes problematic, with the goal of developing, practicing, and refining options for handling these situations in ways that promote physical and emotional well-being.

(3) Coping skills training: The goal of diabetes coping skills training is to help patients overcome attitudinal and emotional barriers to the successful application of new knowledge and skills. Sometimes called a diabetes specific Cognitive Behavioral Model, this

approach, which has been described in detail elsewhere,[20,21] is active and individualized.

(a) Patients learn that certain thoughts or attitudes trigger constructive behavior in difficult situations, while other thoughts and attitudes trigger unconstructive behavior.

(b) Patients are taught how to implement a procedure for achieving a positive approach to those diabetes-related situations that they find particularly troublesome, and they practice this approach.

(c) A final component of coping skills training is relapse prevention — offering protection against the possibility that the inevitable slips in self-care may trigger a full-blown relapse (see Chapter III: Stress Management).

3. The way in which educational and treatment programs are organized or structured can facilitate or hinder change in patients. Educators should keep these structural issues in mind as they design interventions.

a) Multidisciplinary staff: Given the complexity of life with diabetes, patients will generally benefit from educational or treatment interventions that allow them to consult with a multidisciplinary staff that includes physicians, nurses, nutritionists, mental health specialists, exercise specialists, and pharmacists.

(1) Because few clinics can support such a staff, a viable alternative, such as a referral network of experienced specialists in each field, should be considered. Access to specialists tends to minimize barriers to effective self-care, so educators should attempt to develop effective referral networks.

(2) Educators working with physicians should consider "priming" their patients before meetings with the physician. Studies show that a brief intervention focused on training patients to be more active and

assertive during interviews with a physician leads to improvement in glucose control and quality of life.[22]

b) On-call availability and follow-up contact: Most changes involved in maintaining healthy patterns of self-care require continuing support, yet patients typically go for months without consulting health care providers.

  (1) Two options for encouraging more frequent contact (and, potentially, for facilitating behavior change) are on-call availability and follow-up telephone contact.

    (a) It is difficult to get patients to call between scheduled appointments, even when they are having problems with their diabetes. However, concerted efforts to encourage contact, either as circumstances require or at a set time when the educator is available, may be helpful.

    (b) Follow-up telephone contact initiated by the educator may also support effective self-care.

  (2) These contacts can maintain patient motivation to change by addressing specific problems that might lead to relapse, and by facilitating a pattern of open communication that makes it easier for the patient to call if problems do arise.

c) Group support: Whenever possible, the educator should provide opportunities for group experiences with others who have diabetes. Such opportunities can take the form of group education or of formal or informal diabetes support groups. Groups encourage efforts to improve self-care through mutual sharing and encouragement, modeling, positive reinforcement, and personal goal setting.

4. Empowering patients to undertake behavior change is gaining increased support in diabetes education.[23] Given the fact that patients make many important and often complex self-care decisions every day, the goal is to empower people to make these decisions wisely (see Table IV.1).

a) Several key concepts are basic to an empowerment-based practice.

TABLE VI.1:
Four-Step Patient Empowerment Counseling Model

1. *Help patient identify problematic diabetes-related issues.* ("What part of your diabetes regimen is the biggest problem for you?")

2. *Help patient identify thoughts and feelings associated with the problem.* ("What are you thinking and feeling when you are struggling with the problem?")

3. *Help patient identify health-related attitudes and beliefs underlying the problem and establish diabetes self-care goals.* ("What deeper attitudes and beliefs lead you to think and feel as you do when you are struggling with the problem? What is your ultimate goal for dealing with the problem?")

4. *Help patient develop and commit to a plan for achieving the goal.* ("What would be the steps, one by one, that would lead to reaching your ultimate goal?")

Source: Anderson, Funnell, Barr, et al.[23]

---

(1) Emphasizing the whole person: people are more than patients. They are physical, emotional, social, and spiritual beings.

    (a) Every aspect of a person's life interacts and must be taken into account in making diabetes self-care decisions.

    (b) Educators must recognize, respect, and support this holistic dynamic if they are to play a constructive part in the process of change.

(2) Transferring decision making and leadership: the educator should recognize that it is impossible to solve a problem for the patient or to impose a solution.

    (a) The effective educator assumes the role of wise advisor to the patient on subjects related to the treatment of diabetes, offering recommendations

and supporting the generation of potentially useful approaches to a given problem.

  (b) It is the patient's right and responsibility to make decisions.

(3) Educating for informed choice about treatment options: two types of education are crucial to empowerment.

  (a) The first involves providing knowledge about diabetes and its treatment to allow the patient to make wise decisions about diabetes self-care options.[23] This type of education might be called self-management training.

  (b) The second type of education is designed to facilitate patients' self-awareness about the emotional, social, intellectual, and spiritual components of their lives as they relate to the daily decisions the patients must make about their diabetes. This type of education has been called coping skills training.

(4) Viewing treatment plans as ongoing experiments: Treatment plans must be continuously refined in the face of experience. It is critically important that both educator and patient recognize this fact and use it to their advantage. The beauty of an experiment is that it produces information, not success or failure. This information is used to refine the treatment plan and produce more information, which is then used to support further refinement, and so on and so on. Because this process mirrors life with a chronic disease, it is an excellent model for positive coping with diabetes.

b) Empowering patients requires diabetes educators to reevaluate their teaching methods and approach to patient care.

(1) Educators must recognize that patients are in control of their own self-care. Educators often come to this realization "by the back door." That is to say

educators deal every day with patients who refuse to follow the educator's good advice about caring for their diabetes. Although the first and strongest response to this refusal might be frustration, or perhaps disappointment, further thought might lead the educator to see that these patients are telling the educator in no uncertain terms that *they* will decide what they will and will not do.

(a) If patients truly have veto power, and they do, educators must create a coalition for care that helps the patient assume an initiating role rather than a defensive one.

(b) The role of the educator in such a coalition is not to give advice about the "right" or "best" way to accomplish a particular goal, but rather to help patients explore the range of self-care options available to them, and the consequences of implementing each of these options.

(c) Such exploration can be frustrating for the educator when the patient is resistant or "in denial." In such a case, educators must recognize the limits of their ability to effect change.

(2) Many educators have difficulties dealing with the emotional content of patients' problems. This makes it difficult for educators to encourage patients to identify, express, and explore negative emotions that are an inevitable part of life with diabetes. Diabetes educators are trained to be problem solvers; they must learn that emotions are not problems to be solved. Rather, emotions must be recognized, identified, expressed, and accepted, by the patient.

(a) The educator's role is that of thoughtful, compassionate listener.

(b) Educators have no responsibility to "fix" their patients' negative emotions. Recognizing this may help educators feel more comfortable in helping their patients to accept and work with these uncomfortable feelings.

c) Empowering patients offers several potential benefits for educators.

   (1) Accepting that the educator's role is limited to education and counseling can relieve any guilt the educator might feel when patients don't follow healthy self-care regimens. It can be a great relief to say, "I did my job (educating and counseling) as well as I could; getting the patient to change is not part of my job."

   (2) Recognizing that changing patients is not part of the job description may help educators to feel less frustrated with patients who choose to care for their diabetes in ways the educator considers unhealthy.

   (3) When educators spend less energy trying to "motivate" patients, they relieve themselves of a self-imposed burden and free energy for other, more attainable tasks.

REFERENCES

1. Kurtz SMS. Adherence to diabetes regimens, empirical status and clinical applications. Diabetes Educ 1990;16:50-56.

2. Ary DV, Toobert D, Wilson W, et al. Patient perspective on factors contributing to nonadherence to diabetes regimen. Diabetes Care 1986;9:168-72.

3. Skyler JS. Conclusions. Diabetes Spectrum 1988;1:118-20.

4. Funnell MM, Anderson RM, Arnold MS, et al. Empowerment: an idea whose time has come in diabetes education. Diabetes Educ 1991;17:37-41.

5. Becker MH, Janz NK. The health belief model applied to understanding diabetes regimen compliance. Diabetes Educ 1985;11:41--47.

6. Bradley C, Lewis KS, Jennings AM, et al. Scales to measure perceived control developed specifically for people with tablet-treated diabetes. Diabetic Med 1990;7:685-94.

7. Schlenk EA, Hart LK. Relationship between health locus of control, health value, and social support and compliance among people with diabetes mellitus. Diabetes Care 1984;7:566-74.

8. Bandura A. Self-efficacy theory: toward a unifying theory of behavior change. Psychological Review 1977;84:191-95.

9. Rubin RR, Peyrot M. Psychosocial problems and interventions in diabetes. Diabetes Care 1992;15;1640-57.

10. Rubin RR, Peyrot M, Saudek CD. Effect of diabetes education on self-care, metabolic control, and emotional well-being. Diabetes Care 1989;12:673-79.

11. Ingersoll GM, Orr DP, Herrold AJ, et al. Cognitive maturity and self-management among adolescents with insulin-dependent diabetes mellitus. J Pediatr 1986;108:620-23.

12. Glasgow RE, Toobert DJ. Social environment and regimen adherence among type II diabetic patients. Diabetes Care 1988;11:377-86.

13. Ferraro LA, Price JH, Desmond SM, et al. Development of the diabetes locus of control scale. Psychological Rep 1987;61:763-70.

14. Bradley C, Brewin CR, Gamsu DS, et al. Development of scales to measure perceived control of diabetes mellitus and diabetes-related health beliefs. Diabetic Med 1984;1:213-18.

15. Grossman HY, Brink S, Hauser S. Self-efficacy in adolescent girls and boys with insulin-dependent diabetes mellitus. Diabetes Care 1987;10:324-29.

16. Peyrot M, McMurry JF. Psychosocial factors in diabetes control: adjustment of insulin-dependent adults. Psychosom Med 1985;47:542-57.

17. Padgett D, Mumford E, Hynes M, et al. Meta-analysis of the effects of educational and psychosocial interventions on management of diabetes mellitus. J Clin Epidemiol 1988;41:1007-30.

18. Rubin RR, Peyrot M, Saudek CD. Differential effects of diabetes education on self-regulation and lifestyle behaviors. Diabetes Care 1991;14:335-38.

19. Sims D, Sims E. Conclusions. Diabetes Spectrum 1988;2:49-51.

20. Rubin RR, Walen SR, Ellis A. Living with diabetes. J Rational-Emotive Cogn-Behav Ther 1990;8:21-39.

21. Rubin RR, Biermann J, Toohey B. Psyching out diabetes. Los Angeles: Lowell House, 1992.

22. Greenfield S, Kaplan SH, Ware JE, et al. Patients' participation in medical care: effects on blood sugar control and quality of life in diabetes. J Gen Intern Med 1988;3:448-57.

23. Anderson RM, Funnell MM, Barr PA, et al. Learning to empower patients: results of professional education program for diabetes educators. Diabetes Care 1991;14:584-90.

KEY EDUCATIONAL CONSIDERATIONS

Supporting patients in their efforts to initiate and maintain healthy patterns of self-care is a critical responsibility of the diabetes educator. To facilitate the patient's potential to live well with diabetes, keep in mind the following key considerations:

1. *The role of the educator is to facilitate change*; the role of the patient is to make change. Every encounter with the patient should be directed toward empowerment. The key is to ask questions and offer options rather than to issue directives.

2. *The patient's personal model of diabetes*, including health beliefs, locus-of-control orientation, and diabetes self-efficacy, *powerfully influences motivation for change*. Both the patient and educator must learn to identify and understand the effects of these attitudes and, when necessary, how they can be shifted. The power of these attitudes can be demonstrated by discussions which lead to the revelation that the patient's diabetes-related behavior flows directly from these beliefs.

3. *The support a patient receives* from family, friends, and medical staff also *affects patterns of self-care*. The educator should be able to assess and make efforts to influence these factors, as well. The patient should be encouraged to identify gaps in currently available support, and be helped to create plans to fill these gaps.

4. *Behavior-based education is far more effective than knowledge-based education in changing patterns of self-care*, so all interventions should be presented in a practical, experience-based context. Specific self-care skills and more complex problem-solving or self-management skills should all be demonstrated, practiced, observed, and refined in face-to-face interaction.

5. *Coping skills training can be an invaluable component of efforts to improve self-care patterns*. All too often attitudinal and emotional barriers prevent patients from making needed changes in diabetes-related behavior. Patients can be taught a basic approach to managing the emotional side of life with diabetes and this may help them cope more effectively with many common self-care crises.

SELF-REVIEW QUESTIONS

If you are unsure of the answers to the following questions, please review the materials.

1. What do we know about the relationship between self-care behavior and glycemic control?
2. Why is the issue of diabetes self-care even more critically important today than it was 20 years ago?
3. What are some important differences between a compliance-oriented and empowerment-oriented approach to facilitating self-care?
4. What health beliefs seem to be most strongly related to positive patterns of self-care?
5. What are the differences among the following: self-care skills, self-management skills, coping skills?
6. How can the presence of acute or chronic complications of diabetes affect self-care?
7. Identify some organizational or structural factors related to the provision of health care that may influence self-care behavior.
8. Describe the basic approach to diabetes coping skills training described in this chapter.
9. Identify the four steps of the patient empowerment counseling model.
10. Why is it difficult for some educators to deal with patients' diabetes-related emotions?

CASE EXAMPLE

RT is a 57-year-old man diagnosed 3 years ago with non-insulin-dependent diabetes. At the time of diagnosis, RT was hypertensive, weighed approximately 30 pounds (14 kg) above his ideal body weight, did not exercise regularly, and smoked about two packs of cigarettes a day. An oral hypoglycemic agent was prescribed. He was given a calorie-restricted diet, asked to monitor his fasting blood glucose level three times a week, offered a smoking cessation program, and advised to take up some form of regular exercise.

Since his diagnosis, RT has cancelled most of his appointments for medical follow-up of his diabetes, keeping only four appointments in 3 years. Last week he called to complain of increased fatigue, blurred vision, and frequent urination. At his appointment today his blood glucose is 220 mg/dL (12.2 mmol/L), his blood pressure is 160/95, his weight is 10 pounds (4.5 kg) more than it was on diagnosis, and he acknowledges that he is not monitoring his blood glucose levels at home nor is he exercising or eating properly. He is still smoking two packs of cigarettes per day.

When questioned about his diabetes-related behavior, RT offers the following explanations:

"Other than the little problems I had last week, I feel I'm doing fine. After all, I have the milder type of diabetes."

"At my job I'm always on the go. There's no way I could eat the way you say I'm supposed to."

"The cigarettes are my way of relaxing, and they haven't killed me yet."

"My mother died from diabetes when she was 62. I figure it's fate, and it will get me, too, sooner or later. There's nothing I can do about it."

"The exercise, the diet, the blood sugar testing — the whole routine is just more than I can manage. I'm just not a structured sort of person."

"You tell me what to do, like the blood sugar testing, for instance, and I go home thinking I might be able to do it, but when I get home I realize I can't. I can't get the drop on the strip or whatever, so I get frustrated and give up."

"Even when I feel like I'm really going to just do it, like start exercising, right away I flop, because it all gets so complicated, with the timing and making sure I don't go low, and all that. It's just too much to think about."

"I get so mad. It's just unfair. I ask, Why me? When the answer is, there is no reason, I just say to hell with it all. I know that's crazy, but that's just the way my mind works."

QUESTIONS

1. What factors seem to be creating RT's resistance to initiating healthier patterns of self-care?

2. What other factors might you want to assess before beginning to develop an educational intervention for RT?

3. How would you decide which aspect of self-care to address first?

SUGGESTED SOLUTIONS

RT offers a classic, if all too common, example of resistance to change. His attitudes and his lack of skills interact to create a vicious cycle that leaves him stuck. His motivation to change is limited by the fact that he sees his disease as relatively mild, and the consequences of better self-care (coordinating diet and work, giving up cigarettes) as too costly. He also believes that diabetes-related health outcomes are controlled by chance or fate, so there's no reason to pay any significant price to try to affect these outcomes: What will be will be. Beyond this, RT has no confidence that he can manage the self-care regimen, and it's clear that his education to date leaves him without sufficient skill to truly take care of himself. His skills are limited in the realms of specific diabetes self-care skills, problem-solving skills, and coping skills.

An effective approach to RT's problems must begin with the creation of an effective alliance between educator and patient. Such an alliance requires that the educator help RT to identify some of his negative diabetes-related emotions. These feelings must then be acknowledged (if RT is ready). Work may then proceed at both attitudinal and behavioral levels. Using an empowerment approach, even if true empowerment is a long time coming, the educator can ask RT questions about his fatalistic attitude toward diabetes-related health outcomes. Remember, it's crucial to ask questions, not make statements. Given an open, nonjudgmental approach, RT will probably come to see that his mother's fate need not be his own, and that his core beliefs have to do with his lack of self-efficacy, not a belief that diabetes is inherently uncontrollable.

At this point, feelings of inadequacy must be recognized and acknowledged. The practical difficulty of living with diabetes should also be acknowledged, to keep the issue in perspective and maintain some motivation for change. Now RT and the educator are ready to address behavior directly. Again, for purposes of marshaling all available motivation, the educator might ask what aspect of the regimen RT feels he is handling best right now. Even if he's handling nothing very well, this question will usually lead to the acknowledgement that everything isn't totally hopeless. Then it may be possible to identify sources of strength that facilitate the way this issue is handled.

Next, RT should be asked to identify the first issue he'd like to work on. It's important that the choice be his, and he should be encouraged to be both ambitious and realistic in making his choice and setting his goals for change. Reaching a goal that is insufficiently ambitious provides little satisfaction, while an overly ambitious goal is generally unattainable.

It is clear that RT, like so many of our patients, needs intensive, behavior-based skills training. He needs to watch the educator demonstrate important skills, practice them under observation and at home, and then redemonstrate them later. He also needs training in the more complex problem-solving skills, learning how to make use of the various discrete skills in real-life situations. This type of education places considerable demands on the educator, and it is possible to provide such education only where the resources are available. Those in practice settings where such intervention is impossible might refer patients for intensive education. After such an intensive program, effective continuing follow-up will probably be more manageable.

OTHER SUGGESTED READINGS

Aikens JE, Wallander JL, Bell DSH, et al. Daily stress variability, learned resourcefulness, regimen adherence, and metabolic control in type I diabetes mellitus: evaluation of a path model. J Consult Clin Psychol 1992;60:113-18.

Campbell LV, Barth R, Gosper JK, et al. Impact of intensive educational approach to dietary change in NIDDM. Diabetes Care 1990;13:841-47.

Feste C. A practical look at empowerment. Diabetes Care 1992;15:922-25.

Glasgow RE, Osteen VL. Evaluating diabetes education: are we measuring the most important outcomes? Paper presented at the Satellite Symposium on Behavioral Aspects of Diabetes. Va: 14th International Diabetes Federation Congress, June 1991.

Haire-Joshu D. Motivation and diabetes self-care: an educational challenge. Diabetes Spectrum 1988;1:279-82.

Hamera E, Cassmeyer V, O'Connell KA, et al. Self-regulation in individuals with type II diabetes. Nurs Res 1988;37:363-67.

Nagasawa M, Smith MC, Barnes JH, et al. Meta-analysis of correlates of diabetes patients' compliance with prescribed regimens. Diabetes Educ 1990;16:192-200.

Maxwell AE, Hunt IF, Bush MA. Effects of social support group as an adjunct to diabetes training, on metabolic control and psychosocial outcomes. Diabetes Educ 1992;18:303-9.

Padgett DK. Correlates of self-efficacy beliefs among patients with non-insulin-dependent diabetes mellitus in Zagreb, Yugoslavia. Patient Educ Couns 1991;18:139-47.

Polly RK. Diabetes health beliefs, self-care behaviors, and glycemic control among older adults with non-insulin-dependent diabetes mellitus. Diabetes Educ 1992;18:321-27.

Wing RR, Epstein LH, Nowalk MP, et al. Self-regulation in the treatment of type II diabetes. Behav Ther 1988;19:11-23.

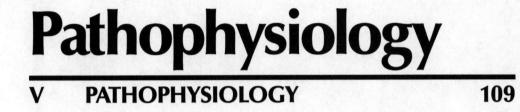

Pathophysiology

PATHOPHYSIOLOGY

V. PATHOPHYSIOLOGY

INTRODUCTION

It is generally recognized that diabetes mellitus encompasses a group of genetically and clinically heterogeneous disorders in which glucose intolerance is a common denominator. Because the syndrome of diabetes mellitus includes many disorders that differ in pathogenesis, natural history, and responses to treatment, it is important that clinicians and researchers use commonly accepted terminology as well as standardized classification and diagnostic criteria.[1]

OBJECTIVES

On completion of this chapter, the learner will be able to:
- define and contrast insulin-dependent diabetes mellitus (IDDM) and non-insulin-dependent diabetes mellitus (NIDDM);
- list three types of diabetes other than IDDM and NIDDM;
- list four symptoms of uncontrolled hyperglycemia;
- discuss the epidemiology of diabetes;
- define the following terms: *glucose toxicity, insulin resistance,* and *gluconeogenesis.*

A. Definition of Diabetes Mellitus

1. Diabetes mellitus can be defined as a heterogeneous group of disorders of intermediary metabolism characterized by glucose intolerance, with hyperglycemia present at the time of diagnosis.

2. Individuals with diabetes are known to have a higher risk of microvascular, macrovascular, and neurologic disorders, and it is widely assumed that chronic hyperglycemia is contributory to the development of these complications.

B. Diagnostic Criteria for Diabetes Mellitus

1. The definitions of the various syndromes of diabetes were standardized in the late 1970s by the National Diabetes Data Group (NDDG).[2]

2. In 1979, the NDDG established several alternative diagnostic criteria for diabetes:

    a) One diagnostic alternative would be the presence of "unequivocal hyperglycemia" now commonly accepted as a random plasma glucose level of 200mg/dL (11.1 mmol/L) or greater, with symptoms of hyperglycemia (such as increased thirst, polyuria, polyphagia, increased urine flow, blurred vision and so forth).

    b) Another option would require multiple tests of the person's glucose level, which could be performed to establish the diagnosis in adult men and in nonpregnant adult women.

        (1) One test criterion would be a fasting venous plasma glucose level at or above 140 mg/dL (7.8 mmol/L) on more than one occasion, OR;

        (2) For adults with a fasting plasma glucose level less than 140 mg/dL (<7.8 mmol/L), sustained elevated plasma glucose levels during at least two oral glucose tolerance tests (OGTT) would confirm the diagnosis of diabetes. Both the two hour plasma glucose level and at least one other between 0 and 2 hours must result in 200 mg/dL (11.1 mmol/L) or greater. Oral glucose tolerance testing is not necessary if the fasting plasma glucose level is 140 mg/dL (7.8 mmol/L) or greater.

    c) Diagnosis of diabetes in children should be restricted to those who have *one* of the following:

        (1) Random plasma glucose levels of 200 mg/dL (11.1 mmol/L) or greater *plus* classic signs and symptoms of diabetes, including polyuria, polydipsia, ketonuria, and rapid weight loss, OR;

(2) Fasting plasma glucose level of 140 mg/dL (7.8 mmol/L) or greater on at least two occasions *and* sustained elevated plasma glucose levels during at least 2 oral glucose tolerance tests. Both the 2-hour plasma glucose and at least one other between 0 and 2 hours after glucose dose (1.75 g/kg ideal body weight up to 75 grams) should be 200 mg/dL (11.1 mmol/L) or greater.

d) Different criteria were specified for pregnant women (see Chapter XV: Pregnancy: Preconception to Postpartum).

e) No mention was made of the use of glycosylated hemoglobin values in the diagnosis of diabetes. Although some recent studies have suggested that the glycosylated hemoglobin level could be useful in establishing the diagnosis, no uniform criteria have been published. It is generally thought that the glycosylated hemoglobin value should be viewed as a supplementary test, rather than a definitive test, with respect to establishing the diagnosis of diabetes.

C. Subclasses and Statistical Risk Classes

1. The NDDG report[2] established subclasses of diabetes.

a) Individuals with *insulin-dependent diabetes mellitus* (IDDM), also called *type I* diabetes, are ketosis-prone and dependent on exogenous insulin to maintain life. Typically, patients with IDDM have the onset of the condition in childhood or as a young adult, although it can occur at any age. In recent years, this condition has been clearly identified as an autoimmune disorder.[3]

b) Individuals who have *non-insulin-dependent diabetes mellitus* (NIDDM), or *type II* diabetes, are not dependent on exogenous insulin, nor are they prone to ketosis.

(1) Typically, patients with NIDDM have the onset of their condition after age 40; many have a family history of diabetes; most are obese, and in these

patients, glucose intolerance is often improved by weight loss.

(2) Many NIDDM patients are treated with supplemental insulin. The addition of insulin supplements to their therapeutic program does not change their disorder from NIDDM to IDDM, despite the unfortunate clinical misunderstanding that has frequently arisen since the publication of the NDDG report.

c) A newer term, *insulin-treated diabetes mellitus* (ITDM), has recently been popularized.[4] ITDM would seem to be a clinically useful term to describe any person with diabetes who is taking insulin as part of their therapeutic regimen, regardless of whether the person has IDDM or NIDDM, or any other variety of diabetes.

d) Diabetes may also occur as a result of other disorders, in which case it is designated as *secondary diabetes mellitus*. Causes include pancreatic disorders, including hemochromatosis, chronic pancreatitis, and pancreatectomy; hormonal disorders, including Cushing's syndrome (excess amounts of corticosteroids), thyrotoxicosis (excess thyroid hormone), and acromegaly (excess growth hormone); and other disorders, including cystic fibrosis, congenital rubella syndrome, and Down syndrome. Treatment of these other disorders may result in amelioration of the diabetes. However, it frequently is impossible to reverse the underlying disorder, and the therapy would be similar to therapy for genetic diabetes, using the modalities of meal planning, exercise, and medications.

e) The diagnosis of *gestational diabetes mellitus* (GDM) applies only to women in whom glucose intolerance develops or is discovered during pregnancy. After pregnancy, the diagnostic classification may be changed to *previous abnormality of glucose tolerance*, IDDM, NIDDM, or *impaired glucose tolerance*. Women whose diabetes predated the pregnancy should not be included in the GDM class. Women with GDM have an increased future risk for progression to NIDDM or rarely IDDM.

   f)   *Impaired glucose tolerance* (IGT) is the term used to describe nondiagnostic fasting glucose levels (<140 mg/dL [<7.8 mmol/L]) and a level of glucose intolerance a degree below that considered definite for diabetes. For example, if an OGTT using 75 g glucose is performed, the results might include a single value above 200 mg/dL (11.1 mmol/L); these results are neither normal or diagnostic of diabetes.

 2.   The NDDG report identified two statistical risk classes for epidemiologic and research purposes.[1]

   a)   *Previous abnormality of glucose tolerance* (PrevAGT) is the diagnostic classification for persons with normal glucose tolerance and a history of transient diabetes mellitus or impaired glucose tolerance.

   b)   *Potential abnormality of glucose tolerance* (PotAGT) is the diagnostic classification for persons who have never experienced abnormal glucose tolerance but have a greater than normal risk of developing diabetes mellitus or impaired glucose tolerance.

 3.   The NDDG report discouraged certain terms, including *juvenile diabetes* and *adult-onset diabetes*. "Borderline" diabetes and "chemical" diabetes are now redesignated IGT, and "prediabetes" has been replaced with either PrevAgt or PotAGT.

D.   Alterations in Fuel Metabolism Relating to Diabetes

 1.   *Glucose* is the principal carbohydrate used for energy production. The process by which glucose is broken down, liberating energy and producing water and carbon dioxide, is called *glycolysis* and is promoted by the hormone *insulin*. After absorption into the cells glucose can be used immediately for release of energy to the cells or it can be stored in the form of glycogen in the liver and muscle.

2. Normal utilization of glucose and other carbohydrates as fuel is dependent on a complex series of chemical reactions. These reactions are primarily modulated by insulin, which is produced by the beta cells of the pancreas. The actions of insulin are opposed by actions of other hormones including *glucagon*, the hormone produced by the alpha cells of the pancreas; *epinephrine*, a catecholamine hormone produced in the adrenal medulla; *growth hormone* (somatotropin), a hormone secreted by the pituitary gland; and *somatostatin*, a hormone produced in the delta cells of the pancreas.

   a) Insulin is *anabolic*. In addition to fostering glycolysis, insulin promotes the synthesis of glycogen from glucose *(glycogenesis)* and the synthesis of proteins and lipids, and opposes the breakdown of glycogen to glucose *(glycogenolysis)*. Thus, after meals, in the fed state, when insulin is present, the processes of glycolysis and glycogenesis predominate, and glycogenolysis is minimal.

   b) The absence of insulin, which would normally occur in the fasting state, is *catabolic*, and results in glycogenolysis, lipolysis, and proteolysis. These catabolic processes are promoted by other hormones; for example, glycogenolysis is stimulated by epinephrine and glucagon.

   c) In the absence of insulin, glucose can be formed from noncarbohydrate sources, such as amino acids and glycerol, to provide glucose during fasting. This process is called *gluconeogenesis*. Glucocorticoids, glucagon, epinephrine, and growth hormone stimulate gluconeogenesis.

   d) When glucose is unavailable (in the fasting state), the breakdown of fats to provide an alternative source of energy (*lipolysis*) occurs, with the production of by-products called *ketones* or *ketone bodies*. In the absence of insulin, excessive ketones are produced and are excreted through the kidneys, and may accumulate in the blood.

3. Decreased insulin secretion causes increasing hyperglycemia due to multiple mechanisms.[5]

   a) Lack of insulin promotes glucose production from endogenous sources (increased glycogenolysis and increased gluconeogenesis).

   b) In the absence of insulin, glucose entering the bloodstream from food is not converted to glycogen (decreased glycogenesis).

   c) There is a decrease in glucose uptake by peripheral tissues during the period following ingestion of food (decreased glucose utilization).

E. Pathophysiology

1. In nondiabetic individuals, insulin is released in two phases. The first phase occurs within the first 5 minutes following glucose ingestion. This represents the release of insulin that had been stored within the beta cell. The second phase represents release of newly synthesized insulin.

2. In patients with IDDM, insulin deficiency occurs because of destruction of the beta cells of the pancreatic islets. Insulin deficiency or relative deficiency also occurs in many patients with NIDDM.

3. Some degree of insulin resistance is present in the vast majority of individuals with IGT, and in essentially all patients with NIDDM who have fasting hyperglycemia of 140 mg/dL (7.8 mmol/L) or more. The severity of the insulin resistance is positively correlated with the elevation of the fasting glucose level. The resistance may be due to the alteration of intracellular events involved in glucose metabolism.

4. There has been considerable discussion about whether diminished tissue sensitivity to insulin or impaired beta cell function is the initial lesion in the patient with NIDDM. It is clear that both insulin action and insulin secretion are markedly

impaired in individuals who have had NIDDM for any length of time.[6]

F. Immunologic Features of IDDM

1. Insulin-dependent diabetes mellitus has been associated with certain genes, called *HLA antigens,* which are part of the major histocompatibility complex of chromosome 6, and help to regulate the body's immune responsiveness. More than 90% of whites with IDDM have one (or both) of the HLA haplotypes (patterns) called DR3 or DR4.[3]

2. Autoantibodies (antibodies directed against normal tissues of the body in an abnormal immune response) have frequently been implicated in causing IDDM.
    a) *Islet cell antibodies* (ICAs) are frequently found before or at the time of diagnosis of IDDM, and serve as a marker for autoimmune attack.
    b) *Insulin autoantibodies* (IAAs) may occur in patients with diabetes who have never received insulin therapy. Why antibodies to a normally secreted product develop is not clear, but these antibodies appear to be a useful predictor of IDDM.
    c) *Anti-GAD* (glutamic acid decarboxylase) and other autoantibodies are also found in IDDM patients.
    d) If persons genetically at risk for IDDM are screened with a combination of ICA and IAA assays, an abnormality may be detected in about 90% of patients prior to establishing the diagnosis of diabetes.

G. Insulin Resistance

1. The role of insulin in the pathogenesis of many disorders, including diabetes mellitus, obesity, atherosclerosis, and hypertension has become a subject of considerable discussion (see comments about syndrome X in Chapter XXIV: Macrovascular Disease). *Insulin resistance* has been defined as

subnormal biologic response to a given concentration of insulin. As used in this context, it refers to the observation that obese people have elevated insulin levels (*hyperinsulinemia*) in the fasting or fed state; it is presumed that such people have some degree of resistance to the effects of insulin at the peripheral level. People with NIDDM, obesity, atherosclerosis, and hypertension tend to have a higher body mass index; higher waist to hip ratios; higher fasting and postprandial glucose levels; higher systolic and diastolic blood pressure readings; higher triglyceride, total cholesterol, and LDL-cholesterol levels; and lower HDL-cholesterol concentrations compared with "normal" subjects.[7] Furthermore, it is sometimes alleged that insulin resistance is a "basic cellular defect" that somehow causes these other disorders. Thus, the terms *hyperinsulinemia* and *insulin resistance syndrome* have sometimes been used to describe the effects of insulin that may ultimately be responsible for adverse effects on the health of the individual who has high insulin levels.

2.   The causes of insulin resistance have been subdivided into several categories.[8]

   a)   Defects intrinsic to the target cells, including mutations of the insulin-receptor gene, problems with the intracellular glucose transporters, and cellular inhibitors of insulin-receptor kinase, have been identified.

   b)   Secondary factors affecting target cells, including abnormal physiologic states (such as stress imposed by fever or sepsis), normal physiologic states (such as pregnancy), and specific hormonal factors (including disorders of glucocorticoids, growth hormone, catecholamines, glucagon, and thyroid hormone), can contribute to insulin resistance.

H.   Glucose Toxicity

1.   *Glucose toxicity* has been identified in animal models of diabetes. It may be defined as hyperglycemia that seems to

contribute to the development of insulin resistance and impaired insulin secretion.[9]

2. In NIDDM (type II diabetes) in humans, accumulating evidence suggests that chronic hyperglycemia leads to progressive impairment in insulin secretion and may contribute to insulin resistance. The precise mechanism of the hyperglycemia-induced decrease in insulin secretion is unidentified.[9] It is assumed that the hyperglycemia provokes reversible adverse effects at the tissue level.

3. Evidence also implicates glucose toxicity in the functional impairment of insulin secretion that occurs during the initial presentation of patients with IDDM (type I diabetes), and this has been postulated to perhaps explain the "honeymoon period" (the period following the initiation of therapy in IDDM during which the diabetes is extremely easy to control, and during which time the insulin requirement may actually decrease to zero for a short while).[9]

I. Etiologic Speculations about IDDM and NIDDM

1. There is general agreement that IDDM is an autoimmune disorder. Several antibodies are frequently observed before deterioration of glucose metabolism, including antibodies to beta cells (usually called islet cell antibodies or ICAs) and occasional antibodies to other endocrine glands, such as the thyroid and adrenal glands. Also, specific HLA patterns are statistically more likely to occur in patients with IDDM than in the general population. Why the autoimmune process is activated is still subject to considerable speculation, and whether the presumed autoimmune destruction of the pancreatic islet cells can be interrupted is undergoing active evaluation in many clinical trials throughout the world.

2. Clearly, NIDDM is a different disorder from IDDM. Some interplay of two or three factors (islet cell malfunction, malfunction of the insulin receptors on target tissues, and/or malfunction of postreceptor function inside the target cells) seems to occur. Without both pancreatic islet cell and peripheral target cell malfunctions simultaneously present, hyperglycemia is much less likely to occur. Exactly what defects occur, and the relationship to heredity, still needs to be studied. One factor that is evident is that the release of insulin in response to the usual stimulus of hyperglycemia is diminished.

J. Epidemiology

1. Differing estimates have been made of the frequency of diabetes in the United States. Estimates have ranged as high as 14 million people with diabetes (based on a survey done in 1980). As of 1993, the American Diabetes Association has refined the estimate to 13 million, including 6.5 million diagnosed cases and 6.5 million undiagnosed cases, based on a 1990 survey.[10] There were 302,613 people diagnosed as having IDDM, about 5% of all diagnosed cases.[10] About 2% of all cases of diabetes are secondary to other conditions; GDM is thought to occur in about 2% to 5% of pregnancies.

2. Genetic, environmental, and lifestyle factors all seem to play a role in the development of diabetes.[11]
   a) The age-adjusted relative risk of having diabetes is higher for minority groups than for the white population.
   b) American Indians are 2.7 times as likely to have diabetes as are whites; Puerto Ricans, 2.2 times as likely; Mexican Americans, 2.1 times as likely; African-Americans, 1.6 times as likely; and Cubans, 1.5 times as likely.[10]

K. Symptoms of Hyperglycemia

1. *Polydipsia* (increased thirst) and *polyuria* (increased urinary frequency with increased urinary volume) are frequently associated with hyperglycemia and are directly attributable to the osmotic diuresis that occurs with glycosuria, and the subsequent volume depletion.

2. *Fatigue* is commonly reported by patients with hyperglycemia.

3. *Abnormalities of healing, polyphagia* (increased appetite), *weight loss*, and increased rate of occurrence of certain *infections,* including those caused by yeasts, are sometimes noticed. These problems are attributed to abnormal carbohydrate metabolism and its effects on the body's tissues.

4. *Visual changes* such as blurry vision may be reported by persons with diabetes. These symptoms are attributed to changes in the lens associated with hyperglycemia and are reversible with control of the glucose level.

REFERENCES

1.   Rifkin H, ed. Physician's guide to non-insulin-dependent (type II) diabetes: diagnosis and treatment. 2nd ed. Alexandria, Va: American Diabetes Association, 1988:4-11.

2.   National Diabetes Data Group. Classification and diagnosis of diabetes mellitus and other categories of glucose intolerance. Diabetes 1979;28:1039-57.

3.   Thai A, Eisenbarth GS. Natural history of IDDM. Diabetes Rev 1993;1:1-13.

4.   Ratner RF, Whitehouse FW. Motor vehicles, hypoglycemia, and diabetic drivers. Diabetes Care 1989;12:217-22.

5.   Seifter S, Englard S. Carbohydrate metabolism. In: Rifkin H, Porte Jr D, eds. Ellenberg and Rifkin's diabetes mellitus: theory and practice. 4th ed. New York: Elsevier Science Publishing, 1990:1-40.

6.   Dinneen S, Gerich J, Rizza R. Carbohydrate metabolism in non-insulin-dependent diabetes mellitus. N Engl J Med 1992;327:707-13.

7.   Ferrannini E, Haffner SM, Mitchell BD, Stern MP. Hyperinsulinemia: the key feature of a cardiovascular and metabolic syndrome. Diabetologia 1991;34:416-22.

8.   Moller DE, Flier JS. Insulin resistance — mechanisms, syndromes, and implications. N Engl J Med 1991;325:938-48.

9.   Rossetti L, Giaccari A, DeFronzo RA. Glucose toxicity. Diabetes Care 1990;13:610-30.

10.   Lipsett LF, Geiss L. Statistics: prevalence, incidence, risk factors, and complications of diabetes [Memorandum]. Am Diabetes Assoc Bull 1993 Apr 9.

11. Maclaren N, Atkinson M. Is insulin-dependent diabetes mellitus environmentally induced? [Editorial]. N Engl J Med 1992;327:348-49.

KEY EDUCATIONAL CONSIDERATIONS

1. People with diabetes need to be taught many new concepts, skills, and behaviors. Traditionally, the definitions and the pathophysiology of diabetes have been among the first topics to be presented to newly diagnosed patients. However, sound learning theory suggests that, for many patients, more immediate needs must be addressed before they will be ready to learn.

2. The pathophysiology of diabetes can be presented using pictures, flip charts, or models to provide a very basic explanation of how glucose is normally used by the body, and why insulin is needed. More sophisticated terminology and concepts can be presented in group or individual question-and-answer sessions, based on the immediate needs of the patient(s).

3. If patients present with blurred vision as a symptom of diabetes, it is important to teach that this is a temporary condition associated with changes in the lens of the eye. Many patients fear that they have permanent eye damage.

4. Often patients whose diabetes is diagnosed on the basis of laboratory values do not have symptoms. This may affect their belief that they have diabetes or that they are susceptible to its complications; this could affect their readiness to learn.

SELF-REVIEW QUESTIONS

If you are unsure of the answers to the following questions, please review the materials.

1. What is the definition of diabetes mellitus?
2. Describe four effects of decreased insulin release on glucose metabolism.
3. What are the two phases of insulin release for the person without diabetes?
4. List three immunologic abnormalities associated with diabetes.

5. List four risk factors for the development of NIDDM.
6. List four symptoms of hyperglycemia and explain the pathophysiology of each.
7. Describe insulin resistance.
8. Describe glucose toxicity.

CASE EXAMPLE

AZ is a 39-year-old obese Hispanic woman. She complains of having felt fatigued for 2 weeks and reports excessive thirst and nocturia. She relates a history of GDM during two pregnancies, and a family history of ITDM. Her sister, who has diabetes, tested AZ's fasting blood glucose level with a blood glucose meter. The result was 187 mg/dL (10.4 mmol/L). The sister insisted that AZ has diabetes and that she should see her physician promptly.

QUESTIONS

1. Is there enough data to state that AZ has diabetes mellitus?
2. If yes, is it more likely that she has IDDM (type I) or NIDDM (type II) diabetes? Why? If no, what additional tests should be performed to establish the diagnosis?

SUGGESTED SOLUTIONS

Any middle-aged person with obesity, appropriate symptoms, and a family history of diabetes is at high risk of developing NIDDM. AZ has many risk factors for NIDDM.

The definitive diagnosis of diabetes, however, must be based upon laboratory determination of blood glucose values. The blood glucose data provided by her sister is not sufficient to label AZ with a lifelong chronic disease, and additional testing is appropriate. Laboratory fasting glucose values over 140 mg/dL (7.8 mmol/L) on two or more occasions, or a random plasma glucose level of 200 mg/dL (11.1 mmol/L), or greater, plus classic signs and symptoms of diabetes would easily suffice to make the diagnosis.

OTHER SUGGESTED READINGS

DeFronzo RA, Bonadonna RC, Ferrannini E. Pathogenesis of NIDDM: a balanced overview. Diabetes Care 1992;15:318-68.

Eisenbarth GS, Pietropaolo M. Prediction and prevention of type I diabetes mellitus. Contemp Int Med 1992;4:15-30.

Herold KC, Rubenstein AH. New directions in the immunology of autoimmune diabetes [Editorial]. Ann Int Med 1992;117:436-38.

Moller DE, Flier JS. Insulin resistance — mechanisms, syndromes, and implications. N Engl J Med 1991;325:938-48.

National Diabetes Data Group. Classification and diagnosis of diabetes mellitus and other categories of glucose intolerance. Diabetes 1979;28:1039-57.

Palmer JP. Predicting IDDM. Use of humoral immune markers. Diabetes Rev 1993;1:104-15.

Rifkin H, ed. Physician's guide to non-insulin-dependent (type II) diabetes: diagnosis and treatment. 2d ed. Alexandria, Va: American Diabetes Association, 1988.

Rifkin H, Porte Jr D, eds. Ellenberg and Rifkin's diabetes mellitus: theory and practice. 4th ed. New York: Elsevier Science Publishing, 1990.

Sperling M, ed. Physician's guide to insulin-dependent (type I) diabetes: diagnosis and treatment. Alexandria, Va: American Diabetes Association, 1988.

Thai A, Eisenbarth GS. Natural history of IDDM. Diabetes Rev 1993;1:1-14.

Therapies

THERAPIES

VI.   NUTRITION

INTRODUCTION

Diabetes is a chronic disease that requires lifestyle changes, especially in the areas of nutrition and exercise. The goal of nutrition care is to assist persons with diabetes to make behavioral changes in nutrition and exercise habits that will improve their overall nutritional status and/or diabetes management, not simply to increase their knowledge.

Nutrition is an essential component of successful diabetes management. Every individual with diabetes should receive education related to diabetes and nutrition, as well as have an individualized meal plan appropriate for personal lifestyle and diabetes management goals. This meal plan and management goals also need modification during the course of treatment.

Achieving nutritional goals requires a coordinated team effort by the Registered Dietitian (RD), nurse educator, physician, exercise specialist, behavioral specialist, and the person with diabetes. Family members and significant others need to be an integral part of the education program and are encouraged to follow the same lifestyle recommendations as the person with diabetes.

Nutritional recommendations from the American Diabetes Association for persons with diabetes are similar to nutritional recommendations from the American Heart Association; National Cancer Institute; the National Cholesterol Education Program for Adults, Children and Adolescents; and the Dietary Guidelines for Americans. The purpose of these recommendations is to improve overall health through optimal nutrition. However, controversy exists about the recommendations and will be discussed in this chapter.

For the person with diabetes, there are additional concerns. A major nutrition goal is to help bring and keep blood glucose levels in as near-normal a range as possible by balancing food with insulin and activity. Diabetes is a major risk factor for morbidity and mortality due to coronary artery disease, cerebrovascular disease, and peripheral vascular disease. Nutrition plays a preventive role in achieving recommended lipid levels.

For persons using insulin, a meal plan based on the individual's usual food intake should be determined, and then insulin therapy can be integrated into the usual eating and exercise patterns. For persons with non-insulin-dependent diabetes, the goal is normalization of blood glucose levels and reduced hyperinsulinemia. This goal can be achieved through moderate weight loss, improved eating habits, caloric restriction, spacing of meals, increased activity levels, and learning new behaviors and attitudes.

OBJECTIVES

On completion of this chapter, the learner will be able to:

- list nutrition goals for diabetes management;
- state the relationship of obesity to hyperinsulinemia and NIDDM;
- define body mass index (BMI) and waist-hip ratio;
- describe the role of insulin in the metabolism of carbohydrate, protein, and fat;
- identify three areas of controversy related to the role of carbohydrate in meal planning for persons with diabetes;
- list guidelines for the use of sucrose and fiber;
- list dietary recommendations for the amount and type of fat to be eaten by persons with diabetes;
- state a realistic protein level for persons with microalbuminuria;
- define the term *acceptable daily intake* (ADI) as it relates to the use of high-intensity sweeteners;
- list guidelines for the use of alcohol;
- list recommendations for the amount of sodium in the diet for persons with and without hypertension;
- describe four steps used to individualize nutrition prescriptions;
- list nutritional guidelines for illness, exercise, and hypoglycemia;
- explain the six exchange lists and their nutritive values;
- describe alternative methods available for teaching meal planning.

A. Goals of Nutritional Therapy

1. Restore and maintain as near-normal blood glucose levels as is feasible by balancing food with insulin and activity levels.

2. Provide assistance in attaining optimal lipid levels (cholesterol, low-density lipoprotein [LDL], triglycerides, very-low-density lipoprotein [VLDL], and high-density lipoprotein [HDL]).

    a) The National Cholesterol Education Program for Adults[1] lipid classification values are:
        Cholesterol levels:
        > Desirable: 200 mg/dL (5.20 mmol/L) or lower
        > Borderline-high: 200-239 mg/dL (5.17-6.18 mmol/L)
        > High risk: >240 mg/dL (6.20 mmol/L) and above
        LDL-Cholesterol levels:
        > Desirable: 130 mg/dL (3.36 mmol/L) or lower
        > Borderline-high: 130-159 mg/dL (3.36-4.11 mmol/L)
        > High risk: 160 mg/dl (4.14 mmol/L) and above.

    b) The National Cholesterol Education Program for Children and Adolescents[2] lipid classification values are:
        Cholesterol levels:
        > Desirable: 170 mg/dL (4.40 mmol/L) or lower
        > Borderline-high: 170-199 mg/dL (4.40-5.15 mmol/L)
        > High risk: 200 mg/dL (5.17 mmol/L) and above
        LDL-Cholesterol levels:
        > Desirable: 110 mg/dL (2.85 mmol/L) or lower
        > Borderline-high: 110-129 mg/dL (2.85-3.34 mmol/L)
        > High risk: 130 mg/dL (3.36 mmol/L)

    c) Recommended triglyceride levels:
        Adults: 150 mg/dL (1.70 mmol/L) or lower[1]
        Children, first decade: <100 mg/dL (1.13 mmol/L)[2]
        Children, second decade: <120 mg/dL (1.35 mmol/L)[2]

3. Provide adequate calories for maintaining or attaining reasonable weights for adults, normal growth and development rates for children and adolescents, and adequate calories and nutrients during pregnancy and lactation.

4. Improve overall health through optimal nutrition.

B. **Strategies for Achieving Nutritional Goals for IDDM**

1. The ideal management plan for persons who require exogenous insulin integrates insulin therapy with usual eating habits. It is not necessary to separate meals and snacks into any artificial or unnatural division. Individuals on conventional insulin therapy need to eat at consistent times, synchronized with the time-actions of insulin, monitor blood glucose levels, and adjust the insulin doses for the amount of food eaten.

2. Individuals can learn to make appropriate insulin adjustments by evaluating blood glucose patterns. (See Chapter IX: Monitoring and Management). After mastering pattern control, individuals can learn a more intensified style of insulin adjustment and can make compensatory and anticipatory changes in regular (short-acting) insulin, based on pre- and/or postprandial blood glucose levels.

3. Individuals on an intensified insulin regimen — multiple injections or continuous subcutaneous insulin infusion (CSII) using an infusion pump — have more flexibility in the timing of meals and snacks, as well as the amount of food eaten.

C. **Strategies for Achieving Nutritional Goals for NIDDM**

1. The nutrition goal for persons with non-insulin-dependent diabetes mellitus (NIDDM), also called type II diabetes, is to achieve and maintain normal blood glucose and lipid levels.

2. Several strategies are available to assist individuals.
   a) Weight loss. Moderate weight loss (10 to 20 lb, or 5 to 9 kg), irrespective of starting weight, has been shown to reduce hyperglycemia, dyslipidemia, and hypertension.[3,4] However, if metabolic parameters have not improved after

moderate weight loss, oral hypoglycemic agents (OHA) or insulin may be needed.

(1) The type of obesity associated with metabolic diseases — NIDDM, impaired glucose tolerance (IGT), hypertension, and lipid abnormalities — is the android or abdominal distribution of adipose tissue. Upper body obesity is associated with hyperinsulinemia and insulin resistance, both risk factors for metabolic disease.[5,6]

(2) Obesity is the excessive accumulation of adipose tissue. Degree of obesity and leanness can be described several ways.[7]

   (a) Relative weight (RW) is the measured body weight divided by the midpoint of the medium-frame, desirable weight recommended in the 1959 or 1983 Metropolitan Life Insurance Company tables. A level of >20% above desirable body weight is associated with increased health risks.

   (b) Body mass index (BMI) is the body weight (in kg) divided by height (in m^2). A BMI of >27 to 30 is used to define overweight and obesity.

   (c) Obesity usually is defined as a percent body fat >25% for men and >30% for women as measured by skinfold measurements or bioelectrical impedance analysis (BIA).

   (d) Morbid obesity is arbitrarily defined as weight twice the desirable weight or 45 kg (100 lb) over desirable weight.

(3) Waist-to-hip ratio (>0.95 for men, >0.8 for women) indicates risk for metabolic diseases. The regional distribution of body fat (abdominal versus hips and thighs) is an important predictor of the risks of obesity and can be easily measured with a tape measure.

b) Moderate calorie restriction. As research continues to elucidate why weight loss is difficult for many persons, the emphasis for persons with NIDDM needs to be shifted from weight loss to achieving and maintaining normal blood glucose levels. A moderate caloric restriction (500 to 1000 calories less than the average daily intake as calculated from the diet history) and a nutritionally adequate meal plan should be initiated to produce a gradual and sustained weight loss.

c) Spacing of meals, eating breakfast and lunch, and avoiding large caloric intakes late in the day and evening. The ideal division of food has yet to be determined. Research is emerging that suggests it may be better to divide total food intake into smaller meals and snacks spread throughout the day.[8] Other recommendations suggest that only three meals should be eaten at four- to five-hour intervals. Long-term comparison studies are needed to determine the ideal spacing of food intake. At this point, the best advice is to individualize the spacing of meals based on the patient's schedule, blood glucose goals, ability to handle food intake, etc.

d) Learning new behaviors and attitudes that will help with long-term lifestyle change.

e) Increasing activity levels.

D. Determining Caloric Needs

1. Calories should be prescribed to achieve and maintain a reasonable body weight. Adult calorie needs vary depending on activity, age, and desired weight change. The most accurate method used to estimate caloric needs is a diet history of usual food intake. See Tables VI.1 and VI.2 for general guidelines that can be used to estimate desirable body weight (DBW) and calorie requirements. DBW, rather than actual weight, is used to determine caloric needs. Weight above DBW is usually from stored fat that does not require calories for maintenance. Short- and long-term weight goals should, however, be based on the individual's determination of a *reasonable weight*, not on ideal or desirable body weight.

TABLE VI.1: Estimation of Desirable Body Weight (DBW)

Build	Adult Women	Adult Men	Children
Medium	100 lbs for the first 5 ft of height 5 lbs per in for each in above 5 ft*	106 lbs for the first five ft of height 6 lbs per in for each in above 5 ft	Consult growth curves
Small	Subtract 10%	Subtract 10%	
Large	Add 10%	Add 10%	

* For conversion to metric system: 2.2 pounds = 1 kilogram; 1 inch = 2.54 centimeter

Reproduced with permission from Nutrition Guide for Professionals: Diabetes Education and Meal Planning. American Diabetes Association, 1988.

TABLE VI.2: Estimation of Maintenance Calories for Adults

	kcal required/ lb DBW	kcal required/ kg DBW
Men and physically active women	~15	~30
Most women, sedentary men, and adults over age 55	~13	~28
Sedentary women, obese adults and sedentary adults over age 55	~10	~20
Pregnant Women		
First trimester*	~13-15	~28-32
Second/third trimester*	~16-17	~36-38
Lactation**	~15-17	~36-38
Gestational Diabetes		
Normal weight 120% DBW	~13-14	~28-30
Obese 120% DBW	~11-12	~24-25

To estimate maintenance calories, multiply desirable body weight (DBW) in pounds by the calories required. To lose 1 lb/wk, subtract 500 cal from daily requirement and/or increase energy expended through exercise. To lose 2 lb/wk, decrease calories by 1000/day and/or increase exercise. To gain weight, do the opposite.

* Follow weight gain on pregnancy weight-gain grids to determine actual needs. Calorie level may need to be increased for women who are >40 lb above DBW. Calories based on DBW may not be sufficient to prevent starvation ketosis and for adequate fetal growth. Consultation between physician and dietitian may be needed for women whose estimated calorie needs are <1800 or >2500.

** Follow weight; actual calorie needs may be less or more.

Reproduced with permission from Nutrition Guide for Professionals: Diabetes Education and Meal Planning. American Diabetes Association, 1988.

2. Calories should be prescribed to provide for normal growth and development in children and adolescents. To determine normal growth and weight profiles, children and adolescents' growth should be monitored on a weight-height growth grid at a minimum of every 3 to 6 months.

   a) Children's calorie requirements should be based on a diet history. It should be emphasized to families that the meal plan is not a restriction of calories but is intended to ensure a reasonably consistent food intake and a nutritionally balanced diet. Two methods can be used to evaluate adequacy of caloric intake.

      (1) Prescribe 1000 calories for the first year of life plus a minimum of 100 calories for each year up to a minimum of 2000 calories at age 11 years. From ages 12 to 15 years, add 100 calories per year for girls and 200 calories per year for boys. For calorie needs after age 15 years (see Table VI.3).

      (2) For other means of determining calorie needs for children and adolescents (see Table VI.3).

E. Insulin and Metabolism

1. The therapeutic goals of diabetes care include not only striving toward euglycemia, but also toward the accompanying return of normal carbohydrate, protein, and fat metabolism.

2. Insulin is a hormone essential for the use and storage of these nutrients.

   a) In the metabolism of carbohydrate, insulin facilitates entry of glucose into cells, stimulates glycogen synthesis, and increases triglyceride stores by facilitating the entry of glucose into cells and its conversion to triglycerides.

   b) In the metabolism of protein, insulin lowers blood amino acids in parallel with a reduction of blood glucose levels; facilitates incorporation of amino acids into tissue protein; and affects hepatic enzymes, causing gluconeogenesis, resulting in an increase of glucose for energy.

TABLE VI.3: Caloric Needs for Children and Young Adults

	kcal/pound of body weight	kcal/kg of body weight
Children		
Age 0-12 months	~55	~120
1-10 years	45 to 36*	100 to 80
Young Women		
11-15 years	~17	~35
16 and older	~15	~30
more with increased activity		
Young Men		
11-15 years	36-20	80-50
	(mean 30)	(mean 65)
16-20 years		
Average activity	~18	~40
Very physically active	~22	~50
Sedentary	~15	~30

* Gradual decline in calories per pound as age increases.

Reproduced with permission from Nutrition Guide for Professionals: Diabetes Education and Meal Planning. American Diabetes Association, 1988.

---

    c)   In the metabolism of fat, insulin promotes lipogenesis by activating lipoprotein lipase, the enzyme that facilitates transport of triglycerides into adipose tissue for storage; inhibits lipolysis; and stimulates hepatic lipogenesis.

    d)   Without insulin, lipolysis occurs rapidly, leading to excessive production of ketones and eventually ketoacidosis.

F.   Prescribing Calories from Carbohydrate in the Diabetes Meal Plan

    1.   The American Diabetes Association (ADA) recommends a range in the percentage of calories from carbohydrate (CHO) that can be prescribed.[9] The average percentage of calories from carbohydrate generally is approximately 45% to 55% of the total daily calories. Controversy exists concerning the ideal percentage of CHO in the diabetes meal plan, especially for the patient with NIDDM. The concern is that consuming 60% of

the calories from CHO might lead to elevated postprandial blood glucose, insulin, and triglyceride levels.[10] However, the ADA recommendations emphasize the need to individualize the amount of CHO in meal plans based on an individual's metabolic parameters, eating habits, changes the person is willing and able to make in usual eating habits, and the impact of the type and level of CHO on blood glucose and lipid levels.

2. It is a commonly held belief that sugars, both added and naturally occurring, are rapidly absorbed and lead to hyperglycemia and increased need for insulin. However, recent studies indicate that sucrose and other sugars do not have more of a deleterious effect on blood glucose levels and are not absorbed more rapidly than starches.[11-15] The ADA position is that sucrose can be used as part of the total meal plan CHO, not additive CHO, and it should be used in the context of an otherwise healthful diet.[9] Sugars and starches, when eaten in equal amounts (eg, 50g carbohydrate) have a wide spectrum of blood glucose responses, with so much overlap that they cannot be distinguished as separate groups. Research also does not substantiate the statement that sugars are absorbed more rapidly into the bloodstream than starches.

    a) The total amount of food, as well as the total amount of carbohydrate, eaten will have more of an effect on blood glucose levels than the source of the carbohydrate. Overeating of any food, even if the food does not contain sugar, can have a detrimental effect on blood glucose levels. Patients still need to be careful of foods that contain significant amounts of added sugars, such as regular soft drinks, syrups, rich desserts, etc. Not only do these foods contain significant amounts of carbohydrate, but they are usually high in calories as well because of their fat content.

    b) A concern has been expressed that sucrose can cause a small increase in both fasting and postprandial triglyceride levels in patients with NIDDM.[16] However, even the Parma conference on the role of carbohydrate concluded that moderate amounts of sucrose (10% or less of total calories) could be substituted or used for a portion of the total carbohydrate in the meal plan and eaten within the context of a healthful diet for most persons with diabetes.[14]

3. The evidence is inconclusive that fiber has a beneficial effect on glycemic control.[9,17] Some research suggests that fiber, especially the soluble variety found in legumes, oats, barley, fruits, and some vegetables, may slow carbohydrate absorption and lessen the postprandial rise in plasma glucose and insulin because it forms a gel within the gastrointestinal tract. Soluble fiber also attenuates potential carbohydrate-induced elevations of plasma triglycerides that may be observed from a high-carbohydrate diet, and reduces serum lipids. In contrast, insoluble fiber found in wheat and corn bran, whole grains, and some vegetables, has no significant effect on either glucose or lipid metabolism. Insoluble fiber is useful for increasing stool bulk, decreasing transient time of the stool, and, thus, may be helpful in the prevention and treatment of constipation. Both types of fiber provide satiety value to the diet.

    a) The average dietary fiber intake for adults is 10 to 30 grams per day, with men averaging 19 grams and women averaging 13 grams.

    b) The ADA's recommendation is to follow the fiber recommendations for the general public related to fiber and a healthful diet.[9] It is good nutritional advice to encourage a gradual increase of dietary fiber with adequate intake of water to minimize side effects.

4. The glycemic index of foods is an attempt to classify foods according to their blood glucose response. The glycemic index of food is defined as the total area under the blood glucose response curve during the 2-hour period after the food is eaten compared with a standard response of an equivalent amount of glucose or bread.[18] Although not generally viewed as a clinically useful tool, patients can use blood glucose monitoring

to determine individual postprandial differences associated with various foods.

    a) Examples of low glycemic foods are legumes, nuts, dairy products, and fruits.

    b) Examples of high glycemic foods are root vegetables (such as carrots and potatoes), cereal, and bread.

5. A major reason that carbohydrate-equivalent foods with similar nutrient content do not produce equivalent glycemic responses appears to be the rate at which foods are digested and the carbohydrate absorbed. Other factors include: size and physical form of food; whether food is cooked or raw; other nutrients such as lectins, tannins, and phytates found in food; blood glucose level before eating; foods eaten in the previous meal; and the body's ability to produce endogenous insulin.

G. Prescribing Calories from Fat in the Diabetes Meal Plan

1. There also is a range in the percentage of calories from fat that can be prescribed. Average percentage of calories from fat generally is 30% to 35% of the total daily calories.

2. Dietary cholesterol intake should be 300 mg or less daily. Saturated fat intake should be no more than 10% of the daily calories, with the remainder of the fat from monounsaturated and polyunsaturated fats.[9] Although it may be difficult to implement, there is some evidence that if the percentage of calories from fat is increased, it should be from monounsaturates.

    a) The prevalence of cardiovascular disease in the population with diabetes is approximately two- to fourfold the prevalence in the population without diabetes. This finding is true even in the absence of other risk factors (hypertension, smoking, and lipid abnormalities).

        (1) Both men and women are affected; females with diabetes have the same risk as males without diabetes. Risk factors are not exaggerated by

diabetes, but the imposition of these factors on the increased risk inherent in diabetes results in a markedly increased overall mortality in persons with diabetes.[19]

(2) Cardiovascular risk is directly proportional to LDL-cholesterol and inversely proportional to HDL-cholesterol. Hypertriglyceridemia, elevated very-low-density lipoproteins (VLDL), and decreased HDL-cholesterol are the most common lipid abnormalities in NIDDM.

b) Risk factors for macrovascular disease in persons with diabetes include: obesity, especially abdominal, with the associated overproduction of lipoproteins; impaired glucose tolerance (IGT) related to hyperinsulinemia needed to keep blood glucose levels in this range; increased VLDL-cholesterol and decreased HDL-cholesterol; poor diabetes control related to an abnormality of lipoprotein lipase that can lead to decreased clearing of triglycerides; glycosylation of LDL- and HDL-cholesterol; and high-saturated fat, high cholesterol, low carbohydrate diets.[19]

c) Several diabetes-related diet factors affect the risk of developing macrovascular disease.

(1) Total fat content causes increased chylomicrons leading to atherogenic remnant particles.

(2) Saturated fats raise blood cholesterol levels. Food sources include animal fats (meat, butterfat, lard, bacon, etc), coconut, palm, and palm kernel oils, dairy-fat-containing foods, hydrogenated vegetable oils.

(3) Polyunsaturated fats (omega-6) have been shown to lower cholesterol levels but have a heterogeneous effect on HDL-cholesterol levels. Food sources are vegetable oils such as corn, safflower, soybean, sunflower, and cottonseed.

(4) Monounsaturated fats lower total cholesterol but do not lower HDL-cholesterol levels. Food sources are

olive, peanut, and canola oil, olives, and nuts (except walnuts, which are polyunsaturated).

    (5)   Omega-3 (fish oils) have an antiplatelet clotting effect and lower triglycerides and cholesterol. Food sources are fish from cold water and fatty fish such as salmon, herring, albacore tuna, mackerel, and sardines. The capsule form of omega-3 has been shown to elevate blood glucose levels, although this effect is still under investigation.[20,21]

    (6)   Dietary cholesterol content affects LDL-cholesterol concentration by competing for cell receptors for LDL-cholesterol. Dietary cholesterol is found only in animal foods. Some individuals appear to be more sensitive to the blood-cholesterol-raising effects of dietary cholesterol than others. Food sources high in cholesterol include egg yolks, organ meats (especially liver), and dairy-fat-containing food products.

    (7)   Excessive calories affect the risk.

    (8)   Water-soluble fibers (legumes, oats, barley) have been shown to have a hypocholesterolemic effect.

   d)   Over 20 fat substitutes currently are being used in food products. They can be classified according to the nutrient from which they are made or according to the number of calories they contribute to the diet. Carbohydrate fat replacements include dextrins, maltodextrins, modified food starches, polydextrose, cellulose, and gums. Protein fat substitutes include microparticulated proteins from egg whites or milk, and texturized proteins. Only one fat substitute from fat (caprenin) is on the market, although others (eg, olestra) are under development or seeking approval from the Food and Drug Administration (FDA).[22]

H.   Prescribing Calories from Protein in the Diabetes Meal Plan

   1.   Protein intake usually makes up 12% to 20% of the total calories consumed — nearly double the required amount. The

ideal percentage of total calories from protein is undetermined.[9] One gram of protein/kg of body weight will meet the protein needs of most adults, and 1.2 g/kg will meet the needs of most children and adolescents.

2. Experimental and clinical studies have shown that protein restriction as an adjunct to blood pressure control slows the progression of renal disease by reducing albuminuria and preserving renal function. With the onset of microalbuminuria, the protein content of the diet should be reduced. Realistically, 0.8 g/kg of body weight per day is feasible with the use of regular foods. In studies with patients with IDDM with persistent albuminuria, reducing the intake of protein to about 0.6 g/kg body weight per day significantly slowed the rate of decline in the glomerular filtration rate although the response was not homogenous. This level of protein intake requires the use of special low-protein foods.[23,24] A further study reported that IDDM patients with early nephropathy ingesting 0.6 g/kg protein per day experienced protein undernutrition during the first 3 months of treatment.[25]

3. The questions of a difference of animal or vegetable proteins on renal function and whether the restriction of dietary protein prior to the onset of microalbumuria is beneficial currently are under investigation.

I. Sweeteners in the Diabetes Meal Plan

1. The use of low-calorie or high-intensity sweeteners (aspartame, acesulfame K, and saccharin) and caloric sweeteners (fructose and sorbitol) is acceptable depending upon metabolic and weight control.[9,26]

2. Nutritive (caloric) sweeteners include fructose, honey, corn syrup, molasses, sorbitol, hydrogenated starch hydrolysates, fruit juice or fruit juice concentrates, dextrose, maltose, and mannitol. Calories from caloric sweeteners must be accounted

for in the meal plan and have the potential to affect blood glucose levels. Patients can be taught to evaluate food labels for the presence of nutritive (caloric) sweeteners.

3. High-intensity or nonnutritive sweeteners currently available include saccharin (Sweet 'n Low®, Sugar Twin®), aspartame (NutraSweet®, Equal®), and acesulfame K (Sunette™, Sweet One™). Other sweeteners pending approval from the FDA include cyclamates, sucralose, and alitame.

    a) For all food additives, including high-intensity sweeteners, the FDA determines an acceptable daily intake (ADI). The ADI is defined as the amount of a food additive that can be safely consumed on a daily basis over a person's lifetime without any adverse effects and includes a 100-fold safety factor.

    b) The FDA established an ADI for aspartame of 50 mg/kg of body weight. Aspartame intake in the general population of individuals who consume aspartame (including children and special subpopulations) is 2 to 3 mg/kg/day, or about 4% of the ADI.

    c) The ADI for acesulfame K is 15 mg/kg of body weight, which is the equivalent of a 60 kg person eating 150 g (36 tsp) of sugar daily.

    d) When saccharin received Generally Recognized as Safe (GRAS) status in 1955, the recommended consumption limits were 500 mg/day for children and 1000 mg/day for adults. However, even when saccharin was the only nonnutritive sweetener available, actual intake for persons with diabetes ranged from 54 to 173 mg/day.[26]

J. **Sodium in the Diabetes Meal Plan**

1. Moderation of sodium intake is recommended. In general, a sodium intake of less than 3000 mg per day is recommended. For persons who are hypertensive 2400 mg or less of sodium per day is recommended.

2. A teaspoon of salt (5g) contains 2300 mg of sodium. Sodium in food products is listed on labels in mg per serving. The Food and Drug Administration defines a low-sodium food as having 140 mg or less of sodium per serving.

K. Precautions Regarding Alcohol Use

1. The same precautions regarding the use of alcohol that apply to the general public apply to persons with diabetes.[9]

2. Alcohol is absorbed from the stomach and small intestine, and because of its toxicity, is metabolized in the liver before other nutrients. Alcohol does not require insulin to be metabolized; in fact, it augments the action of insulin. Alcohol cannot be converted into glucose; it is used as an energy source, or excessive amounts are converted to fats. Alcohol yields 7 calories per gram.[27]

3. If used in moderation, and if diabetes is well controlled, blood glucose levels are not affected by the ingestion of moderate amounts of alcohol.[28,29] Moderation is defined as two equivalents of an alcoholic beverage once or twice a week.[9] The following are an equivalent: 1.5 oz shot of a distilled beverage, 12 oz beer (preferably light), or 4 to 5 oz wine (preferably dry).

4. Alcohol inhibits the release of glucose from the liver (gluconeogenesis) and can cause hypoglycemia when consumed without food.[27] Hypoglycemia can occur at blood alcohol levels that do not exceed mild intoxication, and the hypoglycemic effect may persist from 8 to 12 hours after the last drink.

5. For persons using insulin, two equivalents of an alcoholic beverage (approximately 2 oz of alcohol) can be used in addition to their regular meal plan. No food should be omitted because of the possibility of alcohol-induced hypoglycemia and

because alcohol does not require insulin to be metabolized. If used daily, the calories from alcohol must be counted in the meal plan.[27]

6. For persons concerned with calories, alcohol is best substituted for fat exchanges. Alcohol is high in calories (7 calories per gram) and is metabolized in a manner similar to fat (1 equivalent of alcohol = 2 fat exchanges).[29]

7. Alcohol may potentiate or interfere with the action of other medications.

8. Alcohol may raise triglyceride levels.

L. Vitamin and Mineral Supplementation

1. There is no evidence unique to persons with diabetes that warrants vitamin and mineral supplementation.

2. Supplements may be necessary with very-low-calorie diets (less than 1200 calories/day), during pregnancy, or with other unusual circumstances.[9]

M. Other Nutritional Issues

1. Nutrient caloric values and food sources are a nutritional issue in diabetes management.
   a) Carbohydrates provide 4 calories per gram. Food sources of carbohydrate in the diet are fiber, sugars, and starches (breads, fruits, vegetables, cereals, grains). Carbohydrates provide the major sources of energy.
   b) Protein also contributes 4 calories per gram. Food sources of protein are both animal (meat, milk, dairy products) and vegetable (legumes, starches, and vegetables). Protein is necessary for growth and tissue maintenance, and is a secondary source of energy. Animal proteins are called complete proteins because they contain all of the essential

amino acids. Vegetable proteins are deficient in one or more of the essential amino acids and must be combined to be complete. This deficiency rarely is a concern, as foods deficient in one amino acid are combined naturally with foods that result in complete proteins, for example, rice and beans, wheat (bread) and nuts (peanut butter), and cereal and milk.

c) Fat contributes 9 calories per gram. Food sources of fat are meat fats, oils, dairy-fat-containing foods, and many snack foods. Fats in foods are broken down into triglycerides (three fatty acids attached to glycerol), the form in which fat travels through the bloodstream and is stored in adipose tissue. Fat is used as an energy source in the form of free fatty acids (FFA).

d) Vitamins and minerals do not contribute calories and do not require insulin to be metabolized, although many act as co-factors in the metabolism of carbohydrate, protein, and fat.

e) Although water provides no calories, it is considered an essential nutrient. Water is an important component of body tissue, accounting for between one-half and three-fourths of body weight. Water is important in regulating body temperature and in carrying nutrients to and waste products away from the cells. It is involved in all the chemical reactions in metabolism. Daily water losses need to be replaced from dietary sources, including drinking water, beverages, and water in food. (For additional discussion of fluid needs, see Chapter XII: Managing Diabetes During Intercurrent Illness.)

2. Food labeling is another nutritional issue in diabetes management.

a) New food regulations were announced in 1992, and by 1994, nearly all foods will have nutrition information based on standard portion sizes and listed in common household and metric measures.

b) The following information is required in the new food labeling: calories, calories from fat, total fat, saturated fat, cholesterol, total carbohydrate, sugars, dietary fiber, protein, sodium, vitamin A, vitamin C, calcium, and iron. Label descriptors also have specific definitions, including free, low, reduced, less, light/lite, lean, extra lean, high, more, and good source. The Percent of a Daily Value based on a 2000 calorie diet is listed for total fat, saturated fat, cholesterol, sodium, total carbohydrate, and fiber.

N. Nutritional Guidelines for Special Conditions

1. Illness, especially when nausea and vomiting are involved, requires food adjustments that are specific and unique depending upon whether the person is using insulin or taking oral hypoglycemic agents (OHA) (see Chapter XII: Managing Diabetes During Intercurrent Illness).

    a) If regular foods are not tolerated, carbohydrate-containing liquids or soft foods (such as regular soft drinks, regular jello, fruit juice, etc) should be consumed in small, frequent feedings to prevent starvation ketosis. To prevent starvation ketosis and to prevent any potential problems with hypoglycemia 15g of carbohydrate should be consumed over 1 to 2 hours or 50g of carbohydrate should be consumed every three to four hours.[30]

    b) Drinking fluids also is important. If nausea is a factor, small sips should be consumed every hour or so.

    c) If vomiting, diarrhea, or fever is present, small amounts of salted foods and/or liquids (eg, broth) also are recommended to replace lost electrolytes.

2. Exercise may require additional food and/or insulin adjustments, especially for persons with IDDM. Exercise affects individuals differently, so adjustments must be based on blood glucose levels and previous experiences of the individual. In general, 10 to 15 grams of carbohydrate for every hour of

exercise can be recommended. Because of the danger of postexercise late-onset hypoglycemia, and depending on the time of day and intensity of exercise, it may be necessary to consume additional carbohydrate after exercise[31] (see Chapter VII: Exercise).

a) Persons with IDDM, or nonobese persons with NIDDM who exercise regularly should have a meal plan that provides enough calories to provide for the exercise.

   (1) Individuals with IDDM who exercise sporadically may need to increase food before or after exercise to prevent hypoglycemia. They may also need to decrease insulin.

   (2) In order to prevent postexercise hypoglycemia, carbohydrate should be ingested after completion of exercise to replenish liver glycogen stores that have been utilized during exercise. Blood glucose levels can continue to decline for up to 12 to 24 hours after the completion of exercise.

b) Persons with NIDDM being treated with diet alone or OHA usually do not need supplementary food when exercising.[32]

3. Hypoglycemia (usually defined as a blood glucose level of less than 70 mg/dL or 3.85 mmol/L) requires treatment (see Chapter XIII: Hypoglycemia).

   a) Blood glucose testing is important before, during, and after treating hypoglycemia.

   b) Treatment begins by eating 10 to 15 g of carbohydrate (5 to 10g for younger children).

   c) Blood glucose should be retested in 15 minutes, and 15 g of additional carbohydrate should be eaten if the blood glucose level still is less than 70 mg/dL (3.85 mmol/L) or symptoms do not abate. A snack or the scheduled meal should follow.

   d) The food used to treat hypoglycemia is in addition to the usual meal plan.

e) Frequent episodes of hypoglycemia requiring treatment, and/or overtreatment of hypoglycemia, can contribute to weight gain.

4. For women who are pregnant, changes in macronutrient percentages and distribution of food throughout the day, plus an increase in calories, may be needed. Such changes should be individualized for each woman. Monitoring blood glucose levels, urine ketones, appetite, and weight gain can guide the dietitian in developing a meal plan (see Chapter XV: Pregnancy: Preconception to Postpartum).

5. Sensitivity to ethnic and cultural communication strategies is essential for successful diet counseling. Cross-cultural counseling can be improved by health professionals using a four-step process.
   a) First, health professionals should become familiar with their own cultural heritage.
   b) Second, they should become acquainted with the cultural background of each client.
   c) Third, by using an in-depth cross-cultural interview, they should establish the client's cultural background, food habit adaptations made in the United States, and personal preferences.
   d) Fourth, they should modify the diet based on the unbiased analysis of the dietary data.[33]

O. The Two Phases of Nutrition Education and Counseling[34]

1. Initial education is the information required at the time of diagnosis, when a management regimen changes, or at the time of initial contact with a patient.

2. In-depth/continuing education and counseling is the comprehensive level that includes both management skills (information required to make decisions to achieve management goals and foster self-care) and improvement of

lifestyle (problem-solving skills that allow for a more flexible, self-determined lifestyle). During this second phase, individuals learn to make adjustments in meal planning for a number of situations. Flexibility in meal planning also is addressed. This phase is ongoing (see Table VI.4).

3. Food records are very helpful for all phases of education and counseling (see Table VI.5 for guidelines concerning how to use food records effectively).

P. Calculating a Diet Prescription[30]

1. Assess DBW and caloric needs. See Tables VI.1, VI.2, VI.3.

2. Assess current food intake. Two methods that can be used to assess diet are a diet history taken by the dietitian, or food records (1 to 3 days) kept by the individual. Appropriate diet changes then can be recommended.

3. Based on usual food intake, the meal plan can be divided into meals and snacks.
    a) With increasing use of more flexible insulin regimens, it is not necessary to divide the meal (or carbohydrate) content into various fractions; insulin therapy usually can be adjusted to match the patient's customary food intake. However, meals and snacks still need to be synchronized with the time actions of the insulins the patient is injecting.
    b) For persons with NIDDM, smaller meals spaced throughout the day may require less insulin and assist in achieving blood glucose control.[8]

4. Develop an initial meal plan.

5. Implement initial education emphasizing one or two priorities.

TABLE VI.4: In-Depth Continuing Education Topics

Management Skills (Information required to make decisions to achieve management goals)

Meal planning and insulin adjustments for:
- Illness
- Delay and changes of meals
- Drinking alcoholic beverages
- Sweetener use
- Exercise
- Travel
- Competitive athletics
- Holidays

Reducing and modifying fat intake
Reducing salt intake
Increasing fiber intake

Improvement of Lifestyle (Problem-solving skills)
- Eating out in restaurants
- Eating school lunch in cafeterias
- Fast foods
- Label reading
- Special occasions
- New ideas for snacks
- Recipe modifications
- Vegetarian food choices
- Ethnic foods
- Convenience food use
- Understanding fat substitutes
- Adaptations of favorite recipes
- Canning and freezing

6. Plan for follow-up and continuing education. Ideally, all persons with diabetes should be seen periodically for continuing education, updating of the meal plan, and support.

    a) Adults should be seen every 6 months to 1 year, or if there is any major change in work schedule, activity level, or type of medication for diabetes (especially insulin). Weight management may require more frequent visits.

    b) Children should be seen a minimum of every 6 months, preferably every 3 months. Calories need to be adjusted to accommodate growth and development requirements.

TABLE VI.5: Evaluating Food Diaries

Food diaries have been shown to be a strategy that can help patients make positive eating changes as well as lose weight and maintain weight loss. The patient is asked to write down everything she/he eats with approximate amounts and the circumstances under which it was eaten over a period of time. Food diaries can be kept for one day a week, a few days a month, or for longer periods of time.

Keeping food diaries is time consuming for the patient and may be considered by the patient as another record-keeping chore. Outline the benefits of the food record from the beginning so that the patient sees their value.

These patients might benefit from keeping a food diary:
- Patients starting a new meal plan.
- Patients who need to lose weight.
- Patients who are having problems with blood glucose control.

With the patient look for:
- What, where, and how much food was eaten.
- Improvements that can be made.
- Progress made toward short-term goals.
- Effect of food intake on blood glucose levels. Correlations between foods eaten and blood glucose record can be made.

Assist the patient in analyzing his/her food diary for any of the following problems:
- Unconscious eating or nibbling patterns.
- Portion sizes that are too large.
- Eating for the wrong reasons, such as boredom, being tired, being under stress, etc.
- Skipping planned meals and/or snacks.
- Eating food in places other than at the table.
- Making inappropriate food choices, such as foods high in fat, foods with hidden fats, excessive sweets, etc.
- Getting little or no exercise.

Assist the patient in setting short-term, realistic goals that address some of the identified problems.

Q. Methods for Teaching Meal Planning

1. No single educational tool works in every situation. For each phase of education, different educational tools may be needed — simple tools for beginning counseling and possibly more

complex tools as the counseling process continues. Preplanned printed diet sheets should not be used.

2. Several meal planning approaches are available to teach basic nutrition and diabetes nutrition guidelines. Many of the educational tools are based on some system of grouping foods.

   a) A popular educational tool has been the *Exchange Lists for Meal Planning,* developed and published by The American Dietetic Association and the American Diabetes Association. Food is grouped according to six food categories based on calorie and macronutrient composition (see Table VI.6).[35]

TABLE VI.6: Nutrient Values per Serving for 1986 Exchange Lists

Food Group	Energy (Kcal)	Carbohydrate (g)	Protein (g)	Fat (g)
Starch/bread	80	15	3	1*
Meat and substitutes				
Lean	55	—	7	3
Medium-fat	75	—	7	5
High-fat	100	—	7	8
Vegetable	25	5	2	—
Fruit	60	15	—	—
Milk				
Skim	90	12	8	1*
Low-fat	120	12	8	5
Whole	150	12	8	8
Fat	45	—	—	5

* *In* Exchange Lists *trace is listed. For calculation purposes, 1g can be used.*

Reproduced with permission from Nutrition Guide for Professionals: Diabetes Education and Meal Planning. American Diabetes Association, 1988.

   b) *Meal Planning Approaches in the Management of the Person with Diabetes*[36] describes additional approaches and the situations in which they might be useful. Educational tools are divided into two categories: survival skill nutrition education tools and continuing nutrition education tools.

(1) Survival-skill nutrition education guidelines included in this category provide information about basic nutrition, diabetes nutrition guidelines, and beginning strategies for altering an individual's eating pattern. The following educational tools can be used to negotiate with persons with diabetes to begin changing their eating habits (eg, eating less fat, using more high-fiber foods, etc).

(a) *Dietary Guidelines for Americans* is a basic nutrition guide aimed at all Americans for the purpose of health promotion and the prevention of chronic diseases.

(b) The *Food Guide Pyramid* illustrates the research-based *Dietary Guidelines for Americans* and was developed by the United States Department of Agriculture (USDA), with support from the Department of Health and Human Services (DHHS). The Pyramid, which replaces the basic four food groups, is a general guide or outline of what and how much to eat each day for a healthful diet.

(c) *Healthy Food Choices* is a pamphlet that promotes healthy eating. It is divided into two sections: guidelines for making healthy food choices (eat less fat, salt, sugar) and simplified exchange lists that can be used to give persons a general idea of what to eat and when. This pamphlet also can serve as an introduction to the exchange lists system.

(d) *Eating Healthy Foods* and *Healthy Eating* are two low-literacy booklets that utilize drawings to visually present nutrition concepts. Simplified exchange lists are included.

(2) Meal planning approaches for continuing nutrition education provide information about the process of meal planning.

(a) Individualized menus is a method of meal planning that the educator can use to help persons with diabetes plan menus that specify the foods and appropriate quantities that can be eaten over a period of days.

(b) *The Food Choice Plan* is a method of meal planning based on the development of three different menus that are followed for a period of weeks or months.

(c) *Month of Meals-1, Month of Meals-2, Month of Meals-3* and *Month of Meals-4* are four separate books that provide sample menus and teach a menu-planning approach for persons with diabetes.

(d) *Exchange Lists for Meal Planning* groups foods into six categories called exchange lists. Each list includes a group of measured foods of approximately the same nutritional value. Therefore, foods in each list can be substituted, or exchanged, for other foods in the same list. The exchange lists need to be used with an individualized meal plan that specifies when and how many exchanges from each group can be used.

(e) The *High Carbohydrate-High Fiber* (HCF) exchange lists follows a format similar to the *Exchange Lists for Meal Planning*, except that foods are divided into eight exchange groups. The cereal and bean exchange groups are unique to this meal planning approach, which emphasizes intake of fiber from food sources.

(f) *Calorie Point System* is an approach that can be used for calorie counting. A calorie point is equal to 75 calories. An established number of calorie points are assigned and can be divided between meals and/or snacks.

(g) *Calorie Counting* is another approach that places emphasis on the caloric density of food. A calorie reference book is provided to look up calorie values of food, and food diaries and calorie calculations must be completed.

(h) *Fat Counting* establishes a daily fat allowance. The person with diabetes counts the grams of fat consumed at each meal and snack. The approaches in *Calorie Counting* and *Fat Counting* can be combined.

(i) *Carbohydrate Counting* is used to adjust regular insulin for changes in meals. The amount of insulin given to cover a meal is based in part on the amount of carbohydrate and calories in that meal. Carbohydrate counting can be used to make compensatory or anticipatory adjustments in premeal, regular insulin doses. Patients have a baseline diet (often exchange lists are used) and a base insulin dose to which carbohydrate counting and changes in insulin doses (based on blood glucose monitoring) can be added for fine-tuning of blood glucose control. To fine-tune premeal insulin doses, determinations can be based on the amount of insulin an individual needs to cover the usual amount of carbohydrate, or on a more general guideline, such as 1 unit of regular insulin for 15 grams of additional carbohydrate.

(j) *Total Available Glucose* (TAG) is designed to provide the body with a predictable amount of glucose. Foods are assigned TAG values based on the conversion of protein, carbohydrate, and fat to glucose in the body.

(k) *Constant Carbohydrate* is based on the principle of maintaining a constant level of carbohydrate intake from day to day.

(3) Overall nutritional quality of the diet also must be monitored when using any of the approaches described in (f) through (k).

REFERENCES

1.   Report of the national cholesterol education expert panel on detection, evaluation, and treatment of high blood cholesterol in adults. Arch Intern Med 1988;148:36-68.

2.   Report of the expert panel on blood cholesterol levels in children and adolescents. Pediatrics 1992;89(suppl):525-84.

3.   Watts NB, Spanheimer RG, DiGirolamo M, et al. Prediction of glucose responses to weight loss in patients with non-insulin-dependent diabetes mellitus. Arch Intern Med 1990;150:803-6.

4.   Wing RR, Koeske R, Epstein LH, et al. Long term effects of modest weight loss in type II diabetic patients. Arch Intern Med 1987;147:1749-53.

5.   Bjorntorp P. Metabolic implications of body fat distribution. Diabetes Care 1991;14:1132-43.

6.   DeFronzo RA, Ferrannini E. Insulin resistance. A multifaceted syndrome responsible for NIDDM, obesity, hypertension, dyslipidemia, and atherosclerotic cardiovascular disease. Diabetes Care 1991;14:173-94.

7.   Burton BT, Foster WR. Health implications of obesity: an NIH consensus development conference. Am Diet Assoc 1985; 85:1117-21.

8.   Jenkins DJA, Ocana A, Jenkins AL, et al. Metabolic advantages of spreading the nutrient load: effects of increased meal frequency in non-insulin-dependent diabetes. Am J Clin Nutr 1992;55:461-67.

9.   American Diabetes Association Position Statement. Nutritional recommendations and principles for individuals with diabetes mellitus. Diabetes Care (in press).

10. Coulston AM, Hollenbeck CB, Swislocki ALM, et al. Deleterious metabolic effects of high-carbohydrate, sucrose-containing diets in patients with NIDDM. Am J Med 1987; 82:213-20.

11. Bantle JB. Clinical aspects of sucrose and fructose metabolism. Diabetes Care 1989;12(suppl 1):56-61.

12. Peterson DB, Lambert J, Gerrig S, et al. Sucrose in the diet of diabetic patients — just another carbohydrate? Diabetologia 1986;29:216-20.

13. Loghmani E, Rickard K, Washburne L, et al. Glycemic response to sucrose-containing mixed meals in diets of children with insulin-dependent diabetes mellitus. J Pediatr 1991;119:531-37.

14. Reaven G. Parma symposium: current controversies in nutrition. Am J Clin Nutr 1988;47:1078-82.

15. Franz MJ. Avoiding sugar: does research support traditional beliefs? Diabetes Educ 1993;19:144-50.

16. Coulston AM, Hollenbeck CB, Swislocki ALM, et al. Persistence of hypertriglyceridemic effects of low-fat, high carbohydrate diets in NIDDM patients. Diabetes Care 1989;12:94-101.

17. National Institutes of Health Consensus Development Conference Statement. Diet and exercise in non-insulin-dependent diabetes mellitus. Diabetes Care 1987;10:639-44.

18. Jenkins DJA, Wolever TMS, Jenkins AL. Starchy foods and glycemic index. Diabetes Care 1988;11:149-59.

19. American Diabetes Association Consensus Statement. Role of cardiovascular risk factors in prevention and treatment of macrovascular disease in diabetes. Diabetes Care 1989; 12:573-79.

20. Friday KE, Childs MT, Tsunehara CH, et al. Elevated plasma glucose and lowered triglyceride levels from omega-3 fatty acid supplementation in type II diabetes. Diabetes Care 1989;12:276-81.

21. Hendra TJ, Britton ME, Roper DR, et al. Effects of fish oil supplements in NIDDM subjects. Controlled study. Diabetes Care 1990;13:821-29.

22. Warshaw HS, Powers MA. Ingredients that replace fat: their role in today's foods and challenges in educating people with diabetes. Diabetes Educ 1993;19:419-30.

23. Walker JD, Dodds RA, Murrells TJ, et al. Restriction of dietary protein and progression of renal failure in diabetic nephropathy. Lancet 1989;ii:1411-15.

24. Zeller K, Whittaker E, Sullivan L, et al. Effect of restricting dietary protein on progression of renal failure in patients with insulin-dependent diabetes. N Engl J Med 1991;324:78-84.

25. Brodsky IG, Robbins DC, Hiser E, et al. Effects of low-protein diets on protein metabolism in insulin-dependent diabetes mellitus patients with early nephropathy. J Clin Endocrinol Metab 1992;75:351-57.

26. Position of the American Dietetic Association. Use of nutritive and non-nutritive sweeteners. J Am Diet Assoc 1993;93:816-21.

27. Franz MJ. Alcohol and diabetes: its metabolism and guidelines for its occasional use, parts I and II. Diabetes Spectrum 1990;3:136-44, 210-16.

28. Gin H, Morlat P, Ragnaut JM, et al. Short-term effect of red wine (consumed during meals) on insulin requirements and glucose tolerance in diabetic patients. Diabetes Care 1992;15:46-48.

29. Flatt JP. Body weight, fat storage, and alcohol metabolism. Nutr Rev 1992;50:267-70.

30. American Diabetes Association, American Dietetic Association. Nutrition guide for professionals: diabetes education and meal planning. Alexandria, Va: American Diabetes Association, 1988.

31. American Diabetes Association Technical Review. Exercise and NIDDM. Diabetes Care 1990;13:785-89.

32. American Diabetes Association Position Statement. Diabetes mellitus and exercise. Diabetes Care 1990;13:804-5.

33. Kittler PG, Sucher KP. Diet counseling in a multicultural society. Diabetes Educ 1990;16:127-31.

34. American Diabetes Association. Goals for diabetes education. Alexandria, Va: American Diabetes Association, 1986.

35. Franz MJ, Barr P, Holler H, et al. Exchange lists: revised 1986. J Am Diet Assoc 1987;87:28-36.

36. The American Dietetic Association Diabetes Care and Education Practice Group. Meal planning approaches in the nutrition management of the person with diabetes. Chicago: American Dietetic Association, 1993 (in press).

KEY EDUCATIONAL CONSIDERATIONS

1. *Sugar-free, lite,* and *dietetic* do not mean "free." To teach this concept, use product labels to demonstrate the number of calories, fat, carbohydrate, etc in a common sugar-free product.

2. Use restaurant menus from local restaurants to help patients plan a meal according to their meal plan. Use of a menu allows for patient preferences, variety, and often brings some humor to the teaching session.

3. Use examples of former patients (changing all identifying information) to elicit a patient's past history with dietitians or with weight loss. For example, "I worked with a woman who resisted making the initial appointment because her previous experience with dieting was in a program where she had to weigh in at every visit, measure her food at all times, and eat foods that she did not like. She was amazed that diabetic meal planning was so flexible. What's been your experience?"

4. Use blood glucose monitoring results to teach a patient the relationship between food, exercise, medication, coping skills, etc.

5. To encourage participation, show patients a list of all the nutrition-related topics offered. They can check off what they want to learn at the first session, second session, etc. This technique also removes the unreasonable burden from the educator of trying to teach everything in one visit.

6. Offer samples of products or coupons to encourage a patient to try some new foods. Moving a patient from the usual egg-and-bacon-on-a-roll breakfast may be more successful if the patient has tried and liked a new whole-grain cereal.

7. In a hospital, suggest that patients keep the daily menus as a guide after discharge. Or ask patients to plan a series of menus based on their meal plan that would be realistic for them to prepare.

8. Conduct a supermarket tour to teach flexibility and variety in meal planning. Participants can read the food labels, learn where to find the recommended foods in the supermarket, learn the aisles to avoid, and compare the nutritional content of different brands of foods.

9. Invite patients to teach the educators about the ingredients in cultural/ethnic foods. Combining the patient's cultural expertise with the diabetes and nutrition knowledge of the educator allows for a true exchange of information that will benefit the patient.

10. Using food packages, point out the grams of carbohydrate, protein, fat, and the number of calories per serving. Distribute a small card with exchange values that individuals can take to the grocery store. Help them understand that starch and fruit servings are based on 15 grams of carbohydrate and fat servings on 5 grams of fat.

11. Display a chart or test tubes comparing amounts of sucrose in common foods. Compare the small portions of sucrose in common foods, such as a cookie, frozen yogurt, ice milk, etc with the sucrose in a 12-ounce can of regular soft drink, Jell-O®, fruited yogurt, etc. Point out that small servings of simple desserts often can be substituted for a starch or fruit serving, but foods with large amounts of sucrose are best avoided because it is difficult to substitute for them in a meal plan.

12. Emphasize goals of meal planning for patients with IDDM and NIDDM. The goals are to prevent hyperglycemia and maintain euglycemia by balancing the food eaten with insulin taken by injection, or with insulin still being produced by the pancreas and exercise. Strategies for improving blood glucose control for persons with NIDDM that can be helpful include:
    a) Moderate weight loss. The biggest improvement in blood glucose levels occurs with only a 10 to 20 pound weight loss.
    b) Better food selections and portion sizes (for example, decreasing fat intake).
    c) Distribution of food throughout the day.
    d) Increased activity (exercise) level.

e) Improved eating behaviors. For example, eating breakfast and lunch instead of consuming all calories late in the day.

f) Using blood glucose monitoring to evaluate the success of food and meal changes.

g) Awareness of normal blood glucose ranges and the target blood glucose range.

h) Knowledge that blood glucose levels reach a peak about $1^1/_2$ hours after finishing a meal and should return to preprandial levels in about 4 to 5 hours.

i) An understanding that if these strategies have not been successful in returning blood glucose levels to target ranges, OHA or insulin may need to be adjusted or added to the management plan.

13. Emphasize to patients that they have not failed. A change in therapy may be necessary in order to successfully meet the predetermined short-term goals. Changing medications is a natural progression in the management of diabetes.

SELF-REVIEW QUESTIONS

If you are unsure of the answers to the following questions, please review the materials.

1. List four major goals of nutritional therapy for persons with diabetes.
2. What are the recommended ranges for percentages of calories from carbohydrate, protein, and fat in a meal plan?
3. Name three types of high-intensity sweeteners currently available on the market and four caloric sweeteners that frequently are substituted for sucrose in food products.
4. What is the recommendation for the use of alcoholic beverages for persons with IDDM? How is the recommendation different for the person with NIDDM?
5. How many calories per gram do carbohydrate, protein, fat, and alcohol contribute to the energy content of the diet?
6. Define the glycemic index of foods. List two foods that have a high glycemic index and two foods that have a low-glycemic index.

7. What are the two types of dietary fiber? List two examples of each type. What effect does each type of fiber have on metabolic parameters?

8. List three types of fatty acids found in foods. List three examples of foods containing each type of fatty acid. What is the major effect of each type of fatty acid on blood lipid levels?

9. List two nutritional concerns during illness.

10. What are two major factors in determining a diet prescription?

11. What is a desirable body weight (DBW) for a man 5 ft 11 in tall with a large frame? If he was only moderately active, what would be his approximate caloric requirement per day?

12. List the six exchange lists. Each list is based on how many calories and grams of carbohydrate, protein, and fat?

13. List four other meal planning approaches that can be used to teach meal planning guidelines to persons with diabetes.

14. List six considerations for individualizing a meal plan.

15. Distinguish between initial versus continuing nutrition education.

CASE EXAMPLE 1

LF is a 28-year-old housewife with two children, ages 2 and 4. LF's father has NIDDM. She was diagnosed with IDDM a year ago. Her second child, age 2 years, weighed 10 lb 4 oz at birth, although LF was not tested for gestational diabetes during her pregnancy. She is referred for nutrition and nursing consultations because of frequent problems with hypoglycemia. The most recent episode occurred a week ago when her husband arrived home from work at 5:00 PM and found LF very confused and incoherent and called 911. A blood glucose of 30 mg/dL (1.67 mmol/L) was recorded.

Current laboratory values are a random blood glucose value of 240 mg/dL (13.3 mmol/L), negative urine ketones, hemoglobin A_{1c} of 6.8% (normal = <6%), cholesterol 205 mg/dL (5.30 mmol/L), and triglycerides 180 mg/dL (2.03 mmol/L).

She reports being very fearful of needles and still has difficulty administering her insulin injections. She denies being angry about having diabetes, but admits to a great deal of fear about the potential development of complications. Her father is experiencing painful neuropathy. She reports that her husband is not very supportive, especially regarding her health problems. She expresses feeling very guilty about having developed diabetes, blaming it on her poor eating habits. At the same time, she has very high expectations of herself and is having trouble understanding why she is having so many problems related to her diabetes.

LF is 5 ft 4 in tall, and weighs 108 lb (49 kg), although she reports that her normal weight is between 110 and 115 lb (50 kg and 52 kg). She has very erratic eating habits, frequently skipping breakfast and lunch. Dinner is fairly consistent. She still drinks regular soft drinks, and frequently eats sweets and high-fat foods and snacks. She drinks alcohol only on special occasions, and then limits herself to one or two glasses of wine.

Before the birth of her second child she biked and jogged regularly. However, since that time she has not been exercising regularly. She reports never having a minute to sit down because of running after the two children, housework, and neighborhood activities.

She hasn't been doing blood glucose monitoring because she says she doesn't know what to do with the results. She's been frustrated with the wide fluctuations in values when she does test. At this point, she says she is ready to try anything to make her life go more smoothly!

QUESTIONS

1. What are some suggested short-term educational goals for LF?
2. What are short-term meal planning goals for LF?
3. What information and educational tools might be helpful for LF at this time?
4. What are long-term suggested meal planning goals for LF?
5. How can continued education and counseling be planned and provided for LF and her husband?

SUGGESTED SOLUTIONS

Short-term educational goals to be discussed and planned with LF include: assess LF's usual pattern of symptoms, treatment, and prevention of hypoglycemia; review blood glucose monitoring and the time actions of insulin; target blood glucose levels; introduce pattern control to assist her in making insulin adjustments; and assist her in being more realistic and more patient with her self-expectations.

Short-term meal planning goals should include: consistency in the timing of her meals, regular snacks, fewer sweets, drinking diet soft drinks, and returning to some type of regular exercise.

LF's caloric needs are determined to be about 1800 calories (120 lb DBW x 15 calories per lb of DBW). Although her eating habits are erratic, according to a 3-day food record and diet recall, she eats about 1900 to 2100 calories daily. She is familiar with exchange lists and reports being anxious to have a meal plan she might be able to follow a little more consistently. She agreed to drink diet soft drinks and will try to limit sweets to once a day.

A 1900 calorie meal plan based on exchanges was discussed with her. She agreed to try eating a small breakfast, lunch, simple dessert for her afternoon snack, dinner, and an evening snack. Food models were used to help LF visualize portions of food. She will keep food records and return in 2 weeks for a follow-up visit. She will also try to begin exercising three evenings a week after dinner when her husband has agreed to watch the children.

Long-term goals include: better blood glucose control to be achieved by LF eating more consistently and learning to make insulin adjustments based on blood glucose patterns, acceptance of more realistic self-expectations, and introducing LF to a more intensified form of insulin therapy.

Long-term goals for meal planning include: better overall food choices, more flexibility in meal planning while maintaining blood glucose control, and introducing LF to carbohydrate counting that she can add to her use of exchanges.

LF is planning to attend a week-long education program during the summer when it will be easier to get a sitter for the children. Her husband has agreed to attend with her. In the meantime, she will call the nurse educator with her blood glucose values so she can receive assistance as she begins to make insulin adjustments. She will return for a follow-up consult in 2 weeks. At that time, a letter will be sent to her doctor reporting on her success with short-term goals. She also is going to become involved in a support group sponsored by the local American Diabetes Association affiliate.

CASE EXAMPLE 2

JS is a 35-year-old woman referred for a nutrition-nursing consult for initiation of insulin therapy. She was first seen for a nutrition-nursing diabetes consult 3 years ago. At that time, her fasting blood glucose level was in the 160 mg/dL range (8.8 mmol/L), HbA_{1c} 7.4% (HbA_{1c} normal less than 6.0%), cholesterol 223 mg/dL (5.80 mmol/L), LDL-cholesterol 143 mg/dL (3.72 mmol/L), HDL-cholesterol 49 mg/dL (1.27 mmol/L), triglycerides 137 mg/dL (1.54 mmol/L), weight 243.5 lb (110.7 kg), height 68 inches (172.7 cm). She worked as a nurse's aide in a nursing home and lived at home with her mother and a brother. Her grandmother, mother, another brother, sister, and aunt all have diabetes.

General information on diabetes was reviewed and she was taught blood glucose monitoring. Based on an estimated caloric requirement of 2000 calories (large frame, moderate activity), she was taught about a 1500 to 1600 calorie meal plan, asked to keep food records, encouraged to begin a walking program, and asked to return for a follow-up consult in 3 to 4 weeks. At the 4-week return visit, her weight was 229 lb (104 kg) (decrease of 14.5 lb), fasting blood glucose ranges were 100 to 110 mg/dL (5.6-6.1 mmol/L), HbA_{1c} 6.7% (decrease of .7%), and she was walking 2 to 3 times a week for 20 minutes or more. Examination of her food records revealed excellent adherence to her meal plan of ~1600 calories, 44% carbohydrate, 19% protein, and 37% fat (considerably less than her diet history), with three meals and one snack daily. She was referred back to her primary care physician for ongoing care.

Currently her weight is 238.5 lb (108.4) (increase of 9.5 lb during the past 3 years), fasting blood glucose in the 150 mg/dL range (8.3 mmol/L), HbA_{1c} 8.7%, cholesterol 215 mg/dL (5.59 mmol/L), and triglycerides 214 mg/dL (2.40 mmol/L). JS reported having again lost about 8 lb since realizing her blood glucose levels have been consistently elevated, but her blood glucose values have not improved despite the weight loss. She still is working as a nurse's aide, from 10:30 PM to 7:00 AM for 10 days, followed by 4 days off. On her days off, she goes back to a day schedule, sleeping at night.

The dietitian went over her four schedules: work (nights), transition to days off, days off, and transition back to nights. The nurse reviewed blood glucose monitoring and taught her about insulin and insulin administration.

She maintained contact with the nurse, reporting blood glucose values, and returned for a follow-up consult in 3 weeks. She had again lost 9 lb (229.5 lb [104.3 kg]), and her preprandial blood glucose level the last week ranged from 83 to 129 mg/dL (4.6 to 7.2 mmol/L) with only one recording at 234 mg/dL (13.0 mmol/L). She reported having made major changes in her eating habits. Her HbA$_{1c}$ at this time was 7.7%. She also was back to exercising — walking and strength training at her health club on a regular basis. Her mother accompanied JS and also mentioned that she was eating better and her blood glucose levels also were improved.

Her insulin injection and blood glucose monitoring techniques were very good. JS registered for the week-long diabetes self-management class for the next month. At that time she will be taught pattern control so she will be able to make insulin adjustments based on her blood glucose values. Her mother will attend class with her and will be instructed on how to inject glucagon.

JS was again referred back to her primary care physician for ongoing care. The challenge for her will be to continue to be motivated to maintain the changes she has again made.

QUESTIONS

1. What are suggested short-term educational goals for JS?
2. What are short-term nutrition goals for JS?
3. What are long-term educational goals?
4. What are long-term nutrition goals?
5. How can continued education and support be planned for JS?

SUGGESTED SOLUTIONS

Short-term educational goals for JS include: learning insulin injection techniques; learning the time actions of injected insulin; learning hypoglycemia prevention and treatment; and updating basic information about diabetes, exercise, and blood glucose monitoring techniques.

Short-term nutritional goals include: developing a meal plan with JS that she feels comfortable with and able to follow over an extended period of time; emphasizing the need for consistency in the timing of her scheduled meals, snacks, and insulin injection times; and emphasizing that the primary goal of meal planning is to assist with blood glucose control, with weight loss being a secondary goal.

Name _____JS_____ Date _____

Total Calories _1500 –_ Carbohydrate _170_ gm. Protein _85_ gm. Fat _60_ gm.
_1600_ _40_ % _23_ % _37_ %

	BREAKFAST: Time: 8 AM	LUNCH: Time: 1–2 AM OR NOON	DINNER: Time: 5–6 PM
M	Starch/bread ___2___	Starch/bread ___2___	Starch/bread _2–3_
E	Meat _____	Meat ___3___	Meat _3–4_
A	Fruit _____	Vegetable _1–2_	Vegetable _0–1_
L	Milk _½–1_	Fruit ___–___	Fruit ___–___
S	Fat _0–1_	Milk ___–___	Milk ___–___
		Fat _1–2_	Fat _1–2_

	Morning: Time: _____	Afternoon: Time: 2 PM	Bedtime: Time: 11 PM
S N A C K S		OR 4 AM Starch OR Fruit 1 Fat 0–1	Fruit OR Starch 1

A 1500 to 1600 calorie meal plan based on exchanges — 40% carbohydrate, 23% protein, 37% fat — was discussed with JS. The meal plan still is higher in fat than desired but lower than her diet history and considered realistic by JS. See the above sample meal plan.

Dinner (supper) is with her family (she is living at home) and is fairly consistent at 5 to 6 PM. Breakfast is eaten at 7:30 to 8:30 AM (work) or 8 to 9 AM (days off). Lunch and snacks are "flipped" from days to nights and nights to day depending on her work schedule. She was started on the a

Days		Days to Nights	
7:30 AM	7 R 14 NPH	7:30 AM	7 R
8:00 AM	Breakfast	8:00 AM	Breakfast
Noon	Lunch	Noon	5 R
3:00 PM	Snack	12:30 PM	Lunch
4:30 PM	5 R 5 NPH	4:30 PM	5 R
5:00 PM	Dinner	5:00 PM	Dinner
10:30 PM	Snack	11:00 PM	Snack
Midnight to 7:30 AM	Sleep	1:30 AM	5 R 5 NPH
		2:00 AM	Lunch
		4:00 AM	Snack
		7:30 AM	Breakfast
		8:00 AM to Noon	Sleep
		1:00 PM	Snack
		4:30 PM	7 R 14 NPH
		5:00 PM	Dinner

Work Nights		Nights to Days	
8:00 AM to 2:00 PM	Sleep	4:30 PM	7 R 5 NPH
		5:00 PM	Dinner
2:30 PM	Snack	11:00 PM	Snack
4:30 PM	7 R 14 NPH	Midnight	5 R
5:00 PM	Dinner	12:30 AM	Lunch
11:00 PM	Snack	4:00 AM	Snack
1:00 AM	5 R 5 NPH	7:30 AM	5 R 14 NPH
1:30 AM	Lunch	8:00 AM	Breakfast
4:00 AM	Snack	8:30 AM to 1:00 PM	Sleep
7:30 AM	Breakfast	1:00 PM	Lunch
8:00 AM	Sleep	3:00 PM	Snack
		4:30 PM	5 R 5 NPH
		5:00 PM	Dinner
		10:30 PM	Snack
		Midnight to 7:00 AM	Sleep

a plan for meals and insulin, with frequent blood glucose monitoring especially on the Nights to Days schedule, when she takes insulin, eats breakfast, and goes to sleep. Monitoring will help prevent the potential for hypoglycemia.

The long-term educational goals are to: assist JS in using blood glucose monitoring information to make changes in her insulin doses, achieve target blood glucose levels of 70 to 120 mg/dL (3.9 to 6.7 mmol/L), and achieve a target hemoglobin A_{1C} level <7.0%. Continued support of her family is essential; her mother will attend class with JS.

The long-term goal of nutrition is improved eating habits by making healthier food choices. Her lipid levels need continued monitoring. Short-term changes must become a part of her lifestyle on a consistent, permanent basis.

For long-term goals to be met, JS also will need support and encouragement from her family/friends and health care providers. Strategies for long-term improvement in blood glucose and HbA_{1C} levels include: moderate and realistic weight-loss goals, improved food choices, reduced dietary fat content, consistent schedules and spacing of meals, continued involvement in exercise, and support from family and health care providers. In the past, JS has handled stressful events by overeating. She also needs to learn better techniques for handling stress.

OTHER SUGGESTED READINGS

American Diabetes Association, American Dietetic Association. Nutrition guide for professionals: diabetes education and meal planning. Alexandria, Va: American Diabetes Association, 1988.

American Dietetic Association Diabetes Care and Education Practice Group. Meal planning approaches in the nutrition management of the person with diabetes. Chicago: American Dietetic Association, 1993.

American Dietetic Association Position Statement. Use of nutritive and nonnutritive sweeteners. J Am Diet Assoc 1993;93:816-21.

Beebe CA, Pastors JG, Powers MA, Wylie-Rosett J. Nutrition management for individuals with non-insulin-dependent diabetes mellitus in the 1990s:

a review by the diabetes care and education dietetic practice group. J Am Diet Assoc 1991;91:196-207.

Bertorelli AM, Czarnowski-Hill JV. Review of present and future use of nonnutritive sweeteners. Diabetes Educ 1990;16:415-20.

Connell JE, Thomas-Dobersen D. Nutritional management of children and adolescents with insulin-dependent diabetes mellitus: a review by the diabetes care and education dietetic practice group. J Am Diet Assoc 1991; 91:1556-64.

Cooper NA. Nutrition and diabetes. A review of current recommendations. Diabetes Educ 1988; 14:428-32.

Franz MJ. Diabetes and exercise. In: Haire-Joshu D, ed. Management of diabetes mellitus. St. Louis: Mosby, 1992:80-114.

Franz MJ. Exchanges for all occasions. Minneapolis: ChroniMed Inc, 1993.

Franz MJ, Etzwiler DD, Joynes JO, Hollander P. Learning to live well with diabetes. Minneapolis: ChroniMed Inc, 1991.

Heins JM, Beebe CA. Nutritional management of diabetes mellitus. In: Haire-Joshu D, ed. Management of diabetes mellitus. St. Louis: Mosby, 1992:21-79.

Holler HJ. Understanding the use of the exchange lists for meal planning in diabetes management. Diabetes Educ 1991;17:474-84.

Lyon RB, Vinci SM. Nutritional management of insulin-dependent diabetes mellitus in adulthood: a review by the diabetes care and education dietetic practice group. J Am Diet Assoc 1993;93:309-14,317.

Maryniuk M. Nutrition education: taking it one step at a time. Diabetes Educ 1990;16:26-28.

Pastors JG. Alternatives to the exchange system for teaching meal planning to persons with diabetes. Diabetes Educ 1992;18:57-64.

Powers MA, ed. Handbook of diabetes nutritional management. Rockville, Md: Aspen Publishers Inc, 1987.

Warshaw HS. Alternative sweeteners — past, present, pending, and potential. Diabetes Spectrum 1990;3:335-43.

THERAPIES

VII.   EXERCISE

INTRODUCTION

As early as the 1920s, the effects of exercise in people with diabetes were recognized.[1,2] Today, exercise is regarded as an important part of diabetes management. Much of the morbidity and mortality among persons with diabetes is attributed to cardiovascular disease. Epidemiological evidence suggests that regular exercise and physical fitness are associated with decreased cardiovascular disease in the general population, as well as a decreased occurrence of non-insulin-dependent diabetes mellitus (NIDDM), also called type II diabetes.[3] As individuals with diabetes are living longer, the prevalence of diabetes in the elderly and the number of people with diabetic complications are increasing. The role of exercise consequently becomes of special significance. This chapter presents the benefits, effects, risks, and precautions of exercise for persons with diabetes. Additionally, exercise options for special populations, strategies to avoid problems, developing exercise programs, and increasing adherence are discussed.

OBJECTIVES

Upon completion of this chapter, the learner will be able to:
- discuss the benefits of exercise;
- describe the physiologic response to exercise in nondiabetic and diabetic individuals;
- identify risks associated with exercise and ways to minimize them;
- outline principles of an exercise program for people with diabetes;
- identify appropriate exercise therapies for special populations;
- outline strategies to enhance adherence to exercise programs.

A. Benefits of Exercise

1. Exercise generally is regarded as having a salutary effect for everyone. Although the benefits are many, exercise should not be regarded as a panacea. Such benefits may be the direct or indirect result of exercise. Most of the benefits are a result of

chronic (regular, long-term), aerobic (cardiovascular) exercise. Since persons with diabetes have an increased risk of developing cardiovascular disease, the role of exercise in reducing modifiable risks has primary importance. The benefits of exercise for persons with diabetes include[4-6]:

a) Improved functioning of the cardiovascular system.

b) Improved efficiency of cardiac and skeletal muscle tissue.

c) Improved strength and physical-working capacity.

d) Decreased risk factors for coronary artery disease (CAD), notably a reduction in plasma cholesterol, triglycerides, and low-density lipoproteins (LDL), particularly in the presence of weight loss. Increase in high-density lipoproteins (HDL) is seen.

e) Acute improvement in glucose tolerance.[7]

f) Increased insulin sensitivity.[6,7]

g) Reduced hyperinsulinemia, a proposed risk factor for atherosclerosis.[8-10]

h) Enhanced fibrinolysis. (Hypercoagulability frequently is present in persons with diabetes. Chronic exercise can enhance fibrinolysis and affect other mechanisms responsible for this hypothesized risk factor for atherosclerosis.[11,12])

i) Aid in modifying body composition (reduction of fat and weight, and increase in muscle mass).

j) Adjunct therapy for controlling hypertension.

k) Improved quality of life and self-esteem, and reduced psychological stress.[13]

2. The chronic effects of exercise appear to benefit the person with NIDDM (type II diabetes) by reducing HbA_{1c}, improving insulin sensitivity, assisting in attainment and maintenance of desirable body weight, and decreasing CAD risk factors.[14] Exercise should be a regular part of diabetes treatment. It is difficult to discern whether the lower HbA_{1c} is a result of meal planning, exercise, or a combination of meal planning, exercise, and the increased attention to self-management that often accompanies an exercise program.

3. Exercise should be included as part of overall diabetes management of insulin-dependent diabetes mellitus (IDDM), also called type I diabetes. It is especially important in light of the increased risk for macrovascular disease. Regular exercise in IDDM has not been shown consistently to result in improved diabetes control as evidenced by the HbA_{1c}.[15] This finding may be due to the difficulty of balancing insulin adjustments with food, in concordance with physical activity. Yet, many anecdotal reports show that the addition of a regular exercise program may enhance adherence to diabetes self-management regimens.

B. Physiology of Exercise

1. *Non-diabetic individuals.* Plasma glucose levels in nondiabetic individuals who exercise remain relatively stable due to an intricate regulation between the increase in glucose uptake by exercising muscles and increased hepatic glucose production.[16] This regulation involves a hormonal balance between decreased insulin secretion and increased action of catecholamines, glucagon, growth hormone, and cortisol (counterregulatory hormones).

    a) At the onset of exercise, fuel utilization by muscle progresses from primarily fat (extracted from the bloodstream as free fatty acids [FFA]) at rest, to glucose utilization from intramuscular stores of glucose and triglycerides.[17] As exercise continues, muscle glycogen stores are depleted, causing a shift from local fuels to fat.

       (1) The contribution of carbohydrate (stored as glycogen in the liver and muscles) and fat (stored as triglyceride in adipose tissue) depends upon exercise intensity, duration, fitness level, and time and content of the last meal.[5,18]

       (2) During the first 5 to 10 minutes of exercise, and during high-intensity exercise, glucose that is derived from the breakdown of muscle glycogen (glycogenolysis) is the major but limited source of

fuel for energy. This process is primarily anaerobic. Intramuscular triglycerides also are used.[17]

(3)   As exercise continues past 20 to 30 minutes, the muscle glycogen stores are depleted, and substrates (glucose from the liver and FFA from adipose tissue) in the blood are mobilized from tissue stores. Plasma glucose is maintained as hepatic glycogenolysis occurs when liver glycogen is broken down. Lipolysis occurs as triglycerides are mobilized from adipose tissue.

(a)   Liver glycogenolysis represents the majority of total carbohydrate used during the first 50 minutes of exercise; 25% of hepatic glucose output (HGO) is from gluconeogenesis (eg, the making of new glucose from lactate, glycerol, and amino acids).[19]

(b)   Because hepatic glycogen stores are limited, gluconeogenesis contributes approximately 50% as exercise progresses.[20]

(4)   Use of FFA increases as duration of exercise increases. Exercise of low to moderate intensity relies primarily on FFA as the oxidative fuel for muscle.[5]

(a)   As exercise duration progresses, the contribution of FFA as a fuel increases relative to glucose, from about 35% at 40 minutes of exercise to nearly 70% at 4 hours of exercise.[5,17]

(b)   The oxidation of fat-derived fuels cannot replace the utilization of glucose. When carbohydrate is limited, fat is not completely oxidized and ketone bodies are formed.

(5)   Amino acids contribute little as fuel for muscle during exercise, although they do contribute as gluconeogenic precursors.

b)   Hormonal response to exercise determines substrate utilization during exercise.

(1) Insulin secretion is decreased during exercise as a result of increased activity of the sympathetic nervous system.[21,22] The suppression of insulin secretion facilitates HGO and lipolysis, which allows blood glucose to be maintained.[17,18,23]

(2) Secretion of counterregulatory hormones increases and helps maintain glucose homeostasis.[16,24]

(a) Glucagon increases with exercise, particularly in relation to intensity, and stimulates up to about 75% of HGO.

(b) Epinephrine increases in response to high-intensity exercise, or in response to decreases in blood glucose levels. Epinephrine has a less prominent effect on HGO. Epinephrine stimulates lipolysis from adipose tissue thus providing glycerol for gluconeogenesis and FFA for fuel.[17]

(c) Norepinephrine stimulates liver and muscle glycolysis; it also stimulates lipolysis to a lesser extent.

(d) Growth hormone and cortisol increase with duration of exercise. Their role is to increase lipolysis, decrease insulin-stimulated glucose uptake in peripheral tissues, and increase gluconeogenic precursors during prolonged exercise.[6,17]

c) An ongoing increased uptake of glucose by muscle occurs during the *postexercise* period, as a possible means to replenish glycogen stores.

(1) Replenishment of glycogen stores may take 24 to 48 hours.[5,25]

(2) The postexercise recovery, particularly after exhaustive work, is characterized by enhanced insulin sensitivity.[19,26]

d) Trained athletes demonstrate a reduction in fasting insulin secretion in response to a glucose load.

(1) Accompanying this reduction in insulin secretion is an increase in muscle sensitivity to insulin.[18,27]

(2) Generalized secretion of counterregulatory hormones in trained individuals is less than in sedentary individuals.[21]

(3) Trained athletes utilize less glucose than sedentary individuals during exercise that is similar in intensity and duration. As a result, a slower rate of glycogen usage occurs, as well as a greater reliance upon fats for fuel, which are associated with greater endurance.[6,21,24]

2. *Individuals with diabetes.* A person with diabetes who exercises may have a decreased need for, or better utilization of, insulin, thus resulting in a decrease in required diabetes medications. Acute effects of exercise generally cause a reduction in plasma glucose. Chronic exercise results in improved insulin sensitivity and glucose tolerance, which often is mediated through changes in body composition and the additive effects of daily exercise. The hormonal response to exercise depends upon the degree of diabetes control, medication, time and content of the last meal, fitness level, and type of exercise. Specifically, the response to exercise depends upon the availability of insulin, thus explaining the difference in exercise metabolism between IDDM and NIDDM. Because the person with IDDM does not have a normal compensatory decrease in insulin secretion with exercise, metabolic abnormalities may occur.

a) The most commonly encountered problem is hypoglycemia. In nondiabetic individuals, plasma insulin decreases with exercise. This decrease, along with increases in plasma counterregulatory hormones, allows HGO and lipolysis to match glucose utilization.

(1) In persons taking insulin, the plasma insulin concentration does not decrease. Because the insulin is exogenous in origin, plasma insulin concentration actually can increase due to mobilization from subcutaneous depots.

      (a) A high plasma insulin level during exercise may enhance glucose uptake and further stimulate glucose oxidation in exercising muscle.[6]

      (b) A high plasma insulin level inhibits HGO and FFA mobilization.[23]

      (c) As a result, HGO does not keep pace with peripheral glucose utilization, and blood glucose concentration falls.

  (2) In patients with NIDDM treated with sulfonylureas, hypoglycemia also can result from exercise.

b) Another major concern for all medically treated persons with diabetes, particularly those with IDDM, is postexercise, late-onset hypoglycemia (PEL). PEL generally occurs following exercise of moderate to high intensity with a duration greater than 30 minutes. PEL results from increased insulin sensitivity, ongoing glucose utilization, and repletion of glycogen stores.

c) Occasionally in hyperglycemic and ketotic IDDM, acute exercise may result in a worsening of metabolic control.[6,22] Despite the fact that exercise stimulates glucose uptake, a certain amount of insulin is required. In the absence of adequate insulin, exercise causes increased plasma glucose, FFA, and ketones.

  (1) With onset of exercise, peripheral glucose utilization is impaired because of the low level of insulin.

  (2) The low level of insulin also stimulates excessive glucoregulatory hormones, which enhance HGO, lipolysis, and ketogenesis.

  (3) As a result, a rapid rise occurs in the already elevated blood glucose, as well as increased development of ketosis.

d) Individuals with NIDDM are less prone but able to develop exercise-induced hypoglycemia and very rarely develop hyperglycemia with ketosis. Improvements in insulin sensitivity, insulin secretion, and glucose disposal rates have been well documented in NIDDM, but the mechanisms underlying these improvements have not been clearly explained. Changes in body composition (decrease in fat weight, and increase in muscle mass) aid in increasing sensitivity to endogenous and exogenous insulin. The potential result is a reduction in exogenous insulin and/or oral hypoglycemic agents.

C.   Side Effects of Exercise and Precautions

1.   The primary side effects of acute exercise are hypoglycemia and, occasionally in IDDM, hyperglycemia and ketosis. Blood glucose response to exercise is affected by the type, amount, and intensity of exercise; the timing and type of previous meal and medication; preexercise blood glucose level; and fitness level.[6,16,18] Because of the heterogeneous response to exercise in individuals with diabetes, general guidelines to either increase carbohydrate consumption or decrease medication are not sufficient. Adjustments need to be determined on an individual basis.

2.   Hypoglycemia is a significant threat to persons who exercise while taking insulin or sulfonylureas, whereas persons controlling NIDDM by meal planning and exercise alone are not at risk of developing hypoglycemia when exercising.

  a)   For persons treated with continuous subcutaneous insulin infusion (CSII), hypoglycemia remains a risk with exercise.[28] However, the chances of developing hypoglycemia are less in insulin pump users due to the mechanics of the insulin infusion (eg, continual instead of bolus). The amount of insulin to decrease, or carbohydrate to supplement, depends upon a person's fitness level, and the duration and intensity of the exercise.[29,30] Several options for insulin pump users to maintain euglycemia with exercise include reducing basal infusion rate, consuming additional carbohydrates, or temporarily suspending pump use.[29-32]

  b)   Some controversy exists regarding subcutaneous insulin injection sites for exercise.[33,34] The concern is that insulin injected into a body limb that will be exercised will accelerate hypoglycemia via rapid mobilization of the insulin. Intramuscular injections have a tendency to result in a rapid mobilization of insulin with exercise.[35] Until definitive data are available, it is prudent to advise patients to avoid injecting insulin into body areas likely to be involved in exercise. The longer the interval between injection and onset of exercise, the less significant this effect will be.[6] To minimize the risk of hypoglycemia, patients should be advised to be *consistent* with the timing and sites of injections, and the time and type of exercise.

c) Blood glucose monitoring before and after exercise is required feedback for the patient learning to adjust insulin and/or carbohydrate with exercise. The choice between decreasing medication or increasing carbohydrate will depend upon the goals of the patient and the health care professional (eg, if losing weight is a goal, it is prudent to adjust medication). The amount of additional carbohydrate will depend upon the time of exercise in relation to medication and previous meal; the type, intensity, and duration of exercise; and the preexercise blood glucose level.

(1) Preexercise snacks are recommended if the blood glucose level is less than approximately 100 to 120 mg/dL (5.6-6.7 mmol/L), or if about 90 minutes has passed since the last meal.

(2) For mild-to-moderate exercise of <30 minutes, appropriate snacks (approximately 15 grams carbohydrate) include an 8-oz. glass of low-fat milk, half of a banana, or a small apple.

(3) For moderate intensity exercise longer than 60 minutes, snacks containing roughly 20 to 30 grams carbohydrate should be consumed approximately every 45 minutes.

(a) For exercise longer than 60 minutes, patients should be advised to check their blood glucose level every 45 to 60 minutes. This monitoring frequency will allow them to make adjustments (carbohydrate, medication) as needed.

(b) When exercise is of moderate intensity and long duration (>60 minutes), patients should be advised to sip on a carbohydrate replacement drink.

(c) Consuming foods that contain slow-releasing, complex carbohydrates is recommended to offset postexercise, late-onset hypoglycemia.

d) The safest time for people with diabetes to exercise is about 60 to 90 minutes after a meal. This strategy helps to prevent postprandial hyperglycemia, safeguards against hypoglycemia, and allows people taking insulin to reduce their premeal insulin if necessary.

(1) Patients with a tendency to develop hypoglycemia following exercise often do better exercising in the morning, either before or after medication/breakfast (depending upon individual response). At this time, postexercise hypoglycemia appears to be less prominent, and the patient is better able to detect any ensuing postexercise hypoglycemia during normal waking hours.

(2) Food to ingest while exercising to treat hypoglycemia include 4 to 6 ounces of juice or glucose tablets. Rapid-acting sugars will quickly raise the blood glucose level, which is especially important when hypoglycemia occurs during exercise.

(3) Reducing mealtime insulin may be necessary for individuals who exercise within approximately 90 minutes before or after a meal.

e) The likelihood of developing exercise-induced hypoglycemia can be decreased by avoiding exercise when injected insulin is peaking.

(1) For individuals participating in extended periods of exercise (longer than 2 hours), it often is easier to reduce insulin than to continually supplement with carbohydrate. Depending upon the time and type of

exercise, it may be necessary to reduce the dose of both regular and intermediate- or long-acting insulin.

   (2)   If it is difficult to avoid exercise when medication is peaking, then *consistency* in timing and type of exercise is helpful.

f)   Postexercise, late-onset hypoglycemia is a significant concern to persons treated with insulin, and can occur in persons treated with oral hypoglycemic agents. PEL can be the result of acutely increased insulin mobilization and sensitivity, increased glucose utilization, replenishment of glycogen stores, and defective counterregulatory mechanisms.[16,36] Options to minimize the occurrence of postexercise, late-onset hypoglycemia include: awareness and education about this condition; reduction of the insulin that peaks during the postexercise period, and supplementary carbohydrate during the postexercise phase (approximately 12 to 24 hours, depending upon exercise intensity and duration); avoidance of exercise prior to bedtime because PEL can occur during sleep; and frequent blood glucose monitoring during the postexercise period.[36]

3.   Occasionally, in persons treated with insulin, hyperglycemia and worsening of ketosis can result if exercise is initiated when the blood glucose level is greater than 240 to 300 mg/dL (13.3-16.7 mmol/L).[22] Exercise should be avoided until ketones are negative. If the IDDM patient has a blood glucose level greater than 240 to 300 mg/dL (13.3-16.7 mmol/L) because of a dietary indiscretion, an insulin deficiency may not be indicated; exercise generally will cause a drop in blood glucose levels. Negative urine ketones will confirm the absence of insulin deficiency.

a)   Occasionally in persons with well-controlled diabetes,[37] high-intensity exercise causes an acute rise in blood glucose levels. This phenomenon may be due to excess sympathetic stimulation as a result of high-intensity exercise; catecholamines are released that act on the liver to produce glucose. This interesting phenomena has been observed to cause initial rises, followed by declines, in blood glucose levels. The definition of moderate is relative to one's fitness level, thus a standard exercise recommendation of moderate may be too strenuous for some unfit individuals.

b) Exercise is especially effective in reducing hyperglycemia in individuals with impaired glucose tolerance, hyperinsulinemia, or NIDDM with a fasting glucose level less than 200 mg/dL (11.1 mmol/L).[38] An excellent strategy with these patients is to encourage them to think of exercise as a daily medication. This natural method to reduce blood glucose levels can become a part of daily treatment, resulting in decreased medication requirements.[39] It is best for persons with NIDDM to exercise daily, or at least every other day, in order to take advantage of the glucose-lowering effect of exercise.

D. Other Safety Precautions

1. All persons with diabetes that is treated by medication should carry a fast-acting carbohydrate with them while exercising.

2. Blood glucose monitoring, both pre- and postexercise, is the key to safety and understanding how exercise affects diabetes control.

3. Persons with diabetes should be advised to wear some form of diabetes identification, and to exercise with a buddy who is familiar with their diabetes.

4. Vigorous exercise should be avoided if the environment is extremely hot, humid, smoggy, or cold.

5. To reduce the likelihood of injury, persons with diabetes should have proper equipment and properly fitting exercise shoes.

6. All workouts should include warm-up and cooldown sessions. Stretching exercises should be performed to enhance flexibility and prevent injury.

7. Certain medications can impair exercise tolerance. Beta-blockers may dull the heart rate response to exercise, as well as mask hypoglycemia and the body's counterregulatory response.

8. Hydration should be maintained while exercising.

9. Patients should stop exercising if they feel faint, experience pain, or are unusually short of breath (see Table VII.1).

10. The American Diabetes Association recommends an exercise stress electrocardiogram in all people over age 35 years who want to begin exercising.[38] Special attention should be directed during assessments toward identifying a history of cardiac disease (including silent heart disease), the presence of complications, medications, medical and family history, and degree of diabetes control. Physical activity assessments are useful in designing exercise programs.

E. Components of Physical Fitness

1. *Aerobic exercise,* the preferred type of exercise for persons with diabetes, involves repetitive, submaximal contraction of major muscle groups (eg, swimming, cycling, jogging) and requires oxygen to sustain muscular effort. Aerobic exercise includes the following components:[4,38,40,41]

   a) Duration of exercise should be 20 to 60 minutes per session. Shorter sessions do not produce the desired aerobic and metabolic benefits; longer sessions may result in greater incidence of musculoskeletal injuries.

TABLE VII.1:
Risks of Exercise in Persons with Diabetes

1. Hypoglycemia, if diabetes is treated with insulin or oral agents:
   - Exercise-induced hypoglycemia
   - Postexercise, late-onset hypoglycemia (PEL)

2. Hyperglycemia after very strenuous exercise

3. Hyperglycemia and ketosis in insulin-deficient patients

4. Precipitation or exacerbation of cardiovascular disease:
   - Presence of silent heart disease: arrhythmias, cardiac dysfunction
   - Excessive increments in blood pressure with exercise
   - Angina pectoris
   - Myocardial infarction
   - Sudden death

5. Worsening of long-term complications:
   - Proliferative retinopathy: vitreous hemorrhage, retinal detachment
   - Nephropathy: increased proteinuria
   - Peripheral neuropathy: soft tissue and joint injury, foot ulcers, orthopedic injury
   - Autonomic neuropathy: decreased cardiovascular response to exercise, decreased maximum aerobic capacity, impaired response to dehydration, orthostatic hypotension, impaired counterregulatory response

Source: Adapted from Horton ES. Prescription for exercise. Diabetes Spectrum 1991;4(5):250-57.

---

b) Frequency of exercise should be five times per week to achieve the desired fitness level, or three to four times per week for maintenance. For improvement of glycemic control, exercise is recommended at least every other day.[38]

c) Intensity of exercise should be at a level of 60-85% of the maximal age-adjusted heart rate (comparable with 50% to 70% of maximal oxygen uptake, or VO_2 max). Results of an exercise stress test will allow accurate calculation of training intensity. When this testing is not possible, the following formula is commonly used to calculate maximum heart-rate and target heart-rate zones: 220

minus age equals estimated maximum heart-rate reserve; then multiply the estimated heart-rate reserve by a percentage (usually 60% and 85%) to estimate the training heart-rate range. This procedure may overestimate the maximal heart rate of some NIDDM patients, particularly those with autonomic neuropathy.[38] Due to the high prevalence of occult cardiovascular disease, caution is required when applying standard heart-rate formulas to the diabetic population.

(1) Exercise performed at low levels (<50% HR max) shows less effect on glucose disposal than exercise performed at higher intensities. The effect on glucose disposal during high-intensity exercise is roughly proportional to the total work performed (time x intensity). However, high-intensity exercise may result in transient hyperglycemia and cause an excessive rise in blood pressure.[16]

(2) When initiating an exercise program, it may be necessary to begin at low levels (50%), with brief rest intervals, and progress weekly to higher-intensity, continual exercise.

d) All workouts should include a 5 to 10 minute warm-up and cooldown. The warm-up helps to raise core body temperature and prevent muscle injury; the cooldown will help prevent blood pooling in the extremities and facilitate removal of metabolic by-products.

e) These goals will help achieve aerobic training effects. However, individual factors such as fitness level, age, and medical status can affect the attainment of these goals. Medications (eg, beta-blockers) and the presence of secondary complications may affect exercise prescription and tolerance (see Table VII.2).

2. *Anaerobic exercise*, defined as exercise not requiring sustained oxygen to meet the energy demands, often does not induce the same benefits as an aerobic program. Furthermore, anaerobic exercise may cause excessive rises in blood pressure, cardiac

workload, and intraocular pressure. These reactions could potentiate problems in elderly persons, or those with vascular disease or complications. However, properly designed programs of resistance exercise may improve indices of cardiovascular function, glucose tolerance, strength, and body composition.[42,43]

3.   *Muscle strength*, which often deteriorates as a result of inactivity or neuropathy, needs to be maintained.

4.   *Body composition*, or the lean-to-fat ratio, is essential to overall fitness and optimal diabetes management.

5.   *Flexibility* becomes impaired as muscle collagen becomes glycosylated.[17] Stretching exercises should be done to maintain flexibility and prevent injury.

F.   Special Populations

1.   *Elderly persons*: Physical working capacity (PWC) is known to decline with age, although what percentage is due to organic changes and what percentage is due to inactivity is unknown. Research in aging has shown that increased levels of physical activity are associated with longevity, increased physical working capacity, reduced risk of cardiovascular disease, and favorable influence on health status.[44,45] Special concern in the elderly population needs to be directed toward potential hazards.[45-47]

   a)   Prior to preparing an exercise prescription for elderly persons, a thorough medical exam should be done, with an emphasis on detecting occult heart disease, cardiovascular and/or peripheral vascular disease, joint/bone disease, and secondary complications. The following components of exercise should be included for the elderly.

      (1)   Anaerobic or muscle strength, often is neglected with advancing years. However, certain types of anaerobic training should be recommended for the

TABLE VII.2:
Summary of Exercise Recommendations

Screening	Presence of vascular and neurological complications, silent heart disease, stress ECG (GXT) in patients >35 y
Exercise Program	
Type	Aerobic preferred; anaerobic allowed if no secondary limitations
Intensity	60-85% of maximal heart rate (50-70% of maximum aerobic capacity)
Duration	20 to 60 minutes
Frequency	3 to 4 times per week for maintenance 5 times per week for improvement
Safety Precautions	Warm-up/cooldown
	Careful selection and progression of exercise program
	Patient education
	Blood glucose monitoring pre-/postexercise
	Treatment of hypoglycemia
	Management by medical personnel

Abbreviations: GXT, Graded Exercise Test.

Source: Adapted from ADA Exercise and NIDDM: technical review.[38]

---

elderly. Each major muscle group should be stressed two to three times per week, with an emphasis on the quadriceps, back, abdominals, and arm muscles, where weakness commonly develops.[48] Muscular toning can be accomplished via free weights, strap-on ankle/wrist weights, and traditional strengthening machines (eg, Nautilus). The focus should be on high repetitions with low weights.

(2) The decline of flexibility with age, combined with a tendency for increased muscle collagen glycosylation in persons with diabetes, suggests a need for daily stretching exercises. Caution is needed to avoid

overstretching, especially when sensation is impaired in the presence of peripheral neuropathy.[46]

    (3)   Aerobic fitness is encouraged for older persons. Because of the progressive decline in oxygen transport and functional capacity, an effective training stimulus for this age group may be much less than is needed in a younger person.[45,46] Good choices for aerobic fitness include cycling, brisk walking, swimming, dancing, and rowing. Initial exercise involvement may need to be interspersed with brief rest periods, eventually achieving continuous exercise. Adding 2 to 5 minutes per week to the workout time usually is appropriate for achieving the following desired goals:[46] duration of 30 to 40 minutes; frequency of five to six times per week; intensity based on graded exercise test (GXT), risk factors, medical history (typical training heart rate in the elderly is 60% to 75% of maximal heart rate); and progression and re-evaluation at about 4 to 6 weeks.

    (4)   Additional sources of fitness include chair exercises and water aerobics to improve strength and flexibility.

b)   Individuals with degenerative joint disease or osteoarthritis should avoid orthopedic or musculoskeletal stress.

c)   Exercises that induce excessive increases in blood pressure or involve Valsalva-type maneuvers (an attempt to forcibly exhale when the glottis is closed) should be avoided.

d)   Temperature extremes should be avoided because the elderly are more vulnerable to frostbite and heat intolerance.

e)   Certain medications may impair exercise capacity (eg, beta-blockers can affect heart rate and may mask symptoms of hypoglycemia).

f)   Sedentary individuals have an increased risk for cardiac arrest and cerebral vascular accidents if exercise is too vigorous. Initiate exercise at lower levels, progress slower, and work on gradually increasing duration and frequency of exercise to reach a desired fitness level.

2. *Obese persons:* The effectiveness of combined programs of exercise, meal planning, and behavior modification for obese persons has been demonstrated. The therapeutic approach that emphasizes increased levels of physical activity has the advantage of not only enhancing caloric expenditure but also drawing on the benefits of exercise in influencing blood lipids, diabetes control, blood pressure, mood and attitude.[41] Often, the initial fitness goal in this population is to simply increase the amount of physical activity from an inactive state.

    a) A combination of meal planning plus exercise has been shown to be more effective at long-term weight control than either meal planning or exercise alone. The addition of exercise to a weight-control program may facilitate a more permanent weight loss than total reliance on caloric restriction.[41]

    b) Regular exercise in a weight-control program helps to maintain muscle mass while promoting fat loss. Weight loss achieved by caloric restriction alone may lead to loss of lean muscle mass and less loss of fat.

    c) For the greatest impact on weight loss, continuous aerobic exercise for longer than 45 minutes is recommended.

        (1) There appears to be no selective effect of running, walking, or cycling; each training mode is equally effective in altering body composition.[41]

        (2) As the duration of exercise increases, so does the utilization of fat as a fuel. A longer duration (eg, greater than 45 minutes) has been shown to have a greater calorie-burning and fat-mobilization effect than shorter exercise periods.[5,41]

        (3) Intensity should be at a moderate level (60% to 75% HR max). Because obese persons may not be able to perform moderately strenuous exercise, it is more realistic to recommend a goal of 40 to 60 minutes of moderate exercise.

(4) Frequency of exercise should be a minimum of three times per week. However, a more frequent program would increase weight loss and facilitate better diabetes management.

(5) The most effective exercise options for people who are obese are brisk walking, cycling, rowing machines, simulated cross-county ski machines, and dancing. Less effective options are swimming (less likely to induce weight loss or aerobic effects) and running (too much knee stress in obese individuals).

3. *Complications*: Persons with diabetic complications often fail to take part in any activity programs. Yet it is important for this group to undertake an exercise program to improve or maintain functional capacity, strength, and flexibility.[49] Even though an aerobic program may not be possible, other benefits may be achieved with less strenuous exercise programs. Since persons with diabetes have an increased risk of cardiovascular disease, special assessments may be necessary to determine the most appropriate exercises.

a) *Cardiovascular disease*: Patients with established cardiovascular disease usually require supervision in a cardiac rehabilitation program. Hypertension and exercise-induced hypertension frequently are seen in persons with diabetes. Exercise should be prescribed at an intensity that avoids a hypertensive response. The Working Group on Hypertension and Diabetes[50] recommends limiting exercise intensity to prevent systolic blood pressure from exceeding 180 mmHg for extended periods of time. If the patient is hypertensive, exercises that involve heavy lifting, straining, and Valsalva-like maneuvers should be avoided. Furthermore, exercise that involves the upper body and arms generally induces larger increases in systolic blood pressure than similar workloads performed by the legs alone. Therefore, rhythmic exercises using the lower extremities are recommended, such as walking, light jogging, and cycling.

b) *Peripheral vascular disease*: Assessment of arterial circulation in a diabetic patient with peripheral vascular disease (PVD) should be done before the person engages in a physical activity program. An effective, noninvasive therapy for persons with PVD is an interval training program (eg, 3-minute walk, 1-minute rest, 3-minute walk).[51,52] The distance and duration of the walk should be determined by a pain-limited threshold. Intensity should be kept low because higher intensity demands greater blood supply and induces claudication pain. This suggested walk:rest:walk program results in greater exercise tolerance of pain-limited work capacity. Walking may be the best noninvasive therapy. Other aerobic exercise options include swimming, cycling, or rowing.[49]

c) *Retinopathy*: Caution is urged when recommending exercise for persons with proliferative retinopathy because of the correlation of high blood pressure and retinal damage or hemorrhage. Exercise prescriptions should be based on blood pressure while exercising. Heart rate should not exceed that which elicits a systolic blood pressure response greater than 180 mmHg.[49,52,53] Aerobic exercise choices include low-to-moderate cycling, swimming, jogging, or brisk walking.

(1) Resistive exercises using standard weight-lifting equipment generally are not recommended. If a patient strongly desires this type of exercise, physician approval is requisite and the focus should be on high repetitions (>15) with low resistance.

(2) Avoid exercises that cause breath holding or Valsalva-type maneuvers (eg, any near-maximal isometric contractions or high-intensity work).

(3) Avoid vigorous bouncing that can cause retinal detachment (eg, high-impact aerobics, heavy contact sports).

(4) Avoid exercises that involve lowering the head below waist level, which can cause excessive rise in blood pressure.

(5) Scuba diving is not recommended for people with proliferative retinopathy.

(6) Exercise is contraindicated following recent (<6 weeks) retinal photocoagulation. However, the clearance for exercise depends upon the patient's ophthalmologist.

d) *Visual impairment*: For persons with recent visual impairment and some with longstanding visual loss, aerobic capacity may be reduced due to loss of independent mobility. Suitable choices for exercise include swimming (using lane guides), stationary cycling, running with a partner, tandem cycling, and folk dancing (using the sighted person as an anchor). Various teaching adaptations and organizations have broadened sports participation (snow skiing, track and field competition) for visually impaired individuals.[49]

e) *Nephropathy*: Nearly all known risk factors for coronary artery disease are found in persons with end-stage renal disease, thus underscoring the need for a properly planned exercise program. Although aerobic exercises are preferred, the ability to perform this type of activity depends upon the degree of kidney impairment. These individuals usually have low functional and aerobic capacity. Any recommended aerobic activity should begin at a low level, perhaps using interval work, and follow a gradual, progressive exercise plan.[54] Brisk walking, swimming, and cycling are good choices. If heart and blood pressure response to exercise are normal, some *light* weight-training exercises can be done to improve muscle tone.[54]

f) *Neuropathy*: Peripheral neuropathy can result in sensory losses of pain, touch, and balance. Neuroarthropathy (Charcot's joint) can lead to disarticulations and injury in sensory-impaired individuals. Exercise cannot reverse the symptoms of neuropathy, but it can prevent further loss of muscle strength and flexibility that commonly is seen in these patients. Adaptive shortening of connective tissue can occur due to immobilization or limited proprioception. Thus, daily range-of-motion exercises are recommended.[49] Extra care is needed to avoid injury and overstretching when designing exercise programs for sensory-impaired individuals.[49] Weight-bearing exercises usually are not recommended because of the increased likelihood of soft tissue and joint injury. Avoiding orthopedic stress is important, and exercises such as cycling and swimming are good choices. If balance is not impaired, brisk walking may be another alternative.[49] Jogging is contraindicated because it places a threefold increase on the foot compared with walking. Proper footwear and daily inspection of the feet after exercise is necessary to avoid blisters or injury. For persons with limited mobility, chair exercises may improve flexibility and strength.

g) *Autonomic neuropathy*: Exercise by persons with autonomic neuropathy should be approached with caution because of the role of the autonomic nervous system in hormonal and cardiovascular regulation during exercise.[55,56] In the presence of autonomic neuropathy, high-intensity exercise should be avoided. Physical working capacity is reduced. Recumbent cycling and water aerobics are options for persons with orthostatic hypotension. Frequent blood glucose monitoring also is recommended during exercise for people with defective counterregulatory mechanisms.[49]

G. Guidelines for Exercise Adherence

1. If the physiologic effects of exercise are not immediately apparent, it is helpful to have patients identify the benefits they find personally motivating, and to reinforce these benefits frequently.

2. Goals that are too vague, too ambitious, or too distant do not provide enough motivation to maintain long-term interest.

Realistic and practical goals should be established at the beginning of an exercise program and reassessed regularly.

3. Social support from the family, class members, or a buddy system is essential for exercise adherence.

4. Using rewards, such as accumulating points for a large reward (eg, buying new clothes) or a small reward (eg, time off to engage in fun activities) can help promote adherence to an exercise program.

5. Regular feedback in the form of assessments (self-administered or done by the health care team) can encourage exercise adherence. For example, have patients compare the time it now takes to walk 2 miles with the time required to walk this distance at the beginning of their exercise program. A particularly effective method of feedback for people with diabetes is to keep a log of pre- and postexercise blood glucose levels, or to chart HbA_{1c} for the duration of the training program.

6. To prevent boredom with an exercise program, help patients identify alternative physical activities.

7. Establishing routine activities is helpful for all persons with diabetes because it fosters lifestyle changes and allows for exercise to become habitual. Routine is especially important for elderly persons.

8. Adherence to exercise programs is enhanced when exercise is convenient (eg, close to home or work).

9. Patients who may be self-conscious because of their weight or fitness level should be encouraged to find a group or class of similar status and with comparable goals. A significant deterrent for many overweight people is joining an exercise class comprised of people who are lean and relatively fit.

10. Be certain that patients participate in an activity that they enjoy and will do on a regular basis. Anecdotal reports suggest that individually designed programs enhance enjoyment and promote better adherence.

REFERENCES

1.   Allen FM, Stillman E, Fitz R. Total dietary regulation in the treatment of diabetes. Exercise 1919; Monograph 11.

2.   Lawrence RH. The effects of exercise on insulin action in diabetes. Br Med J 1926;1:648-52.

3.   Helmrich SP, Ragland DR, Leung RW, Paffenbarger RS Jr. Physical activity and reduced occurrence of non-insulin-dependent diabetes mellitus. New Engl J Med 1991;325(3):147-52.

4.   Pollock M, Wilmore J, Fox S. Exercise in health and disease. Philadelphia: WB Saunders, 1984.

5.   Astrand P, Rodahl K. Textbook of work physiology. St Louis: Macmillan, 1977.

6.   Horton ES. Role and management of exercise in diabetes mellitus. Diabetes Care 1988;11:201-11.

7.   Bogardus C, Ravussin E, Robins DC, Wolfe RR, Horton ES, Sims EAH. Effects of physical training with diet therapy on carbohydrate metabolism in patients with glucose intolerance and non-insulin-dependent diabetes mellitus. Diabetes 1984;33:311-18.

8.   Stout RW. Insulin and atheroma: 20 year perspective. Diabetes Care 1990;13(6):631-54.

9.   Fontbonne AM, Eschwege EM. Insulin and cardiovascular disease: Paris prospective study. Diabetes Care 1991;14(6):461-69.

10. Schneider SH, Ruderman NB. Exercise and physical training in the treatment of diabetes mellitus. Compr Ther 1986;12(1):49-56.

11. Colwell JA. Effects of exercise on platelet function, coagulation and fibrinolysis. Diabetes Metab Rev 1986;1(4):501-12.

12. Hornsby WG, Boggess KA, Lyons TJ, et al. Hemostatic alterations with exercise conditioning in NIDDM. Diabetes Care 1990;13(2):87-92.

13. Rodin J. Physiological effects of exercise. In: William RS, Wallace AG, eds. Biological effects of physical activity. Champaign, Ill: Human Kinetics, 1990.

14. Schneider SH, Amorosa LF, Khachadurian AK, et al. Studies on the mechanism of improved glycemic control during regular exercise in type II diabetes. Diabetologia 1984;26:355-60.

15. Zinman B, Zuniga-Guajardo S, Kelly D. Comparison of the acute and long-term effects of exercise on glucose control in type I diabetes. Diabetes Care 1984;7:515-19.

16. Vittug A, Schneider S, Ruderman NB. Exercise in type I diabetes. In: Pandolf KB, ed. Exercise and sport sciences reviews. New York: Macmillan, 1988;16:285-304.

17. Franz MJ. Exercise and diabetes: fuel metabolism, benefits, risks and guidelines. Clin Diabetes 1988;May/June:58-70.

18. Vranic M, Berger M. Exercise and diabetes. Diabetes 1979;28:147-63.

19. Ahlborg G, Felig P. Lactate and glucose exchange across the forearm, legs and splanchnic bed during and after prolonged leg exercise. J Clin Invest 1982;69:45.

20. Wahren J, Felig P, Hagenfeldt L. Physical exercise and fuel homeostasis in diabetes metabolism. Diabetologia 1978;14:213-22.

21. Hartley LH, Mason JW, Hogan RO, et al. Multiple hormonal responses to graded exercise in relation to physical training. J Appl Physiol 1972;33:602-6.

22. Berger M, Berchtold P, Cuppers HJ, et al. Metabolic and hormonal effects of muscular exercise in juvenile type diabetics. Diabetologia 1977;13:355-65.

23. Zinman B, Vranic M, Albissar AM, et al. The role of insulin in the metabolic response to exercise in the diabetic man. Diabetes 1979;28(suppl 1):76-81.

24. Winder WW. Regulation of hepatic glucose regulation during exercise. In: Terjung RL, ed. Exercise and sport sciences reviews. New York: Macmillan, 1985;13:1-32.

25. Wahren J. Glucose turnover during exercise in healthy man and in patients with diabetes mellitus. Diabetes 1979;29(suppl):82-88.

26. Richter EA, Canneto LP, Goodman M, Ruderman N. Muscle glucose metabolism following exercise in the rat. J Clin Invest 1982;69:785.

27. Mondon CE, Dolkas CB, Reaven GM. Site of enhanced insulin sensitivity in exercise-trained rats at rest. Am J Physiol 1980; 239(Endocrinol Metab 2):E169.

28. Koivisto VA, Tronier B. Postprandial blood glucose response to exercise in type I diabetes: comparison between pump and injection therapy. Diabetes Care 1983;6:436-40.

29. Sonnenberg GE, Kemmer FW, Berger M. Exercise in type I diabetic patients treated with continuous subcutaneous insulin infusion. Diabetologia 1990;33:696-703.

30. Schriffin A, Parikh S. Accommodating planned exercise in type I diabetic patients on intensive treatment. Diabetes Care 1985;8:337-42.

31. Walsh JA, Roberts R. Pumping insulin. Sylmar, Calif: Minimed Technologies, 1989.

32. Nathan D, Madnek S, Delahanty L. Programming preexercise snacks to prevent postexercise hypoglycemia in intensively treated insulin dependent diabetics. Ann Int Med 1985;102:483-86.

33. Koivisto VA, Felig P. Effects of leg exercise on insulin absorption in diabetic patients. N Engl J Med 1979;298:79-83.

34. Kemmer FW, Berchtold P, Berger M, et al. Exercise-induced fall of blood glucose in insulin-treated diabetics unrelated to alteration in insulin mobilization. Diabetes 1979;28:1131-37.

35. Frid A, Ostman J, Linde B. Hypoglycemia risk during exercise after intramuscular injection of insulin in thigh in IDDM. Diabetes Care 1990;13(5):473-77.

36. MacDonald MJ. Postexercise late-onset hypoglycemia in insulin dependent diabetic patients. Diabetes Care 1987;10(5):584-88.

37. Mitchell TH, Abraham G, Schriffin A, et al. Hyperglycemia after intense exercise in IDDM subjects during continuous subcutaneous insulin infusion. Diabetes Care 1988;11(4):311-17.

38. American Diabetes Association. Exercise and NIDDM: technical review. Diabetes Care 1990;13(7):785-89.

39. Kemmer FW, Tacken M, Berger M. Mechanism of exercise-induced hypoglycemia during sulfonylurea treatment. Diabetes 1987;36:1178-82.

40. American College of Sports Medicine. Resource manual for guidelines for exercise testing and prescription. Philadelphia: Lea & Febiger, 1988.

41. McArdle WD, Katch F, Katch V. Exercise physiology. Philadelphia: Lea & Febiger, 1981.

42. Durak EP, Jovanovic-Peterson L, Peterson CM. Randomized crossover study of effect of resistance training on glycemic control, muscular

strength and cholesterol in type I diabetic men. Diabetes Care 1990;13(10):1039-43.

43.   Goldberg AP. Aerobic and resistive exercise modify risk factors for coronary heart disease. Med Sci Sports Exer 1989;21:669-74.

44.   Paffenbarger RS, Wing AL, Hyde RT. Physical activity as an index of heart attack risk in college alumni. Am J Epidemiol 1978;108:161-75.

45.   Shephard RJ. Prescribing exercise for the senior citizen: some simple guidelines. In: Pandolf KB, ed. Exercise and sport sciences reviews. Baltimore, Md: Williams & Wilkins, 1989:xv-xxiii.

46.   Graham C. Exercise and aging: implications for persons with diabetes. Diabetes Educ 1991;17(3):189-95.

47.   Schwartz RS. Exercise training in treatment of diabetes mellitus in elderly patients. Diabetes Care 1990;13(2):77-85.

48.   Smith EL, Gilligan C. Physical activity prescription for the older adult. Physician Sports Med 1983;11(8):91-101.

49.   Graham C, Lasko-McCarthey P. Exercise options for persons with diabetic complications. Diabetes Educ 1990;16:212-20.

50.   The Working Group on Hypertension in Diabetes. Statement of hypertension in diabetes mellitus. Final report. Arch Int Med 1987;147(5):830.

51.   Boyd CE, Bird PJ, Teates CD, et al. Pain-free physical training in intermittent claudication. J Sports Med 1984;24:112-22.

52.   Greenlee G. Exercise options for patients with retinopathy and peripheral vascular disease. Practical Diabetol 1987;6(4):9-11.

53. Bernbaum M, Albert SG, Cohen JD, Drimmer A. Cardiovascular conditioning in individuals with diabetic retinopathy. Diabetes Care 1989;12:740-42.

54. Painter P. Exercise in end-stage renal disease. In: Pandolf KB, ed. Exercise and sport sciences reviews. New York: Macmillan, 1988;16:305-40.

55. Hilsted J, Galbo H, Christensen NJ. Impaired responses of catecholamines, growth hormone, and cortisol to graded exercise in diabetic autonomic neuropathy. Diabetes 1980;29:257-62.

56. Hilsted J, Galbo H, Christensen NJ, et al. Hemodynamic changes during graded exercise in patients with diabetic autonomic neuropathy. Diabetologia 1982;22:318-23.

KEY EDUCATIONAL CONSIDERATIONS

1. Design an exercise program with the patient, agreeing on recommendations and goals. Reevaluate the program every few weeks and establish new goals as necessary to help reinforce the effects, benefits, and principles of the exercise program.

2. Have the patient identify barriers to their exercise program. Review these barriers together, and plan alternative strategies/exercise options to overcome the barriers. For example, to overcome a fear of hypoglycemia, you can discuss ways to prevent this barrier; or you can discuss activities for an indoor exercise program to overcome the barrier of bad weather.

3. Ask the patient to check blood glucose levels pre- and postexercise, and to record results along with information about medication, nutritional intake, and the type and time of any symptoms that develop during or after exercise. By reviewing these records with the patient, the educator can discuss the effects of exercise and recommend needed adjustments in management. Furthermore, record keeping may enhance adherence to an exercise program.

4. To maintain commitment to an exercise program, have the patient perform self-assessments, comparing current level of physical activity to the amount of exercise that could be performed at the beginning of the exercise program. For patients who are more ambitious and able to undertake a more involved exercise program, the health care team also could monitor weight, blood glucose control, or lipid levels as additional factors that reflect progress with the exercise program.

SELF-REVIEW QUESTIONS

If you are unsure of the answers to the following questions, please review the materials.

1. List the benefits of regular exercise for individuals with diabetes.

2. Discuss the mechanisms for exercise-induced hypoglycemia.

3. What precautions can be taken to help prevent exercise-induced hypoglycemia, including postexercise, late-onset hypoglycemia?

4. For persons with IDDM, when and why can exercise result in a worsening of hyperglycemia and ketosis?

5. Describe components and give examples of aerobic exercise.

6. Discuss strategies to improve adherence to an exercise program.

7. What are the potential risks of exercise for persons with type I (IDDM) and type II (NIDDM) diabetes?

8. Briefly discuss and identify exercise that would be recommended or contraindicated for persons with retinopathy and neuropathy.

CASE EXAMPLE

AB is a 41-year-old female with a 26-year history of IDDM. She has come to the diabetes center because she wants to start an exercise program. During assessment she tells you, "I have retinopathy and my feet are a little numb, but otherwise, my diabetes is well controlled." AB is 5 ft 4 in tall, weighs 170 lb (76.5 kg), and her HbA_{1c} is >11% (normal <6.2%). She is on a split dose of regular and NPH insulins at breakfast and dinner. She checks her blood glucose levels in the morning, with results around 100 mg/dL (5.6 mmol/L). She states that she hasn't seen her doctor in awhile. AB is very enthusiastic to start using some new exercise equipment, but she needs to know where to start.

QUESTIONS

1. What questions would you ask AB about her diabetes and medical management?

2. What should be the goals of AB's exercise program?

3. What kind of program would you recommend to AB (eg, exercise type, intensity, duration, restrictions)?

SUGGESTED SOLUTIONS

AB states that her diabetes is fine, despite an elevated glycosylated hemoglobin level. This finding, together with her comments about her eyes and feet, indicate to the diabetes educator that AB's diabetes probably is not well controlled, that complications could be well established, and that AB may not be adequately educated regarding her diabetes management. Since AB has not seen her physician for some time, she is encouraged to do so prior to initiating an exercise program.

Due to her age and duration of diabetes, the physician should perform an exercise stress electrocardiogram (sometimes called a graded exercise test, or GXT) prior to initiating an exercise program. The results of the GXT allow accurate and safe determinations of exercise tolerances and limitations. The medical exam also should include a plasma lipid profile and blood chemistries, kidney function tests, and a comprehensive eye exam. These assessments are important in view of AB's history and will be helpful in preparing an exercise prescription.

Results of the GXT show no cardiac dysfunction during exercise, but reveal a poor tolerance to exercise, indicating a deconditioned state. When AB walked on the treadmill, her exercise systolic blood pressure was >200 mmHg when her heart rate was 145 beats per minute. Maximal exercise heart rate was 165 beats per minute. Further assessments show elevated lipids and a low HDL:LDL ratio (risk factors for CAD), slight proteinuria, and stable background retinopathy. AB's doctor decides that she should continue with the same insulin regimen, perform more frequent blood glucose monitoring, re-evaluate her meal plan with the assistance of a dietitian, and begin an exercise program. AB is referred to an exercise specialist.

The goals of an exercise program for AB are: a weight loss of about 40 lb (18 kg) (combined with a meal plan), improved lipid profile, improved aerobic capacity, improved overall diabetes management (combined with an education program), and increased feelings of control and self-worth.

An aerobic exercise program is recommended. However, because treadmill walking at a heart rate of 145 beats per minute resulted in an elevated systolic blood pressure, AB's recommended intensity will be based on blood pressure response to exercise. Due to the correlation of elevated blood pressure to increased proteinuria and retinopathy, the exercise will be performed at an intensity that does not induce large systolic changes. AB's training intensity is 165 (HR max) x 0.60 to 0.85 = 99-140 beats per minute. At 132 beats per minute, her systolic blood pressure was 160 mmHg, which is an appropriate training intensity. However, because AB has been inactive and is obese, she will need to initiate her exercise program at a lower training intensity (eg, 110 beats per minute). She may need to have some brief rest periods during the workout, performing only 15 minutes of exercise at a time. However, alternating weekly additions of time and intensity to the workout will help accomplish the ultimate goal (within 6 to 8 weeks) of continual exercise for 45 to 60 minutes at a heart rate of 130 beats per minute. AB should perform the exercise five times per week. Focusing on increasing duration, instead of only intensity, will aid in fat mobilization and favorably alter the lipid profile. Prior to initiating the exercise prescription, her blood glucose profile showed late-afternoon hyperglycemia. Consequently, the best time for AB to exercise is between 2 to 4 PM, when her blood glucose levels are high. Exercising at this time will control her late-afternoon hyperglycemia. Her NPH insulin may be peaking at this point, or even waning if she takes human insulin. Therefore, AB will monitor pre- and postexercise blood glucose levels at this time of day to determine her blood glucose response to exercise. Her late afternoon blood glucose level may improve, in which case adjustments in insulin will be made.

Because AB's feet are a little numb, jogging, stair climbing, or heavy weight-bearing exercises are not appropriate choices. Swimming, cycling, walking, or rowing would be good aerobic options. Anaerobic weight-lifting programs would not be appropriate for AB due to her complications and medical history, and desired goals of the exercise program.

OTHER SUGGESTED READINGS

General Exercise Physiology
American College of Sports Medicine. Guidelines for exercise testing and prescription. 4th ed. Philadelphia: Lea & Febiger, 1991.

American College of Sports Medicine. Resource manual for guidelines for exercise testing and prescription. Philadelphia: Lea & Febiger, 1988.

McArdle WD, Katch F, Katch V. Exercise physiology. 3rd ed. Philadelphia: Lea & Febiger, 1991.

Exercise and Diabetes

Franz MJ, ed. Exercise: its role in diabetes management. Diabetes Spectrum 1988;1(4):218-52.

Horton ES. Role and management of exercise in diabetes mellitus. Diabetes Care 1988;11:201-11.

Maynard T. Exercise: Part I. Physiological response to exercise in diabetes mellitus. Diabetes Educ 1991;17(3):196-204.

Maynard T. Exercise: Part II. Translating the exercise prescription. Diabetes Educ 1991;17(5):384-93.

Vranic M, Berger M. Exercise and diabetes. Diabetes 1979;28:147-63.

Wallberg-Henriksson H. Exercise and diabetes mellitus. In: Holloszy JO, ed. Exercise and sport sciences reviews. Baltimore, Md: Williams & Wilkins, 1992;20:339-368.

Exercising Special Populations

Artal R, Wiswell RA, Drinkwater BL, eds. Exercise in pregnancy. 2nd ed. Baltimore, Md: Williams & Wilkins, 1991.

Graham C, Lasko-McCarthey P. Exercise options for persons with diabetic complications. Diabetes Educ 1990;16:212-20.

Schwartz RS. Exercise training in the treatment of diabetes mellitus in elderly patients. Diabetes Care 1990;13(2):77-85.

Shephard RJ. Prescribing exercise for the senior citizen: some simple guidelines. In: Pandolf KB, ed. Exercise and sport sciences reviews. Baltimore. Md: Williams & Wilkins, 1989:xv-xxiii.

THERAPIES

VIII. PHARMACOLOGIC THERAPIES

INTRODUCTION

Treatment of diabetes mellitus traditionally has included a triad of diet, exercise, and medication. This chapter will present an update of pharmacologic therapy for people with diabetes. Expansion of insulin products through species and purity improvements has generated new treatment choices. Second-generation oral hypoglycemic agents have provided treatment options with fewer side effects than first-generation agents.

OBJECTIVES

On completion of this chapter, the learner will be able to:
- describe the physiologic effects of insulin;
- list and differentiate insulin preparations based upon species/source, type, purity, and concentration;
- describe proper administration and storage guidelines for insulin;
- explain the limitations for insulin mixing;
- compare and contrast potential insulin therapy regimens, including the use of subcutaneous infusion pumps, and indications for specific insulin products;
- discuss the mechanism(s) of action of oral hypoglycemic agents;
- compare and contrast the oral hypoglycemic agents in terms of their clinical usefulness;
- discuss the clinical use of glucagon.

A. Physiologic Effects of Insulin and Indications for Its Use

1. The following describes the physiologic actions and release of insulin.

    a) Insulin, a hormone produced in the beta cells of the islets of Langerhans in the pancreas, is formed from a substance called proinsulin (see Figure VIII.1). The proinsulin is cleaved when stimulated, usually by an elevated blood glucose level, yielding insulin and connecting peptide (C peptide), which enter the bloodstream in equimolar

FIGURE VIII.1:
Biochemical Formation of Proinsulin

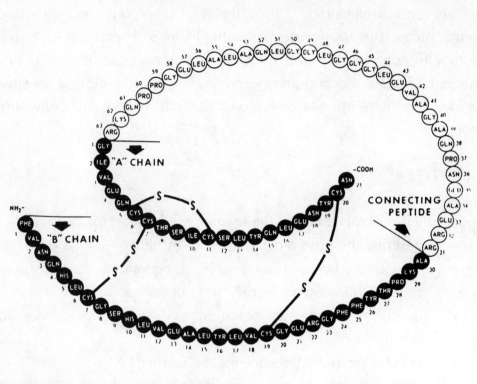

Reprinted with permission: Eli Lilly and Co.

amounts. Some proinsulin also enters the blood. The C peptide levels can be used as a clinical monitor of endogenous insulin production, and also may be used to rule out factitious insulin use as a cause of unexplained hypoglycemia. Since insulin and C peptide have different biologic durations, C peptide levels may not accurately reflect endogenous insulin levels.

b) Insulin exerts varied effects upon body tissues. Insulin stimulates the entry of amino acids into cells, enhancing protein synthesis. Insulin enhances fat storage and prevents the mobilization of fat for energy. Insulin stimulates the entry of glucose into cells for utilization as an energy source and promotes the resulting storage of glucose as glycogen in muscle and liver cells.

c)   Endogenous insulin is insulin that is supplied from the pancreas, while exogenous insulin refers to injected pharmaceutical insulin.

2.   Insulin is indicated as therapy for some specific patients with diabetes.

a)   All patients with insulin-dependent diabetes mellitus (IDDM), also called type I diabetes, require exogenous insulin. The production of insulin by their beta cells is completely or largely lost.

b)   Certain patients with non-insulin-dependent diabetes mellitus (NIDDM), also called type II diabetes, may require insulin if other forms of therapy do not adequately control blood glucose levels or if they experience physiological stress such as surgery.

c)   Patients with gestational diabetes may require management with insulin if diet alone does not adequately control blood glucose levels.

d)   Patients who receive parenteral nutrition or who require high caloric supplements to meet increased intermittent energy needs may require exogenous insulin to maintain normal glucose levels during periods of insulin resistance or increased insulin demand.

e)   Insulin is necessary in the treatment of diabetic ketoacidosis.

f)   Insulin is sometimes needed in the treatment of hyperglycemic hyperosmolar nonketotic syndrome.

g)   Certain patients with secondary diabetes may require insulin. For example, diabetes secondary to pancreatitis may severely diminish beta cell production of insulin.

B.   **Insulin: Species/Source, Type, Purity, and Concentration**

1.   This section differentiates insulin preparations by specific product characteristics.

TABLE VIII.1:
Insulins Available in the United States

PRODUCT	MANUFACTURER	NPH/REG (% ratio)
SHORT ACTING		
Beef		
Semilente	Novo Nordisk	
Pork		
Iletin II regular	Lilly	
regular	Novo Nordisk	
Purified Pork regular	Novo Nordisk	
Velosulin	Novo Nordisk	
Beef/Pork		
Iletin I regular	Lilly	
Human		
Humulin R (regular)	Lilly	
Novolin R (regular)	Novo Nordisk	
Velosulin Human R (regular)	Novo Nordisk	
INTERMEDIATE ACTING		
Beef		
Lente	Novo Nordisk	
NPH	Novo Nordisk	
Pork		
Iletin II Lente	Lilly	
Iletin II NPH	Lilly	
Purified Pork Lente	Novo Nordisk	
Purified Pork NPH	Novo Nordisk	
Insulatard NPH	Novo Nordisk	
Beef/Pork		
Iletin I NPH	Lilly	
Iletin I Lente	Lilly	
Human		
Humulin L (Lente)	Lilly	
Humulin N (NPH)	Lilly	
Novolin L (Lente)	Novo Nordisk	
Novolin N (NPH)	Novo Nordisk	
Insulatard NPH Human	Novo Nordisk	
LONG ACTING		
Beef		
Ultralente	Novo Nordisk	
Human		
Humulin U (Ultralente)	Lilly	
FIXED COMBINATIONS		
Pork		
Mixtard	Novo Nordisk	70/30
Human		
Humulin 70/30	Lilly	70/30
Novolin 70/30	Novo Nordisk	70/30
Mixtard Human 70/30	Novo Nordisk	70/30
Humulin 50/50	Lilly	50/50

2.   Identified in Table VIII.1 are specific insulin products, including each of the characteristics discussed.

   a)   The three species/sources for insulin are beef, pork, and human. The six product types are beef, pork, beef-pork combinations isolated from animal pancreas glands, biosynthetic human insulin derived from bacteria (*E coli*), biosynthetic human insulin derived from fungal cells (*Saccharomyces cerevisiae*), and semi-synthetic human insulin.

      (1)   Beef insulin (see Table VIII.2) differs from human insulin at three amino acid sites, while pork insulin differs at only one amino acid site. Because of these differences, beef insulin induces more antigenic reactions than pork insulin. Beef-pork combination products generally are thought to induce the most antigenic reactions.

TABLE VIII.2:
Amino Acid Sequence Differences
Between Various Insulin Species

| Species | A Chain | | B Chain |
	A-8	A-10	B-30
Bovine	Alanine	Valine	Alanine
Porcine	Threonine	Isoleucine	Alanine
Human	Threonine	Isoleucine	Threonine

Source: Adapted from Insulin. In: Waife SO, ed, Diabetes mellitus. Indianapolis: Lilly Research Laboratories, 1980:37.

      (2)   Human insulin is manufactured by using recombinant-DNA technology (biosynthetic) or by chemical conversion of pork insulin to human insulin (semi-synthetic). Human insulin is less antigenic than beef insulin and slightly less antigenic than pork insulin.

(3) Human biosynthetic NPH, Lente and Ultralente insulins, appear to be absorbed faster and therefore act more quickly than animal-derived insulins, even though the pharmacologic effects are similar. Commercially prepared human insulins are effective and chemically identical to endogenous human insulin. In most market areas, human insulin is less expensive than purified pork insulin.

(4) Patients whose treatment is converted from animal insulin to human insulin may require dosage adjustment because of the shorter duration of action and lower antigenicity (less potential for antibody production) with human insulin.

(5) Human insulin provides an option for vegetarians, Moslems, Orthodox Jews, and Hindus who refuse to use pork or beef insulins. There virtually are no contraindications to human insulin, although there are rare instances of hypersensitivity.

(6) Animal-derived insulins may induce insulin antibody formation to a greater degree than human insulins. When insulin is bound to insulin antibodies, the predictability of the peak effect and duration of action of the insulin will be altered.

b) Five types of insulin are manufactured and are categorized by their peak effect and duration of action, as noted in Table VIII.3. The rapid-acting insulins are regular and Semilente. The intermediate-acting insulins are NPH and Lente. The long-acting insulin is Ultralente.

(1) Regular insulin is the only clear insulin or solution of insulin; all the others are suspensions. Regular insulin is the only insulin product appropriate for intravenous administration.

(2) NPH contains protamine and some zinc, while the Lente insulins have high zinc levels to prolong the duration of action.

TABLE VIII.3:
Onset, Peak, and Duration of Different Insulins

	Onset	Peak	Duration Therapeutic*	Duration Pharmaceutic**
Rapid-Acting (Regular, Semilente)	$\frac{1}{2}$ - 1 hr	2 - 4 hrs	6 - 8 hrs	5 - 12 hrs
Intermediate-Acting (NPH, Lente)	1 - 4 hrs	8 ± 2 hrs	10 - 16 hrs	16 - 24 hrs
Long-Acting (Ultralente)	4 - 6 hrs	18 hrs	24 - 36 hrs	36+ hrs

* Therapeutic (or Effective Duration of Action) — the amount of active insulin needed to keep blood glucose levels in normal limits.

** Pharmaceutic (or Pharmacokinetic) — the action of insulin on "entrance" into and "exit" from the body.

Source: Adapted from Campbell RK. Diabetic management: insulin, oral agents, and intensified insulin therapy (module 9). Chicago: American Association of Diabetes Educators Continuing Education Self-Study Program, 1985: table 3; and Diabetes Treatment Center, Care and control of your diabetes. Wichita, Kan: St Joseph Medical Center, 1988:59.

(3) Both protamine and zinc occasionally have been implicated as the causative agents of immunologic reactions, such as urticaria, at the injection site.

c) Purity of insulin is expressed as parts per million (ppm) of proinsulin, the primary contaminant after extraction from the pancreas. Concern about purity is a less significant issue in insulin therapy today than previously, as all insulins are now highly purified.

d) The concentrations of insulin currently available in the United States are U-100 and U-500. U-100 concentration is the insulin of choice for nearly all patients. Patients who require large doses of insulin may use U-500 regular insulin, which is available only by prescription. The onset and duration of action of U-500 is not the same as U-100 regular. U-40 insulin still is utilized in some countries, a point important to those traveling to foreign countries. Not all countries use U-100 insulin so patients should be instructed to take extra supplies when traveling.

    e)   Certain insulin preparations are preferred for insulin pump users. These preparations of regular human insulin contain phosphate buffers that prevent crystallization of the insulin in the infusion tubing.

C.   Administration and Storage Guidelines

1.   Administration of insulin requires the correct equipment, preparation, and consistent use of proper technique.

2.   Insulin should be stored according to the manufacturer's recommendations.

    a)   Insulin should be refrigerated at 36° to 46° F (2° to 8° C).

    b)   Insulin may be kept at a controlled room temperature of 59° to 68° F (15° to 20° C) if the entire contents of the vial will be used within one month. Older studies that supported storage of insulin at room temperature were based on radioimmunoassay determinations of potency. More sensitive assays demonstrate that insulins stored at room temperature beyond one month have been shown to deteriorate, with a loss of potency, especially if the insulin is stored at temperatures of over 86° F (30° C).[1-3]

    c)   Penfill and disposable pen storage guidelines differ.[2] Penfill regular can be stored at room temperature for 30 days after puncture. Penfills 70/30 and NPH can be stored at room temperature for 7 days after puncture.

    d)   Prefilled syringes of either single formulations or mixtures of insulins should be kept refrigerated and used within 21 days[3] to 30 days.[4]

    e)   To limit local irritation at the injection site that often occurs when injecting cold insulin, patients are advised to roll the prepared syringe between the palms, bring the bottle of insulin to room temperature, or date the vial of insulin stored at room temperature and discard after one month.

f)   When stored according to the manufacturer's recommendations, the expiration date denotes the last date on which that vial of insulin should be used.

g)   Availability of insulin and supplies may vary, so insulin and supplies should be put in carry on luggage when traveling. Due to temperature variations, insulin should not be left in a car or checked through in airline baggage (see Chapter X: Special Issues in Management).

h)   The vial of insulin should be examined for sediment or other visible changes before withdrawing the insulin into the syringe. Cloudiness or discoloration of clear insulin, clumping of insulin suspensions, or flocculation (frosting) of insulin suspensions indicates that the insulin should not be used but should be returned to the pharmacy for exchange. The incidence of frosting may be minimized if temperature is stabilized through refrigeration and if agitation or shaking of the vial is minimized.

3.   Various equipment is used in the administration of insulin.

a)   Needles of disposable syringes used for insulin injections are quite thin and sharp, resulting in comfortable, less traumatic injections. For ease in measuring the insulin dose, 1 cc, $\frac{1}{2}$ cc, and $\frac{3}{10}$ cc syringes are available.

b)   The reuse of syringes and needles can be done safely, although this issue still remains somewhat controversial. Syringe reuse may carry an increased risk of infection for some individuals.[5] Patients who choose to reuse syringes should be advised that the markings on the syringe may rub off and that the needle becomes dull with repeated use.

c)   The patient should be taught to follow a specific routine for insulin injections, including a consistent technique, accurate dosage, and site rotation. Injections are made into the subcutaneous tissue. Most individuals are able to lightly grasp a fold of skin and inject at a 90° angle. Thin individuals or children may need to pinch the skin and inject at a 45° angle to avoid intramuscular injection, especially in the thigh area. Routine aspiration (drawing back on the injected syringe to check for blood) is not necessary.[5]

d)   Alternative equipment to the traditional syringe-needle units is available. The variety of injection devices includes automatic needle injectors, automatic needle and insulin injectors, pen injectors, and needle-free jet injectors. The needle-free jet injectors propel insulin through the skin by air pressure.

e)   Insulin pumps, also known as Continuous Subcutaneous Insulin Infusion (CSII), are used to program a constant infusion of insulin subcutaneously. This method provides a more physiologic pattern of insulin delivery. Pump users are required to monitor their blood glucose frequently. Candidates for insulin pumps need to be screened carefully (see Chapter X: Special Issues in Management). Insulin pumps intended for daily use by the patient utilize an open-loop system of insulin dose adjustment where the patient tests the blood glucose with a meter and uses the pump to deliver insulin over 24 hours. With the insulin pump, a continuous basal dose is programmed, and the patient adjusts pre-meal bolus doses of insulin based on blood glucose levels.

4.   Insulin absorption may vary, depending upon several parameters. Abdominal injection provides the most rapid absorption, followed by the arm, leg, and hip sites.[6,7] Deeper intramuscular (IM) injections induce faster absorption and a shorter duration of action, as does exercise of the injected muscle immediately before or after the injection. High levels of insulin antibodies can inhibit insulin action following injection.

a)   Massaging the injection site following the injection seldom is recommended. Site massage induces more rapid absorption and action from a dose of insulin.[8]

b)   Recommended sites are shown in the diagram (see Figure VIII.2). They are chosen because of the low potential for adverse reactions. These sites are specifically designated areas of the body.

c) The injection sites are rotated to prevent local irritation and reactions. Many people now advocate rotating injections in one area, then moving to another area. This procedure allows an area several weeks of "rest" between uses.

d) Areas for injection must be individualized, considering scar tissue, areas with less subcutaneous fat, and patient preference.

e) Areas used for injection should be assessed at every opportunity. Written patient education materials cannot give a three-dimensional perspective, and patients often inject in areas of poor absorption, such as the inner thigh.

5. Various problems or complications may arise from insulin impurity, species source, and improper injection technique. The most significant problems with insulin therapy can be attributed to incorrect dosage or improper monitoring of the patient.

a) The major complication of insulin therapy is hypoglycemia. Virtually all persons who inject insulin experience hypoglycemia at some time. If a person injects too much insulin, does not eat enough, or exercises more than usual, the blood glucose level may fall low enough to cause hypoglycemia, or an insulin reaction. The patient can reduce the risk of hypoglycemia by routine monitoring of blood glucose levels, recognizing and quickly treating hypoglycemia, preparing for exercise, and following consistent meal patterns (see Chapter XIII: Hypoglycemia).

b) Lipodystrophies include atrophy and hypertrophy. Atrophy, a concavity or pitting of the fatty tissue, is an immune phenomenon that occurs in a small number of patients and usually is related to the species source or purity of the insulin. Use of highly purified insulins, such as human insulin or purified pork insulin, will reduce the occurrence of atrophy. Patients who develop this problem

FIGURE VIII.2:
Multiple Injection Sites

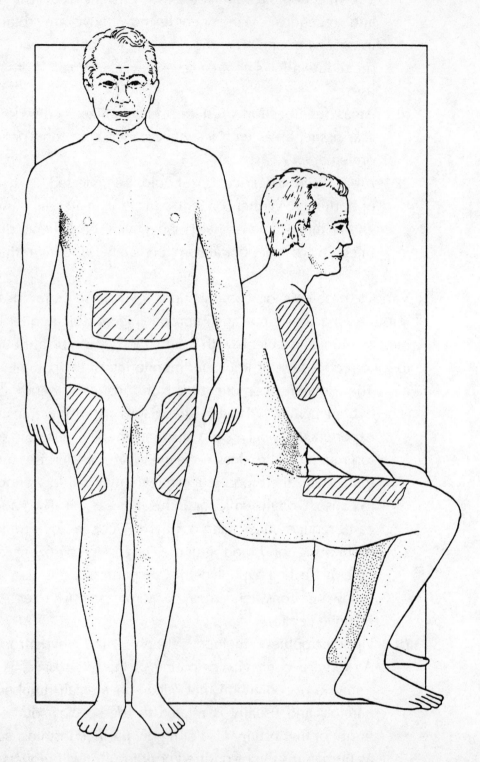

Reprinted with permission: Michigan Diabetes Research and Training Center, University of Michigan, 1988.

230 A Core Curriculum for Diabetes Education

may benefit from injection of insulin in and around the atrophied areas.[9] It is important to assess for hypertrophy, a fatty, tumorous thickening of the lipid tissue, at every opportunity. The causes of hypertrophy are not fully understood.

c) Prescription and nonprescription medications can affect daily blood glucose levels. Whenever a new medication is initiated, frequent monitoring and careful observation of unusual symptoms are important. Medications associated with hypoglycemia and hyperglycemia are listed in Tables VIII.4 and VIII.5.

d) Allergies to insulin are rare but always possible. They can be divided into local (rash, urticarial cutaneous reaction) and systemic (serum sickness, anaphylaxis) reactions.

(1) Prior to insulin purification, local cutaneous reactions were more common. Zinc or protamine in the insulin, preservatives, and rubber or latex stoppers all have been implicated in inducing allergic reactions.

(2) Both local and systemic reactions appear to be immunologically mediated through induction of high titers of IgG and IgE antibodies.

(3) When an allergy occurs, changing from animal insulin to a purified or human insulin often is necessary. If a systemic reaction occurs, desensitization to the insulin also will be necessary.

D. Mixing Limitations

1. Organizing the necessary materials prior to insulin injection will limit errors. This planning also will make administration more routine for traveling purposes.

2. Mixing and prefilling guidelines are listed in Table VIII.6. These standards are based on published data.[10] When mixing Lente and regular insulin, varying the time delay for injection after mixing may result in a different insulin action. As a general rule, the two insulins being mixed should be from the same

TABLE VIII.4:
Drugs Associated with Hypoglycemia:
Mechanisms of Action and Relative Clinical Significance

Drug	Mechanism of action	Clinical Significance
Alcohol	Impairs gluconeogenesis and increases insulin secretion	+++
Anabolic steroids	Unknown	+
Beta-adrenergic antagonists	Inhibit glycogenolysis; attenuate signs and symptoms of hypoglycemia	++
Dicumarol	Inhibits hepatic clearance of tolbutamide (Orinase) and chlorpropamide (Diabinese)	++
Chloramphenicol (Chloromycetin)	May inhibit metabolism of sulfonylureas	++
Chloroquine (Aralen)	Unknown	++
Clofibrate (Atromid-S)	Unknown	+
Disopyramide (Norpace)	Unknown	++
Pentamidine isethionate (NebuPent, Pentam 300)	Causes cytolytic response in pancreas accompanied by release of insulin	+++
Phenylbutazone (Azolid, Butazolidin)	Reduces clearance of sulfonylureas	++
Salicylates	Increase insulin secretion and sensitivity; may alter pharmacokinetic disposition of sulfonylureas	++
Sulfonamides	Alter clearance of sulfonylureas	+

Source: From White J, Hartman J, Campbell RK. Drug interactions in diabetic patients. Postgrad Med 1993;93:132.

manufacturer. The recommended order for mixing insulins is regular insulin drawn up first, followed by the intermediate-acting insulin. This order limits the potential for contamination of the regular insulin, resulting in less dose variance. Consistency in the order of mixing insulins is very important.

3.   Commercially prepared premixed insulins (70/30 and 50/50) are manufactured and stabilized by altered buffering. The common target users for premixed insulin are the patients who

TABLE VIII.5:
Drugs Associated with Hyperglycemia:
Mechanisms of Action and Relative Clinical Significance

Drug	Mechanism of action	Clinical Significance
Alcohol	Chronic ingestion increases metabolism of tolbutamide (Orinase)	+
Asparaginase (Elspar)	May be related to inhibition of insulin synthesis	++ (diabetic ketoacidosis has been reported)
Beta-adrenergic antagonists	Inhibit insulin secretion	++
Calcium channel antagonists	Inhibit insulin secretion	+/-
Combination oral contraceptives	Unknown	++
Diazoxide (Hyperstat IV, Proglycem)	Inhibits insulin secretion	+++
Diuretics	May be related to hypokalemia	++
Glucocorticoids	Increase gluconeogenesis; depress insulin action	+++
Glycerol	Unknown	++ (hyperglycemic hyperosmolar nonketotic coma has been reported)
Lithium salts (Eskalith, Lithane, Lithobid)	May decrease insulin secretion	+
Niacin	Unknown	++
Pentamidine isethionate (NebuPent, Pentam 300)	Promotes pancreatic toxicity	+++
Phenytoin sodium (Dilantin)	Inhibits insulin secretion	++
Rifampin (Rifadin, Rimactane)	Enhances metabolism of tolbutamide	+
Sympathomimetics	Increase glycogenolysis and gluconeogenesis	++

Source: From White J, Hartman J, Campbell RK. Drug interactions in diabetic patients. Postgrad Med 1993;93:137.

TABLE VIII.6:
Guidelines for Mixing Insulin and/or Prefilling Syringes

Regular and NPH
- Mixture stable in any ratio
- Mixture of choice, if rapid and intermediate combination is needed
- Extemporaneously prepared syringes which are refrigerated are stable for at least one month
- Prefilling is acceptable

Regular and Lente
- Binding of Regular begins immediately
- Binding continues for 24 hours
- Activity of Regular is blunted
- Velosulin should not be mixed with Lente insulins
- If mixed or prefilled, the interval between mixing the insulins and administering the insulin should be standardized

Commercially Prepared Premixed Insulins
- Prefilling is acceptable

Semilente, Lente and Ultralente
- Mixture stable in any ratio
- Mixture stable for 18 months
- Prefilling is acceptable

Source: Adapted from White J, Campbell RK.   Guide to mixing insulins.   Hosp Pharm, 1991;26:1046-48.

---

cannot tolerate the complexity of mixing two vials of insulin, or the patients whose insulin needs correspond to these ratios.

E.   Insulin Therapy Regimens

1.   Dosing schedules vary for individuals with IDDM (type I) and NIDDM (type II) receiving insulin. Physiologically, insulin and glucagon are released throughout the day in frequent bursts in response to a variety of stimuli. Such a natural pattern is difficult to achieve with infrequent injections of insulin. The apparent half-life of free insulin has been reported to be approximately 5.2 ($\pm$0.7) minutes and may be increased in patients with diabetes having high insulin antibody titers. The pharmacology and the pharmacokinetics of insulin require that

people receive a small amount of insulin continuously, with boluses of insulin before meals and snacks, if complete normalization of blood glucose is to be achieved.

2. The treatment protocol for insulin administration for the purpose of normalizing blood glucose levels theoretically is simple and easy to describe. Implementing the treatment protocol with the goal of normalizing blood glucose levels may be more challenging.

3. Insulin therapy is indicated for individuals with IDDM and for some individuals with NIDDM. Many authors have developed sophisticated algorithms that advocate various approaches to optimize glycemic control.[11] The evolution of insulin management in America clearly is moving from single-injection, intermediate insulin therapy to multiple injections of human insulin.

4. The starting dose of insulin for an adult patient with IDDM usually is between 0.5 to 1.0 unit/kg/day. There is no formula for arriving at the appropriate insulin dose. The process can include the following steps:
   a) Determine the target blood glucose range.
   b) Start with a small dose based on weight and adjust the dose, using rapid- and intermediate-acting insulins based on the results of blood glucose monitoring.

5. Because patients differ in their response to insulin and in their daily habits regarding diet, exercise, medications, and emotional factors, the dose of insulin required for satisfactory control will vary considerably among individual patients. In other words, there is no typical dose.
   a) Some individuals are managed on one injection daily, usually administered in the morning or sometimes at bedtime. This regimen usually utilizes an intermediate-acting insulin, but could include a commercially prepared premixed insulin. Patients with NIDDM may attain

reasonable glycemic control with this approach, although this regimen generally is not recommended in patients with IDDM since it rarely produces glycemic control[12] (see Figure VIII.3).

FIGURE VIII.3: Time Action of Insulin

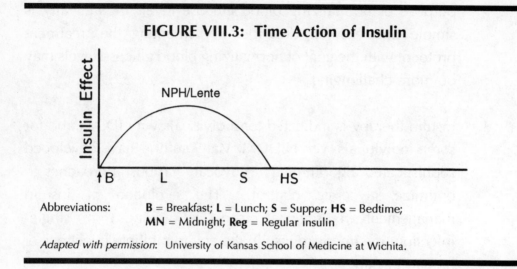

Abbreviations: **B** = Breakfast; **L** = Lunch; **S** = Supper; **HS** = Bedtime;
                    MN = Midnight; **Reg** = Regular insulin

Adapted with permission: University of Kansas School of Medicine at Wichita.

b)   Some individuals are managed on two injections daily (morning and evening). This regimen could include only intermediate-acting insulin, or mixed doses of regular with intermediate-acting insulin. This split-mixed dosage is considered conventional therapy. Usually two-thirds of the total daily dose of insulin is given before breakfast, and one-third is given before the evening meal (see Figure VIII.4).

c)   Some individuals are managed on three injections daily, using any one of a number of protocols. Multiple injections of insulin (three or more) are one component of the system called intensive insulin therapy.

(1)   Administer a combination of rapid- and intermediate-acting insulin before breakfast, a rapid-acting insulin before the evening meal, and an intermediate-acting insulin around 10 PM. This protocol may extend the coverage of biosynthetic human insulins, treat the dawn phenomenon, and also allow for "sleeping in" in some cases (see Figure VIII.5).

FIGURE VIII.4: Time Action of Insulin

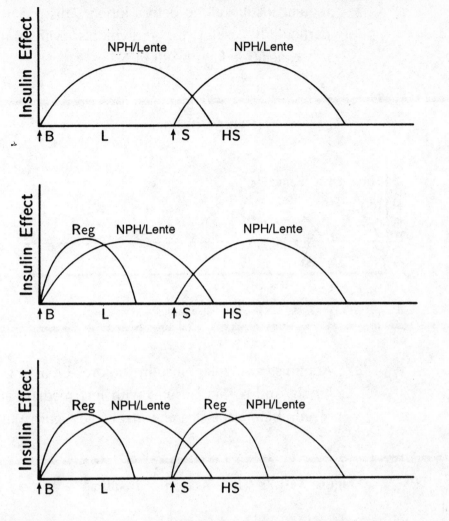

Adapted with permission: University of Kansas School of Medicine at Wichita.

FIGURE VIII.5: Time Action of Insulin

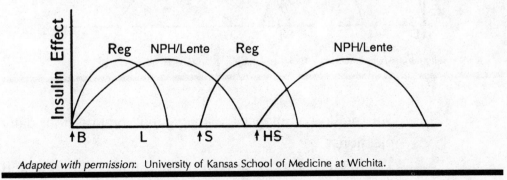

Adapted with permission: University of Kansas School of Medicine at Wichita.

(2) Administer Ultralente insulin combined with regular insulin before breakfast and the evening meal, and regular insulin alone before lunch. This protocol is particularly useful for individuals with unusual schedules (see Figure VIII.6).

FIGURE VIII.6

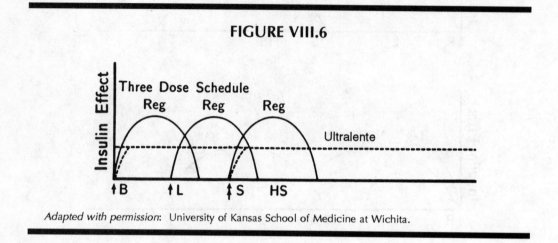

Adapted with permission: University of Kansas School of Medicine at Wichita.

(3) Administer regular insulin before breakfast and lunch, and regular insulin with intermediate-acting insulin before the evening meal (see Figure VIII.7).

Figure VIII.7: Time Action of Insulin

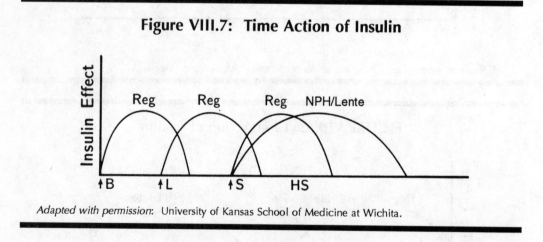

Adapted with permission: University of Kansas School of Medicine at Wichita.

d) One method of intensive management includes four daily injections.

(1) Regular insulin is given before breakfast, lunch, and dinner, and an intermediate- or long-acting insulin

(NPH, Lente, or Ultralente) at bedtime (see Figure VIII.8).

FIGURE VIII.8: Time Action of Insulin

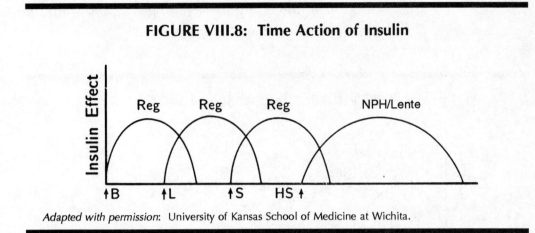

Adapted with permission: University of Kansas School of Medicine at Wichita.

(2) Some patients on this regimen may require the addition of an intermediate-acting insulin with the morning regular insulin. The rapid-acting doses of regular insulin provide for post-meal needs, while the intermediate- or long-acting dose insures a low, steady rate of insulin throughout the day (see Figure VIII.9).

FIGURE VIII.9: Time Action of Insulin

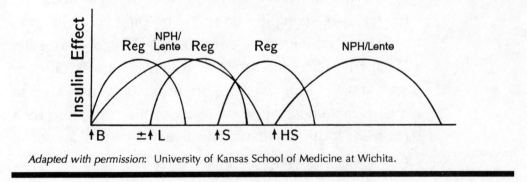

Adapted with permission: University of Kansas School of Medicine at Wichita.

(3) Four injections of regular insulin given about 6 hours apart may be indicated for some patients. Imminent ketoacidosis or illness may mandate using regular

insulin. Formulas for calculating dosages vary, but about 33% of the total daily dose is given before breakfast, a slightly smaller amount at lunchtime, about 30% preceding the evening meal, and about 15% at midnight (see Figure VIII.10).

FIGURE VIII.10: Time Action of Insulin

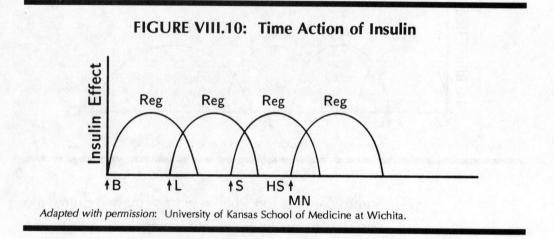

Adapted with permission: University of Kansas School of Medicine at Wichita.

e) With infusion pump therapy, a continuous, basal amount of insulin (0.5 to 1.0 units per hour) usually is administered, in addition to bolus doses given before meals.

f) Some patients with NIDDM may be treated with a combination of oral hypoglycemic agents and insulin. Those patients who do not respond to therapy with oral agents alone may be treated with a small dose of intermediate-acting insulin in the evening, in addition to their usual oral agent (referred to as BIDS-Bedtime Insulin Daytime Sulfonylureas). Conversely, patients already treated with insulin who are not responding may have an intermediate dose of an oral sulfonylurea added to their regimen.[13] The long-term effectiveness of this approach remains to be proven (see Figure VIII.11).

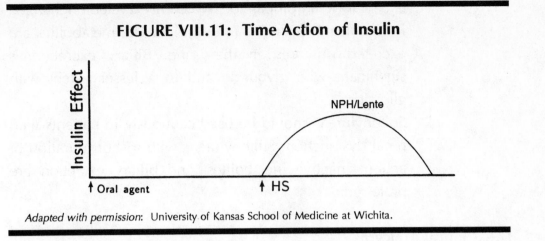

FIGURE VIII.11: Time Action of Insulin

Adapted with permission: University of Kansas School of Medicine at Wichita.

F. Oral Hypoglycemic Agents

1. Oral hypoglycemic agents are believed to have a number of actions on the body.

   a) The mechanisms of action for oral hypoglycemic agents (sulfonylureas) have been well studied. The mechanisms are complex and involve a number of effects on different organ systems, including an increased release of insulin from the pancreas.

   b) An enhanced performance of and increased numbers of insulin receptors on muscle and fat cells also contribute to the hypoglycemic action, as does accelerated glucose transport into cells at the post-insulin receptor site.

   c) Hepatic glucose production is reduced by these products. Oral hypoglycemic agents probably work through a combination of all of the described effects.

2. Hypoglycemic agents can be classified as first- and second-generation agents as shown in Table VIII.7. The first-generation agents are further divided into rapid-, intermediate-, and long-acting products because of the half-life differences.

   a) Absorption generally is quite rapid and fairly complete for the oral agents.

   b) The method and path the body uses to metabolize and eliminate these agents varies greatly. Most oral agents are metabolized in the liver to active or inactive metabolites, except for chlorpropamide, which is excreted unchanged in significant quantities in the urine. The metabolites are excreted primarily in the urine. Biliary excretion is significant with glyburide and to a lesser extent with glipizide.[14]

c) Sulfonylureas should be used cautiously in patients with renal dysfunction. Sulfonylureas with a short duration of action, inactive metabolites, and biliary excretion are preferred.

G. Clinical Concerns

1. Side effects associated with oral hypoglycemic agents vary.

   a) Hypoglycemia is the most serious complication of sulfonylurea therapy. An age-related decline in renal function can contribute to susceptibility to hypoglycemia in the elderly.[15]

   b) Skin rashes occur in about 2% of all patients.

   c) Gastrointestinal disturbances occur in approximately 5% of cases.

   d) Metabolic disorders such as a renal syndrome of inappropriate antidiuretic hormone (SIADH) can occur with the use of oral hypoglycemic agents.

   (1) SIADH (vasopressin), manifested by hyponatremia and water retention, occurs in 4% of people who receive chlorpropamide.

   e) When used with alcohol, chlorpropamide may induce disulfiram-like effects (eg, flushing) in about 35% of patients. This reaction rarely has been reported with the second-generation sulfonylureas. Additionally, alcohol in combination with sulfonylureas may cause severe hypoglycemia, particularly if the patient does not consume food with the alcohol.

   f) Hepatic changes are rare, but may be seen with chlorpropamide use.

   g) Hematologic changes are rare.

2. Treatment failures occur when the pancreas is insensitive to the effects of oral hypoglycemic agents.

   a) Primary failure of the oral agents is found in individuals who show no response to oral agents from the start of therapy. This type of treatment failure occurs in 20% of patients.

   b) Secondary failure of the oral agents occurs in individuals whose diabetes initially responded to a given agent but now is refractory to that drug. These patients are candidates for insulin.

3. The dosage of these preparations is listed on the product chart (see Table VIII.7). Note the variations in the relative weight potency between first- and second-generation agents, although their maximum hypoglycemic effect is quite similar.

4. Some medications can either increase or decrease blood glucose levels by themselves, or interact with sulfonylureas to enhance or decrease the effect of the sulfonylureas (see Tables VIII.4 and VIII.5). Protein-binding displacement can occur when hypoglycemic agents are used in conjunction with drugs such as phenylbutazone, warfarin, etc. Interactions with glyburide and glipizide appear to be substantially decreased because these drugs are bound to protein by a nonanionic-type bond. The first-generation drugs can be easily displaced from protein binding, which would enhance the effect of the sulfonylureas and result in hypoglycemia for the patient.[16] Additionally, sulfonylureas may be affected by medications that alter the hepatic metabolism or the renal excretion of these agents.

5. Oral agents are used individually, with initial product choice determined as previously noted. The agent of choice is given at a low dose, with gradual increases to obtain the desired control. Chlorpropamide should be used with caution in the elderly because of its potential for accumulation. Chlorpropamide and acetohexamide may accumulate in pa-

TABLE VIII.7:
Oral Hypoglycemic Agents

Drug	First Generation				Second Generation	
	Tolbutamide (Orinase)	Acetohexamide (Dymelor)	Tolazamide (Tolinase)	Chlorpropamide (Diabinese)	Glyburide (DiaBeta, Micronase, *Glynase Prestabs)	Glipizide (Glucotrol)
Recommended Dose	0.5 to 3.0 g divided doses	0.25 to 1.5 g single or divided doses	0.1 to 1.0 g single or divided doses	0.1 to 0.5 g single dose	1.25 – 10 mg single or divided dose *0.75-1.2 mg	2.5-20 mg single or divided dose
Maximum Dose	2 to 3 g	1.5 g	0.75 to 1.0 g	0.5 g	20 mg *12 mg	40 mg
Half-life (h)	5.6	5	7	35	Biphasic 3.2+10 hrs	3.5 to 6
Onset (h)	1	1	4 to 6	1	1.5	1
Duration (h)	6 to 12	10 to 14	10 to 14	72	24	12 to 16
Metabolism & Excretion	Totally metabolized to inactive form; inactive metabolite excreted in kidney.	Metabolite's activity equal to or greater than parent compound; metabolite is excreted via kidney.	Absorbed slowly; metabolite active but less potent than parent compound; excreted via kidney.	Previously thought not to be metabolized, but recently found that metabolism may be quite extensive; significant percentage excreted unchanged.	24% absorbed; completely metabolized in liver to nonactive derivatives; excreted in urine & bile 1:1	Metabolized in liver to inactive metabolites; excreted primarily in urine.
Comments	Most benign; least potent; short half-life; especially useful in kidney disease.	Essentially no advantage over tolbutamide, although a few patients who fail on tolbutamide are controlled.	Essentially no advantage over tolbutamide; said to be equipotent with less severe side effects.	Longest duration; caution in elderly patients and those with kidney disease; disulfiram-like reactions may occur with alcohol; hyponatremia may be a problem.	50 to 200 times more potent than other agents no disulfiram-like reaction; low toxicity; caution in elderly.	Needs to be taken on an empty stomach; low toxicity; no disulfiram-like reaction; caution in elderly.

Source: Adapted from Campbell RK. How oral agents are used in the treatment of type II diabetes. Pharm Times 1987;53(10):32-40.

tients with renal dysfunction and should be avoided in these cases.

a)   The second-generation agents usually are the medications of choice. These drugs interact less frequently with other agents, have fewer significant side effects, and have alternate routes of excretion.

b)   Glyburide has the advantage that it can be taken on either an empty stomach or with food.

c)   A single daily dose may be the initial approach for treatment. Dosage adjustments for patients with hepatic or renal dysfunction may be required.

H.   Glucagon

1.   Commercial preparations of glucagon are available and are useful for treating patients who develop a severe hypoglycemic reaction requiring assistance from another person, or for patients who lose consciousness.

a)   Glucagon stimulates hepatic glucose release.

b)   This product is used for severe insulin reactions in situations in which patients are unconscious or uncooperative, and cannot take oral fluids.

c)   If hospitalized patients develop hypoglycemia and are unconscious, and an intravenous line is not running, glucagon is the initial treatment of choice until intravenous access can be obtained.

d)   Glucagon use is effective if adequate hepatic glycogen (stored glucose) is available and may not be beneficial for patients with inadequate glycogen stores (eg, patients with alcoholic hepatic disease).

2.   The dosage can vary depending on the patient's age and clinical condition, and is given by subcutaneous or intramuscular injection.

a)   Adults and children over 5 or 6 years of age usually should receive 1.0 mg.

        b)   Children under 5 years of age should receive 0.5 mg.

        c)   Infants probably should be given 0.25 mg.

3.   For the glucagon emergency kit, the dose is mixed by adding the diluent from the prefilled syringe in the emergency kit to the vial's contents, and refilling the syringe with the reconstituted glucagon. For the two-bottle package of glucagon, the dose is mixed by filling a 1 cc syringe with the diluent in bottle number one, adding the diluent to the contents of bottle number two, and refilling the syringe with the reconstituted glucagon.

4.   Both the glucagon emergency kit and the two-bottle glucagon package can be stored at a room temperature of 59° to 86° F (15° to 30° C) prior to reconstitution.

5.   Each dose requires 15 to 20 minutes for full onset of action.

6.   Patients should be protected from self-injury or aspiration if hypoglycemic seizures occur. A common side effect of glucagon is nausea, and possibly vomiting, as the patient returns to consciousness. (Turn the patient on the side to prevent aspiration.)

7.   Liquids containing glucose should be given when the patient becomes conscious to prevent hypoglycemia from returning. A snack containing carbohydrate and protein should follow when nausea subsides. An additional snack may need to be repeated because glycogen reserves may take 8 to 12 hours to be replenished.

REFERENCES

1. Product information and recommendations. Indianapolis: Eli Lilly & Co, 1987.

2. Product information and recommendations. Princeton, NJ: Novo Nordisk Pharmaceuticals, 1993.

3. Anderson JH, Campbell RK. Mixing insulins in 1990. Diabetes Educ 1990;16:380-87.

4. White JR, Campbell RK. Guide to mixing insulins. Hosp Pharm 1991;26:1046-48.

5. American Diabetes Association. Position statement: insulin administration. Diabetes Care 1993;16(2) suppl:31-34.

6. Koivisto VA, Felig P. Alterations in insulin absorption and in blood glucose control associated with varying insulin injection sites in diabetic patients. Ann Intern Med 1980;92:59-61.

7. White J, Campbell RK. Pharmacologic therapies in the management of diabetes mellitus. In: Haire-Joshu D, ed. Management of diabetes mellitus. St. Louis: Mosby Year Book, 1992:132.

8. Linde B. Dissociation of insulin absorption and blood flow during massage of a subcutaneous injection site. Diabetes Care 1986;9:570-74.

9. Bolognia JL, Braverman IM. Skin and subcutaneous tissues. In: Lebovitz HE, ed. Therapy for diabetes mellitus and related disorders. Alexandria, Va: American Diabetes Association, 1991:215.

10. White J, Hartman J, Campbell RK. Drug interactions in diabetic patients. Postgrad Med 1993;93:131-39.

11.   Hirsch IB, Farkas-Hirsch R, Skyler JS. Intensive insulin therapy for treatment of type I diabetes. Diabetes Care 1990;13:1265-83.

12.   Insulin treatment. In: Sperling MA, ed. Physician's guide to insulin-dependent (type I) diabetes. Alexandria, Va: American Diabetes Association, 1988:33.

13.   Lebovitz HE. Combination therapy for hyperglycemia. In: Lebovitz HE, ed. Therapy for diabetes mellitus and related disorders. Alexandria, Va: American Diabetes Association, 1991:146.

14.   Lebovitz HE. Sulfonylurea drugs. In: Lebovitz HE, ed. Therapy for diabetes mellitus and related disorders. Alexandria, Va: American Diabetes Association, 1991:114.

15.   Halter JB. Geriatric patients. In: Lebovitz HE, ed. Therapy for diabetes mellitus and related disorders. Alexandria, Va: American Diabetes Association, 1991:159.

16.   Jackson JD, Bressler R. Pharmacology of sulfonylurea hypoglycemic agents. Clin Drugs 1981;22:221-45, 295-320.

KEY EDUCATIONAL CONSIDERATIONS
FOR INSULIN

1. Based on the principles of adult learning, patients should inject themselves first with insulin or saline in order to allay their anxiety. After giving the first injection, the patients then may be ready to learn how to fill the syringe. The educational assessment would help the educator determine the patient's readiness.

2. Educators should see a demonstration of a patient's injection technique, assess injection sites, and review timing of injections at every opportunity. The technique for mixing insulins also should be reviewed because many patients are never taught how to mix insulins. Literature and illustrative diagrams are especially helpful to reinforce the skill.

3. Keep expired glucagon and glucagon emergency kits available for demonstrations. Many family members hesitate to use glucagon when necessary because of their inexperience. Anyone instructed in glucagon administration should also be observed giving an injection.

4. Patients with NIDDM (type II diabetes) commonly harbor fearful misconceptions about insulin therapy. The educator must skillfully position insulin as another treatment method and focus on short-term benefits. Refrain from using insulin as a threat.

5. Patients who require U-500 insulin need specific written instructions for dosage because there is no U-500 syringe. One method is to prescribe the insulin in cc's rather than units.

6. Educators should emphasize the individualized nature of an insulin regimen and that the patient and health care professionals can work together to fine-tune the regimen. It is helpful to reinforce the idea that it may take several days to experience the full effect of a new regimen, and even longer to fine-tune it.

KEY EDUCATIONAL CONSIDERATIONS
FOR SULFONYLUREA USE

1. Educators should reinforce that oral agents are not a substitute for diet and exercise.

2. Many patients assume that sulfonylureas are "oral insulin" and become confused by what they hear about insulin.

3. It is common for patients who take sulfonylureas to state that they have a "touch of sugar" or "mild diabetes." This information is part of the educational assessment and can direct the educator to include content relevant to the patient's perception of diabetes.

4. Many patients with NIDDM (type II diabetes) who take oral agents are unaware that they are vulnerable to hypoglycemia. Many patients will skip meals in an effort to lose weight and may become symptomatic of hypoglycemia.

5. The potential problems of using alcohol with sulfonylureas should be reinforced periodically. Many people consume alcohol on social occasions only and may not remember the potential interaction.

6. Teaching patients to inform all health care providers about any changes in their medication regimen protects against the potential for drug interactions when new medications are combined with sulfonylureas.

SELF-REVIEW QUESTIONS

If you are unsure of the answers to the following questions, please review the materials.

1. Describe the effects of insulin on fat, protein, and glucose utilization.
2. List four categories of patients who are candidates for insulin therapy.

3. List the six product types and sources of insulin.
4. How is the purity of insulin expressed?
5. What concentrations of insulin are available and which concentration is most commonly used in the United States?
6. State the guidelines for insulin storage.
7. List three factors that can alter the absorption of insulin.
8. Name three complications of insulin therapy.
9. Compare and contrast the first- and second-generation oral hypoglycemic agents regarding side effects and potential drug interactions.
10. Which long-acting oral hypoglycemic agent commonly interacts with alcohol to produce a flushing reaction?
11. List three medications that may interact with oral hypoglycemic agents and induce an increased blood glucose level.
12. List the indications for use of glucagon.

CASE EXAMPLE 1

WJ, age 38 years, was diagnosed with IDDM at age 24 years. She recently moved to a different state and was referred by her new physician for continued diabetes education. WJ's usual dose of human insulin was NPH 24 units, regular 2 units after breakfast, and NPH 8 units, regular 3 units before supper. The physician reviewed the proper timing of the injection with WJ, plus the action and duration of the insulins.

WJ had been monitoring using a newer model meter and she demonstrated accurate technique. She presents with carefully recorded blood glucose results that demonstrate fluctuations in the readings with no obvious patterns. She began taking her injections one-half hour before meals, but she is anxious regarding her visit with the diabetes educator because she is not familiar with the concept of team management.

QUESTIONS

1. What issues relating to insulin would be part of your initial assessment?

SUGGESTED SOLUTIONS

You may begin with a brief explanation that diabetes is best managed with the skills of many experts, and that WJ is the central and most important expert. One particular focus of the diabetes educator is the practical aspects of daily insulin management, including insulin administration, storage, site rotation, and syringe disposal.

When WJ demonstrated her technique for mixing insulins, she contaminated the NPH insulin with regular insulin. She used one bottle of NPH insulin per month and one bottle of regular insulin every 6 months. She would store these and all 6 to 8 bottles of insulin that she received from her prescription plan at room temperature.

WJ was open to learning an accurate method for mixing insulins, and she decided to store all her unopened bottles of insulin in the refrigerator. WJ wanted the freedom of carrying her insulin with her during the day without worrying about refrigeration. The diabetes educator offered the following choices to WJ.

1. Prefill the evening dose of insulin and carry the syringe in a specially designed prefilled syringe case.
2. Keep the open bottles of NPH and regular insulin at room temperature. Date the bottle of regular insulin and discard it after 30 days.
3. Purchase a small, discreet carrying case for insulin that is designed to keep the insulin cold.

WJ didn't know about the guidelines for prefilling syringes and chose option number one.

When reviewing the areas used for injection, WJ described one favorite spot that she used for all injections. Because there was some early evidence of hypertrophy, WJ decided to try other areas of injection. The diabetes educator reviewed the syringe disposal guidelines of their state.

WJ was pleased with the specific feedback about her daily routine and made an appointment with the dietitian.

CASE EXAMPLE 2

AH is a 57-year-old white male referred to the diabetes clinic for evaluation of glycemic control. He was diagnosed with non-insulin-dependent diabetes mellitus (NIDDM) about 15 months ago. He is obese and, despite numerous attempts with diet control, fails to have satisfactory weight reduction. His fasting blood glucose concentrations have risen lately, ranging from 170 to 185 mg/dL (9.4-10.3 mmol/L) over the last few weeks. He complains of weakness, fatigue, increased urination, and increased thirst.

His past medical history includes hypertension for 10 years treated with hydrochlorothiazide (HCTZ) 50 mg qd, KCl 40 mEq qd, and propranolol 40 mg qd. His family history includes hypertension and NIDDM. He continues to smoke one-half to one pack of cigarettes per day and has a 40 pack year history of smoking. He consumes three to four beers with his evening meal.

At 5'8" (170 cm), AH weighs 198 pounds (90 kg) and has gained 6.5 pounds (3 kg) since his last visit. His blood pressure is 154/94 (previous readings range from 150/92 to 160/96), with normal pulse and respirations.

QUESTIONS

1. How do the antihypertensive agents impact on his blood glucose level?
2. Should the patient be started on a regimen of oral hypoglycemic agents?
3. Which oral hypoglycemic agent might be appropriate for this patient?
4. What nonpharmacologic alternatives should the patient and health care team discuss?

SUGGESTED SOLUTIONS

It would be appropriate to begin by substituting new drugs in the patient's regimen for those that worsen glucose tolerance (HCTZ, propranolol). This patient's hypertension might be better treated with an ACE-inhibitor or a calcium-channel blocker. If the HCTZ is discontinued, the potassium supplement probably should be discontinued as well. The effects of HCTZ and propranolol on glucose tolerance may resolve after several weeks. In the interim, the patient's hyperglycemia should be treated with oral agents or low-dose insulin, since the patient is symptomatic. In choosing sulfonylureas for this patient, chlorpropamide would be ruled out immediately because the patient consumes alcohol. One would need to check for previous drug allergies and also evaluate the patient's renal function. If the patient's renal function is good, any of the oral agents could be used. The choice of the best agent in this case could be based on cost and the patient's level of adherence. Most patients are more adherent when their regimens are simple, hence a once-a-day agent such as glyburide or glipizide might be more effective. One should be aware that as the effects of the propranolol and HCTZ decrease, the patient's need for the sulfonylurea may diminish or even disappear.

Nonpharmacologic issues of importance to this patient's blood glucose and blood pressure control include weight loss, exercise guidelines, smoking cessation, and the effect of alcohol on lipids and blood glucose and as a source of non-nutritive calories. AH also would benefit from self-monitoring of his blood glucose to learn about both the impact of the oral agents and lifestyle changes on his blood glucose.

OTHER SUGGESTED READINGS

Ahrens ER, Gossain UU, Rovner DR. Human insulin: its development and use. Postgrad Med 1986;80:181-87.

Bailey TS, Mezitis NHE. Combination therapy with insulin and sulfonylureas for type II diabetes. Diabetes Care 1990;13(6):687-95.

Brogden RN, Hell RC. Human insulin: a review of its biological activity, pharmacokinetics, and therapeutic use. Drugs 1987;34:350-71.

Campbell RK. How oral agents are used in the therapy of type II diabetes. Pharm Times 1987;53(10):32-40.

Genuth S. Insulin use in NIDDM. Diabetes Care 1990;13(12):1240-64.

Hirsch IB, Farkas-Hirsch R, Skyler JS. Intensive insulin therapy for treatment of type I diabetes. Diabetes Care 1990;13(12):1265-83.

Hollander P. Pre-mixed insulins. Postgrad Med 1991;89(4):52-64.

Krosnick A. Newer insulin, insulin allergies, and the clinical use of insulins. In: Bergman M, ed. Principles of diabetes management. New Hyde Park, NY: Medical Examination Publishing Co, 1987:123-35.

Ferner RE. Oral hypoglycemic agents. Med Clin North Am 1988;72(6):1323-35.

Gerich J. Oral hypoglycemic agents. N Engl J Med 1989;321(18):1231-45.

Lebovitz HE. Second generation sulfonylureas: what are they and what is their value? Clin Diabetes 1984;2(4):84-85.

Lebovitz HE, ed. Physician's guide to type II diabetes: diagnosis and treatment. 2nd ed. Alexandria, Va: American Diabetes Association, 1988.

Peragallo-Dittko V. Buyers' guide to injection devices. Diabetes Self-Manage 1990;Jan/Feb:6-12.

Peragallo-Dittko V. Straight shooting: a critical look at injection technique. Diabetes Self-Manage, 1992; May/June:8-10.

Peterson CM. Diabetes management in the 1980s. New York: Prager Publishers, 1982.

Schade D, Santiago J, Skyler J, Rizza R. Intensive insulin therapy. Geneva: Excerpta Medica, 1983.

Skyler JS, Skyler DL, Seigler DE, O'Sullivan MJ. Algorithms for adjustment of insulin dosage by patients who monitor blood glucose. Diabetes Care 1981;4:311-18.

Skyler JS. Insulin dependent diabetes mellitus. Postgrad Med 1987;81(6):163-74.

Skyler JS. Strategies in diabetes mellitus. Postgrad Med 1991;89(6):45-63.

Sotsky M, Shamoon H. Human insulin: a second revolution? Clin Diabetes 1986;4(2):25, 27, 28, 33, 46.

Waldhausl WK. The physiological basis of insulin treatment-clinical aspects. Diabetologia 1986;29:837-49.

White J, Campbell RK. Guide to mixing insulins. Hosp Pharm 1991;26:1046-48.

THERAPIES

IX. MONITORING AND MANAGEMENT

INTRODUCTION

The technology explosion has changed the lives of people with diabetes. The advent of the small, portable glucose meter in the early 1980s may be the single greatest breakthrough for self-care in decades.[1] The ability to do precise self-testing at home, work, or school allows the person with diabetes independence, security, and immediate feedback.

Self-monitoring by the person with diabetes is an essential component of the monitoring and management process. With careful technique, capillary blood glucose monitoring can offer a significant contribution to the management of diabetes.

Monitoring provides both patients and members of the health care team with information needed to continually adjust the therapeutic regimen. Research indicates that monitoring is a major adjunct in achieving euglycemia, thus preventing hypoglycemia and hyperglycemia and reducing the long-term complications of diabetes.[2-4] This chapter will address the rationale for and methods of various monitoring techniques.

OBJECTIVES

Upon completion of this chapter, the learner will be able to:
- identify situations in which self-monitoring of blood glucose (SMBG) is indicated;
- list the advantages and disadvantages of SMBG;
- describe quality assurance concerns for glucose monitoring;
- list indications for urine testing for glucose, ketones, and protein;
- identify various long-term glucose monitoring methods;
- list advantages and disadvantages of pattern management and sliding scale management.

A. Self-Monitoring of Blood Glucose (SMBG)

1. SMBG is a critical element in the management of diabetes. It is recommended for all people with insulin-requiring diabetes[5]. Most endocrinologists recommend blood glucose monitoring for

all patients, with the only distinction being the suggested frequency of testing.

2. Many situations affect blood glucose levels, reinforcing the need for accurate monitoring.[6-10]

    a) In cases of insulin-dependent diabetes mellitus (IDDM), also called type I diabetes, minimizing fluctuations of blood glucose can be difficult. Insulin is provided primarily from exogenous sources. Accurate blood glucose values are required to adjust insulin dosage, caloric intake, and levels of physical activity.

    b) With non-insulin-dependent diabetes mellitus (NIDDM), also called type II diabetes, blood glucose monitoring is essential for adjusting dosages of insulin or oral hypoglycemic agents, adjusting the overall meal plan, understanding the effect of food choices on glycemic control, and recognizing the effect of activity and exercise on glycemic control.

    c) The blood glucose results can be used to learn more about meal planning, meal composition, glycemic response of certain food products, etc. People with IDDM and NIDDM may have individual and varying responses to certain foods. Food combinations may have a different glycemic effect than individual food items. Blood glucose testing provides valuable information about these individual variations.

    d) Stressors in the patient's life can trigger the release of stress hormones that tend to aggravate glycemic responses. Accurate blood glucose monitoring and record keeping can help the individual with diabetes identify stressors and respond accordingly.

    e) Physical activity can affect blood glucose levels. Exercise increases the sensitivity of the body to insulin and increases glucose utilization. The continued lowering of blood glucose may extend for several hours after the physical activity. Blood glucose monitoring provides the information needed to adjust insulin dosages and/or food intake to the level of physical activity. Testing blood glucose before and after exercise permits precise caloric replacement based on glucose levels.

f)   Hypoglycemia can be diagnosed and treated appropriately with values obtained from SMBG. SMBG allows for follow-up assessment to determine whether the person is responding promptly to the hypoglycemic treatment.

g)   Beta-blocking medication may mask adrenergic hypoglycemic responses, thus eliminating easily identifiable symptoms associated with changes in blood glucose values. The information obtained through SMBG is critical for maintaining the patient's ability to safely engage in the tasks of daily living.

h)   Illness can cause the level of glucose in the blood to change rapidly. Gluconeogenesis, stress (physical and emotional), lack of exercise, and erratic eating all contribute to physiologic alterations that cause hyperglycemia and often ketosis. Careful and frequent blood glucose evaluations enable prompt adjustment of insulin and caloric intake so that hospitalization can be prevented. Testing every 4 to 6 hours for glucose and ketones will provide valuable information to assist the patient and health care team in calculating an accurate supplemental dose of regular insulin.

i)   Travel may involve crossing time zones and dealing with irregular meal times. During these times, glucose monitoring is critical to maintaining glycemic control. Converting treatment to multiple injections of regular insulin may increase flexibility and glycemic control during travel.

j)   Patients who use an insulin infusion pump (Continuous Subcutaneous Insulin Infusion, or CSII) need the results of blood glucose monitoring to adjust basal and bolus insulin dosages. Testing six or more times per day is common.

k)   Pregnancy requires an intense monitoring schedule of four to six times per day. Blood glucose monitoring to facilitate normoglycemia should begin prior to conception and continue during pregnancy. Elevated blood glucose levels can adversely affect fetal outcome. Urine glucose monitoring is contraindicated due to lowered renal threshold during pregnancy.

l) Surgery is a time of increased stress, decreased exercise, altered caloric intake, and unpredictable pathological situations, all of which can contribute to erratic glucose excursions. Blood glucose values are necessary for titrating insulin infusions or subcutaneous injections, as well as intravenous dextrose infusions.

B. Advantages and Disadvantages of Blood Glucose Monitoring

1. Advantages of SMBG include accurate, immediate results which are especially useful in diagnosing hypoglycemia and hyperglycemia; follow-up information after self-management changes are implemented to enhance accurate regimen adjustment; and enhanced patient independence and confidence.[5]

2. Disadvantages of SMBG include cost of reagents and disposable supplies, especially if insurance reimbursement is not available; discomfort encountered when lancing the finger to obtain blood; complexity of some testing procedures, especially for people with diminished mental acuity and dexterity; potential malfunction of equipment that could contribute to a sense of insecurity with the process or to inaccurate decisions affecting treatment; unreliable results with certain meters, especially for people with very high or very low hematocrit values; and false results due to inaccurate technique that may affect treatment decisions.

C. Selection of Blood Glucose Meters

1. The choice of a meter for glucose testing may be influenced by the individual features of the instruments. In general, the meters

are small, portable devices that are less technique-dependent than earlier models.

2.   The patient's ability to accurately perform the procedure is one of the most important factors in determining which meter is appropriate.

3.   The following other factors should be considered when selecting a blood glucose meter: hematocrit range for patients with high or low hematocrits (eg, renal patients, pregnancy, anemia), because certain meters may yield unreliable results; complexity of operating the meter, because manual dexterity may be an issue for some patients; financial considerations; lifestyle considerations (eg, meter beeps, portability, temperature control, memory capability); and the patient's ability to secure an adequate sample size matched to the reagent's requirements.

D.   Accuracy and Precision of Blood Glucose Monitoring

1.   Several factors may affect test results. Obtaining a large, hanging drop of blood to assure adequate coverage of the test strip is essential. It is critical to get adequate blood cover for each reagent strip. Getting sufficient blood may require extra help. The following suggestions may be useful.

   a)   Wash hands in warm soapy water.

   b)   Shake the hand to be pricked as if you were shaking down a thermometer.

   c)   Briefly tourniquet the finger to be pricked using a firm grasp by the fingers of the other hand.

   d)   Prick the side of the finger with firm pressure.

   e)   Squeeze the finger gently while holding the hand down below the waist.

   f)   Use an end cap that will allow a deeper puncture.

2. Precise timing is essential for accurate glucose determination in monitors that require the user to initiate a timing component. Some meters automatically initiate the timing process.

3. A clean optic window allows the meter to accurately convert from color to numerical results. Certain meters require cleaning, and the manufacturer's recommendations must be followed carefully. Care must be taken not to scratch the glass covering of the optic window.

4. Temperature stability of the meter and reagents will enhance accuracy. Conversely, meters and reagents exposed to high temperatures, usually above 86° F (30° C), may give false readings and will shorten reagent stability from the stated expiration date. Performing a control test on newly opened strips is important to assure strip viability.

5. Manufacturers provide the hematocrit range that yields the most accurate results. Some products correct for hematocrit.

E. **Other Considerations**

1. Blood glucose meters register a wide enough range of values to allow diagnosing hypoglycemia and hyperglycemia in the home and hospital setting. Although these meters should not be used to diagnose diabetes without laboratory confirmation, they are very useful in preliminary testing.

2. Computer analysis of data aids the clinical team or sophisticated patient in making management changes. The computer's ability to convert multiple readings to averages and display them as bar graphs or data plotting helps make the adjustment decisions more objective.

3. Visual blood glucose testing can be done with fairly good accuracy if patients are not color-blind. The patient's confidence in the results can be increased by practicing visual

testing with meter verification of results. When it is inconvenient or impossible to use a meter to determine glucose results, visual testing is a valuable alternative. Some people become very adept at fine color discrimination and do quite well with visual blood glucose monitoring.

4.   Individuals who are visually impaired may benefit from special meters or adaptors with audio cues (see Chapter XX: Adaptive Diabetes Education for Visually Impaired Persons).

F.   Quality Assurance in Blood Glucose Monitoring

1.   Quality assurance is a mandatory concern that must be addressed by health professionals today.[11,12]

a)   The Joint Commission for the Accreditation of Health Care Organizations (JCAHO) and the Health Care Financing Administration (HCFA) require hospitals to have quality assurance programs for bedside blood glucose monitoring.

b)   Proficiency testing, use of control solutions, staff training, and correlational studies comparing bedside results with hospital laboratory values are an essential part of the quality assurance process.

c)   The Clinical Laboratory Improvement Act of 1988 (CLIA '88) placed additional restrictions on blood glucose monitoring done outside of the hospital setting.[13] Blood glucose meters must have verified accuracy, and the physician's office must complete additional paperwork and submit fees for a waivered test, which provides exemption from all of the requirements.

d)   Although meters have internal factory calibration, the user must program each lot number of reagents into the meter. Control solutions are used to verify strip viability, technique accuracy, and meter functioning. Each manufacturer makes available control solutions specific to their meters. Manufacturer recommendations must be followed for greatest accuracy.

e) Blood-transmitted diseases are of concern to educators involved with blood glucose monitoring. Policies from the American Association of Diabetes Educators,[14] the Centers for Disease Control, and the American Hospital Association currently recommend universal precautions for the procedure. It is imperative that disposable lancets, platforms, and gloves be used and changed for each patient in an institutional setting.

f) Some lancing devices have a feature that ejects the used lancet and reduces the chance of accidental puncture by contaminated lancets. Various disposable lancing devices accomplish the same goal. Lancets should be disposed of in appropriate sharps containers.

G. Urine Testing

1. Urine glucose testing was the original method of monitoring diabetes control. Tasting the sweet urine of the person with diabetes predates any other testing procedure. However, urine testing no longer is the preferred method for testing glucose values. Urine testing still is used to monitor for ketone and protein excretion.

2. The results of any urine glucose testing should be reported in percent values and not plus (+) values for continuity of results from one method to another. Urine glucose results also may be obtained with the copper reduction method.

   a) Urine testing for glucose offers several advantages: it is less expensive than blood glucose monitoring, and it is noninvasive.[15]

   b) Urine testing for glucose has several distinct disadvantages: an elevated renal threshold (>180 mg/dL [10 mmol/L]) will give false negative results; false results (positive or negative) may occur with ingestion of certain medications (eg, cephalosporin, large amounts of acetylsalicylic or ascorbic acid); urine testing can be awkward to do when away from home; and urine testing may give a delayed picture of what is happening in the blood.

3. Testing urine for acetone (ketones) is a way to determine impending acidosis.[15] Three ketone bodies are formed from the conversion of free fatty acids in the liver: acetone, acetoacetic acid, and betahydroxybutyric acid.

   a) Acetone can be evaluated by placing a drop of urine, blood, or serum on a tablet (Acetest).

   b) Acetoacetic acid can be measured by use of a urine dipstick.

   c) Urine ketone testing for patients with IDDM should be done when the blood glucose is consistently elevated (>240 mg/dL [>13.3 mmol/L]), during illness,[6] and during pregnancy.

   d) Some clinicians recommend urine ketone testing for people involved in weight loss programs. Ketone is a waste product of fat metabolism. When ketones are present (and blood glucose is normal), the patient can be assured that weight loss is occurring.

4. The presence of proteinuria in the absence of symptoms may be an indication of microvascular changes in the kidneys. Basement membrane thickening and other structural changes of the microvasculature allow abnormal protein leakage.

   a) Dipstick methods for protein screening can be done in the physician's office. Patients frequently are asked for a urine sample for this purpose.

   b) Testing for microalbuminuria, which usually precedes the overt proteinuria identified by conventional dipstick methods, is being done with increasing frequency to detect early renal changes. The presence of microalbuminuria may indicate the need for further testing and management changes.

H. Glycosylated Hemoglobin and Other Tests

1. The measurement of glycosylated hemoglobin in the blood is widely used. This assay gives some correlation with the patient's blood glucose measurements and an average indication of overall glycemic levels over a 3-to 4-month period.[16-18]

2. Glycosylation occurs as glucose in the plasma attaches itself to the hemoglobin component of the red blood cell. This process is irreversible. The more glycosylation, the higher the values. Because the red blood cell has a life span of 120 days, this test reflects the blood glucose concentration over that period of time.

3. HbA_1 is an evaluation of a combination of all fractions of the hemoglobin molecule: HbA_{1a}, HbA_{1b}, and HbA_{1c}. The HbA_1 measurement will have slightly higher normal values than the HbA_{1c} fraction alone. Test procedures and consequent test results vary from laboratory to laboratory. Upper normal values for HbA_1 may be in the range of 8% to 9%. Check the normal values used by the laboratory when advising patients about glycosylated hemoglobin results. As with all monitoring tools, glycosylated hemoglobin results must be interpreted by the health care team and the patient. Tracking the trends in the glycosylated hemoglobin results over time is another useful way to evaluate metabolic control.

4. HbA_{1c} is a measurement of glycosylation of the "c" fraction only. The values are lower because only one fraction is measured. The normal value usually is in the range of 4% to 7%.

5. Glycosylated albumin (fructosamine), a glycosylated serum protein test, reflects blood glucose control over the preceding 7 to 10 days.[18,19] The reliability and clinical applicability of these tests continue to be evaluated.

I. Using the Blood Glucose Monitoring Results

1. Results of blood glucose monitoring in combination with other tests, such as glycosylated hemoglobin or fructosamine, are necessary for data analysis when adjusting insulin or oral agent dosages. Health care professionals must have glucose results that are accurate and data that can be analyzed to determine trends. Patients must have comprehensive education on diabetes, insulin action curves, and blood glucose record interpretation to be competent with insulin adjustment.[20,21]

2. Patterned management of blood glucose is a logical and methodical retrospective assessment of diabetes control that allows consistent problems to be identified and preventive action to be taken.[20-22]

   a) For example, the insulin-treated patient with consistently elevated prelunch blood glucose values would examine the events that contribute to that test result. Some of the major adjustable factors causing the elevated blood glucose level at lunch are breakfast foods, morning snack, morning activity, interval between insulin injection and meal consumption, injection site chosen, evidence of lipodystrophy, dose of regular insulin before breakfast, or the dose of ultralente insulin taken at dinner the previous night. Pattern management suggests that the patient should identify the contributing factors to high prelunch glucose results and try changing one factor, such as the composition of breakfast (eg, substitute whole fruit for juice at breakfast). Increasing morning activity or increasing the prebreakfast dose of regular insulin also would be considerations. Increasing the time interval between injection and breakfast would allow the regular insulin more time to begin working and might impact on prelunch readings.

   b) The benefits of patterned management are: patients learn more about factors that affect blood glucose (eg, food, injection site, activity level, insulin time actions);

consistent problems can be identified and corrected; and fluctuations in blood glucose levels that occur when a number is treated instead of identifying the factors that contributed to that number can be prevented.

  c) The disadvantages of patterned management include: the extra time needed to correct patterns; adjustment difficulties for patients who are used to doing something when their blood glucose is high; and the need for patients to be able to emotionally tolerate a few days of hyperglycemia.

3. According to the sliding scale method of insulin adjustment, when a high blood glucose level occurs, an extra supplement of regular insulin would be given. Many clinicians offer specific details on how much insulin to give depending on how high the blood glucose level is.

  a) The advantages of the sliding scale method are: immediate lowering of blood glucose; and, insulin adjustment to compensate for strenuous exercise, acute illness, working rotating shifts, and traveling to different time zones.

  b) The disadvantages of the sliding scale method are: patients do not learn about factors that affect blood glucose; the problem is chased rather than prevented; may contribute to blood glucose fluctuations; weight gain may occur due to overinsulinization; and, the need to adjust intermediate (basal) insulin dosages may be masked.

4. Patients treated with CSII use a combination of pattern management and sliding scale insulin adjustment. Acute care inpatient issues often are addressed by a modified sliding scale method. Outpatient management may incorporate greater use of patterned management.

5. Consistently low blood glucose levels must be corrected carefully.

  a) One option for patients with consistently low blood glucose readings is to reduce the overall insulin or oral agent dose. Insulin is an anabolic (storage) hormone. Extra calories that are consumed to correct hypoglycemia will contribute to weight gain. Modest reductions in the insulin or oral agent dose can be made in conjunction with careful, frequent blood glucose testing. If blood glucose levels remain low, another dose reduction may be indicated.

b) The patient's caloric intake also must be assessed. If the patient's food record reflects inadequate caloric consumption, then the meal plan may need to be adjusted to meet the patient's needs.

c) Any change in activity or exercise may contribute to consistently low blood glucose levels. Insulin or oral agent doses may need to be adjusted accordingly.

6. Gradually increasing or consistently high blood glucose levels in a well patient may be caused by consuming too much food, reduced or insufficient exercise, insufficient dose of diabetes medication, expired insulin, unrecognized illness, prescription or nonprescription medication, change in injection site, change in daily schedule (weekends), or chronic stress. Identifying the cause of the problem is an important step toward management.

7. Data management is crucial to analyzing any problems. Readings that are stored in the memory of the meter do not replace log books. Some meters with memory can be interfaced with computer systems in the physician's office or diabetes center, thus providing a manageable and time-efficient way to review the data. In addition, a patient's charting records of blood sugar levels can provide a picture of trends, which aids in self-management. Computer-assisted self-care is available in several formats to encourage independence in persons with diabetes.[23]

REFERENCES

1.   Peterson CM, ed. Diabetes management in the 1980s: the role of home blood glucose monitoring and new insulin delivery systems. New York: Praeger Publishers, 1982:184-97.

2.   The Diabetes Control and Complications Trial Research Group. The effect of intensive treatment of diabetes on the development and progression of longterm complications in insulin-dependent diabetes mellitus. New Engl J Med 1993;329(14):977-86.

3.   Carlson A, Rosenqvist U. Diabetes care organization, process, and patient outcomes: effects of a diabetes control program. Diabetes Educ 1991;17:42-48.

4.   Hanssen KF, Dahl-Jorgensen K, Lauritzen T, Feloh-Rasmuessen B, Brinchmann-Hansen O, Deckert T. Diabetic control and microvascular complications: the near-nomoglycemic experience. Diabetologia 1986;29:677-84.

5.   American Diabetes Association. Consensus statement. Self-monitoring of blood glucose. Diabetes Care 1987;10:95-99.

6.   American Diabetes Association. Physician's guide to Insulin Dependent (Type I) Diabetes: diagnosis and treatment. Alexandria, Va: American Diabetes Association, 1988:41-45.

7.   Koivisto VA, Felig P. Effects of leg exercise on insulin absorption in diabetic patients. New Engl J Med 1978;298:79-83.

8.   Koivisto VA. Saung-induced acceleration in insulin absorption from subcutaneous injection site. Br Med J 1980;280:1411-13.

9.   Shade DS, Santiago JV, Skyler JS, Rizza RA. Intensive insulin therapy. Princeton, NJ: Excerpta Medica, 1983:175-93.

10. Nathan DM. Monitoring diabetes mellitus. In: Lebovitz HE, ed. Therapy for diabetes mellitus and related disorders. Alexandria, Va: American Diabetes Association, 1991:86-91.

11. Levine A, Sotomayor G. Bedside glucose monitoring: in compliance with regulatory standards. Diabetes Educ 1991;17:279-83.

12. Walker EA, Paduano DJ, Shamoon H. Quality assurance for blood glucose monitoring in health-care facilities. Diabetes Care 1991;14:1043-49.

13. American Diabetes Association. CLIA guidelines implemented. Diabetes Rev 1993:1:130.

14. American Association of Diabetes Educators. Infection control guidelines for patient education as a means of preventing blood-borne disease transmission during diabetes self-care procedures. Diabetes Educ 1991;17:259.

15. Guthrie D, Guthrie R, Hinnen D. Urine tests: still useful after all these years. Diabetes Forecast 1985;38(2):43-45.

16. Garlick RL, Mazer JS, Higgins PJ, Bunn HF. Characterization of glycosylated hemoglobin. J Clin Invest 1983;71:1062-72.

17. Singer DE, Conley CM, Samet JH, Nathan DM. Tests of glycemia in diabetes mellitus. Ann Intern Med 1989;29:677-84.

18. Gebhart SSP, Wheaton RN, Mullins RE, Austin GE. A comparison of home glucose monitoring with determinations of hemoglobin A_{1C}, total glycated hemoglobin, fructosamine, and random serum glucose in diabetic patients. Arch Intern Med 1991;151:1133-37.

19. Steen G, Weber RF. Clinical usefulness of serum fructosamine and HbA_1 as markers for metabolic control in patients with changing insulin regimens. Diabetes Res 1990;13(4):177-82.

20. Skyler JS, Skyler DL, Seigler DE, O'Sullivan MJ. Algorithms for adjustment of insulin dosage by patients who monitor blood glucose. Diabetes Care 1981;4:311-18.

21. Skyler JS, Ellis GJ, Skyler DL, Lasky IA, Lebovitz FL. Instructing patients in making alterations in insulin dosage. Diabetes Care 1979;2:39-45.

22. Albisser AM, Sperlich M. Adjusting insulins. Diabetes Educ 1992;18(3): 211-22.

23. Albisser AM. Beyond the insulin pump: computer-assisted diabetes self-care through specialized centers. In: Davidson JK, ed. Clinical diabetes mellitus: a problem oriented approach. 2nd ed. New York: Thieme, 1991:330-40.

KEY EDUCATIONAL CONSIDERATIONS

1. A variety of meters are available, and each one is unique. Carefully assess the patient's visual acuity and dexterity skills before recommending a specific meter. Let the patient practice using the meter. Demonstration meters and supplies are available from the manufacturer's representative. You, the diabetes educator, are the pivotal person in guiding the patient's meter selection. Be sure you help your patients select the meter that is most appropriate for them and one for which they easily can obtain supplies.

2. Patients should bring their meter and all supplies to each visit. The meter can be cleaned, the reagents and control solution can be tested, codes can be verified, and an actual blood test can be performed. Comparing their test to a lab test can be additional verification of accuracy. Expect the results from venous serum blood tests to be 10% to 15% higher than the results from capillary whole blood samples.[10]

3. Make sure your patients have the toll-free customer service number for the manufacturer of their meter. Experts are available at this number for the majority of the day to answer questions and provide assistance.

4. Careful and safe disposal of used lancets is critical. Teach patients to place used lancets in a puncture resistant container. When patients monitor blood glucose away from home, they can place used lancets in an empty pill container or 35 mm film canister.

5. Consider the cost of supplies when determining with patients the frequency of monitoring. Be familiar with local suppliers who charge reasonable prices. Refer patients to a social worker or community agencies when appropriate.

6. Conceptually, patients may not realize that they are allowed to adjust their own calories or insulin/oral agents. Work with the

physician to determine adjustment protocols prior to the patient teaching appointment.

7. Teach patients how to use the blood glucose results in a way that is appropriate for their level of understanding and cognitive skills. If you determine that they cannot competently do insulin adjustment themselves, be sure they know when to call the doctor. JCAHO requires follow-up and discharge information following hospitalization. Check that the patient has the doctor's telephone number and pager number.

8. Utilize patient records or log books that list glucose levels for a certain time of day in a linear and vertical fashion. This format allows simple visual interpretation of the results.

9. Recording blood glucose levels on a graph, as well as having a numerical listing, provides a valuable visual aid when doing pattern management. Offer graphs for patient record-keeping, and demonstrate how to use them.

10. Use actual blood sugar records of common patterns when teaching self-management.

11. Have small groups discuss and role play situations from their lives. Ask realistic and practical questions, and wait for patients to answer.

12. Provide simple, written summary instructions for self-management.

13. Have patients practice urine testing for ketones during your teaching appointment.

14. A supply sheet, signed by the physician, can be an organizational aid for the patient and the pharmacist, and may serve as a prescription.

SELF-REVIEW QUESTIONS

If you are unsure of the answers to the following questions, please review the materials.

1. List five considerations for using blood glucose meters.
2. What are two disadvantages and two advantages of using blood glucose meters?
3. What are the key factors that affect the accuracy of blood glucose monitoring?
4. What are the elements of quality assurance regarding blood glucose meters?
5. Define the term *glycosylated hemoglobin.*
6. Compare and contrast pattern management and sliding scale management.

CASE EXAMPLE 1

FG, who has NIDDM treated with second-generation oral agents, was admitted to the hospital for treatment of pneumonia. The diabetes educator is called for consultation. Your assessment includes some clues that FG has not been monitoring his blood glucose for awhile. A family member brings FG's meter to the hospital. The battery is dead, and the reagent strips are expired and out of the container. FG tells you that he stopped monitoring because he couldn't get blood from his finger.

QUESTION

1. How would you approach your first teaching session with FG?

SUGGESTED SOLUTIONS

After greeting FG and determining that he feels well enough for a brief teaching session, you begin by building on his clue about inadequate blood supply. You offer to share some of the tips you have learned to secure an adequate blood sample. Hopefully, FG will consent to an extra fingerstick so that he can demonstrate the new techniques. (Some hospitalized patients receive many fingersticks and will not consent to one more. If so, you will need to arrange for another opportunity to demonstrate the new techniques.)

In discussing the cost of supplies, you uncover that FG is paying twice the usual price for his reagents. You provide FG with a list of suppliers who offer reasonable prices. If you have access to manufacturers' samples, you could provide FG with a fresh supply and written instructions concerning storage of reagents, a reminder to purchase a new battery, and the manufacturer's toll-free number.

You notice that FG is tiring so you end the session and make another appointment to review the use of blood glucose monitoring results and sick- day management.

CASE EXAMPLE 2

JT presents at a clinic visit 18 months after receiving initial education for initiation of insulin. The initial dose prescribed was 20 units of 70/30 insulin. The patient's goal for this visit is to obtain a prescription for syringes.

JT has gained 35 pounds since his last visit. Among other things, you note that he tests only his fasting blood glucose level and changes his insulin dose for the day based on the FBS reading. Today his FBS was 296 mg/dL (16.4 mmol/L) and he took 65 units of 70/30 insulin. He is referred to you for education.

QUESTIONS

1.   What went wrong?
2.   How would you start when the patient's goal is to secure a prescription?
3.   What would be the initial assessment and plan?

SUGGESTED SOLUTIONS

It may be helpful to use the time to introduce yourself again and listen to JT's perceptions of living with diabetes. The initial assessment indicates that JT has learned only the skills of self-injection and blood glucose monitoring. He does not see any difficulty with managing diabetes ("I just take my shot"), and reports no episodes of hypoglycemia. JT does mention that he is upset about gaining weight.

The weight gain issue could be your opportunity to explain how insulins work, when to monitor based on 70/30 insulin-action curves, and some of the factors that affect blood glucose. You introduce the concept that diabetes management involves more than taking an injection. Because you do not want to overwhelm JT, you try to give a broad perspective and constantly invite his comments and perceptions. JT agrees to return for individual instruction, and together you outline his learning needs. JT realizes his need for meal planning guidelines and agrees to keep a food record. From JT we learn the importance of both medical and educational follow-up.

OTHER SUGGESTED READINGS

American Diabetes Association. Implications of the diabetes control and complications trial; Position Statement. Diabetes Spectrum 1993;6(4):225-27.

Fox MA, Cassmeyer V, Eaks GA. Blood glucose self-monitoring usage and its influence on patients' perceptions of diabetes. Diabetes Educ 1984;10(3):27-31.

Nathan DM. Glycosylated hemoglobin: what is it and how to use it. Clin Diabetes 1983;1:1-7.

National Steering Committee for Quality Assurance in Capillary Blood Glucose Monitoring. Proposed strategies for reducing user error in capillary blood glucose monitoring. Diabetes Care 1993;16(2):493-98.

For a listing of currently available meters, refer to Diabetes Forecast: Buyers Guide (annual issue), and Diabetes Self-Management.

Management

MANAGEMENT

X. SPECIAL ISSUES IN MANAGEMENT

INTRODUCTION

Managing diabetes to attain euglycemia presents challenges that are only beginning to be understood. When dealing with special issues, the health care team must assess all aspects of a patient's life. Obtaining accurate information about the patient's self-care practices is especially important. This chapter will call attention to a variety of special issues pertinent to diabetes management.

OBJECTIVES

Upon completion of this chapter, the learner will be able to:
- describe the "honeymoon" (remission) period;
- identify special concerns for travel;
- identify various alternative insulin administration methods, such as insulin pumps;
- describe the challenges of unusual schedules;
- identify hygiene issues with special relevance for the person with diabetes;
- discuss the impact of smoking, alcohol, and drugs on diabetes.

A. Honeymoon (Remission)

1. The "*honeymoon*," or remission, is a time after the initial diagnosis of insulin-dependent diabetes mellitus (IDDM), also called type I diabetes, during which the beta cells of the pancreas continue to produce some insulin. During remission, blood glucose values remain near normal most of the time, although there may be periods of low blood glucose levels.

    a) If insulin is necessary, very low insulin doses can be prescribed during this time.

    b) In the treatment of young children, the use of diluted insulin (U-50 or U-25) allows for more accurate dosage.

        (1) Very minute but precise dose alterations are possible with diluted insulin.

        (2) Half-unit alterations can be made by using half strength or U-50 insulin.

c) Blood glucose monitoring should continue during the remission phase.

2. Laboratory evaluation of C peptide levels can determine whether endogenous insulin production remains. Usually, however, clinicians assume that remission has ended when blood glucose values begin to climb even though no change in caloric intake, exercise, or growth has occurred.

B. Dawn and Somogyi Phenomena

1. Fasting morning hyperglycemia may be a common problem for persons with diabetes, and its pathogenesis has been the subject of much interest and debate.

2. The term *dawn phenomenon* has been used to describe an increase in blood glucose levels and/or rise in the amount of insulin required to reach euglycemia in the pre-breakfast hours.
   a) For patients with insulin-dependent diabetes mellitus, a decline in plasma insulin levels during the night is probably an important cause of fasting hyperglycemia.
   b) Considerable evidence suggests that the anti-insulin effect of nocturnal growth hormone may be responsible.[1]

3. The hypothesis that nocturnal hypoglycemia causes hyperglycemia the next day was proposed by Michael Somogyi, an American biochemist. This effect is referred to as the *Somogyi phenomenon.* Although the existence of this hormone-mediated response has been confirmed,[1] the clinical relevance of the Somogyi phenomenon has been challenged.[2]

4. Nocturnal hypoglycemia is a common clinical concern in insulin-treated diabetes. For the treatment of nocturnal hypoglycemia (see Chapter XIII: Hypoglycemia).

C. Travel

1. Travel for the person with diabetes requires careful pretrip planning.

    a) Lists of supplies and emergency medical contacts should be available to patients before departure.

        (1) Supplies for the patient to carry when traveling can include:

            (a) Extra bottles of insulin or extra oral hypoglycemic pills;

            (b) Extra syringes;

            (c) Carbohydrate for hypoglycemia;

            (d) Snacks to cover late or delayed meals

            (e) Glucose meter and supplies;

            (f) Glucagon emergency kit;

            (g) Signed letter from patient's doctor regarding need for syringes;

            (h) Medical identification bracelet or necklace;

            (i) Prescriptions for generic forms of all medications taken;

            (j) Name of diabetes health care professional or diabetes center at destination;

            (k) Name of English-speaking doctor if patient is traveling abroad.

        (2) Health care professionals should provide patients who are traveling abroad with information about how to locate an English-speaking doctor. The International Association for Medical Assistance to Travelers publishes a directory of English-speaking doctors (716-754-4883).

    b) In case insulin vials are lost or broken, patients should be encouraged to explore ahead of time the availability of insulin supplies at their destination. Insulins of various strengths and with unfamiliar names are available in other countries.

    c) Some diabetes care equipment is temperature sensitive.

(1) When traveling, patients should carry their glucose meter, strips, insulin, and extra syringes with them in carry-on luggage.

(2) Insulin should also be protected from temperatures in excess of 86°F (30°C). Insulated travel kits are readily available.

2. Different types of travel make different demands on the patient with diabetes.

a) Airline travel poses special problems.

(1) If the trip requires crossing times zones, normal meal and sleep schedules will be disrupted. Erratic meal schedules may best be handled by having the patient convert to multiple injections of rapid-acting insulin on travel days.

(2) Letters to confirm that the traveler has diabetes and must carry medical supplies through customs should be signed, not stamped, by the patient's doctor.

b) Patients driving long distances need some specific guidelines.

(1) Meal and snack times should be as consistent as possible.

(2) Patients who have to drive in heavy traffic should monitor their blood glucose before starting out to be sure it is at a safe level.

(3) When driving, patients should keep an extra source of carbohydrate (eg, commercial glucose preparations or snacks) in the glove box to treat unexpected hypoglycemia.

(4) Drivers with diabetes who are traveling long distances should stop every few hours for a walk to help them stay alert.

c) Patients with diabetes who backpack may need to store their insulin, meters, and strips next to their body at night to prevent freezing.

d) Snow skiers with diabetes should take special precautions.

(1) Diabetes supplies must be kept from freezing.

(2) High altitude may depress the appetite, therefore skiers should make a conscious effort to eat extra snacks between runs.

(3) Less insulin may be required, so blood glucose levels should be monitored regularly.

D. Alternative Insulin Administration Methods

1. *Continuous subcutaneous insulin infusion* (CSII) using an open loop *insulin pump* is a technology that delivers insulin in a more physiologic fashion (more like the way beta cells secrete insulin) (see Figure X.1).

   a) A small, externally worn computerized device houses a syringe/reservoir containing regular insulin. Twenty-four to 42 inches of tubing connect the insulin reservoir to a 27-gauge needle that the patient inserts subcutaneously and secures. The patient is advised to change the insertion site at a minimum of every 48 hours.

   b) The continuous basal infusion is complemented by a premeal bolus infusion delivered at the direction of the patient.[3]

2. Intensive insulin therapy (multiple daily injections of insulin) and CSII may provide a metabolic advantage over conventional therapy; however, pump therapy must be considered carefully for each potential candidate before implementation.

   a) CSII candidates might include pregnant women with diabetes,[4] metabolically unstable individuals, and postrenal transplant patients.

   b) Highly motivated individuals who want to improve or stabilize their glycemic control, increase their lifestyle flexibility, or participate more fully in self-care are also likely candidates.[5]

   c) Patients who work erratic schedules or variable shifts, or who must travel extensively may also want to consider insulin pump therapy.

FIGURE X.1: Insulin Pump

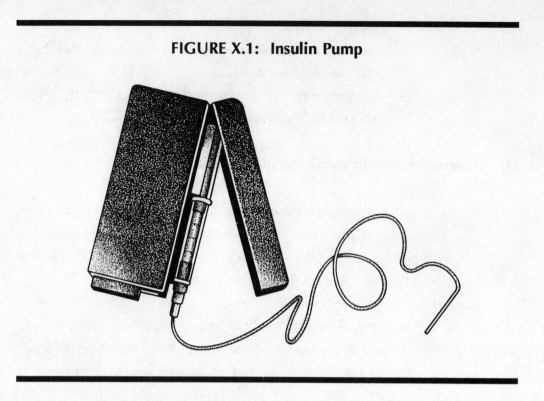

3. To determine if a patient is a candidate for CSII therapy, the diabetes team — including the doctor, nurse, dietitian, and counselor — should make a careful evaluation to ascertain the patient's metabolic condition, general ability to learn, and motivation. The patient's financial resources must also be considered.

   a) The patient's knowledge about diabetes, previous self-management history, and current self-management practices should be determined.[5]

   b) Insulin pumps are expensive and monthly supplies may run $100 or more. Thus cost may rule out patients with inadequate resources.

4. Because of the intensive nature of CSII therapy, the patient needs an emotional support system as well as access to a knowledgeable health care team at all times.

5. Insulin pump therapy has some potential risks.

   a) The onset of hypoglycemia is more subtle.

   b) Mechanical failure may rapidly precipitate ketoacidosis.

       c)   Cutaneous infections may occur at the needle site.

    6.   The potential benefits of CSII therapy are twofold.
        a)   Patients experience a more flexible lifestyle and an improved sense of well-being.
        b)   CSII and intensive insulin therapy may provide better metabolic control.

    7.   An implantable infusion device with a similar computer technology is currently being tested as an alternative to the externally worn device.

E. Hygiene

    1.   Prevention of complications through education and self-care is a major goal of diabetes management.

    2.   The person with poorly controlled diabetes may have a higher risk of infection than the nondiabetic population.

    3.   Among the factors contributing to this potential problem are altered circulation from micro- and macrovascular disease, hyperglycemia, which may increase glucotoxicity of the tissues, and diminished platelet functioning, immunologic responses, and white blood cell activity.[6(pp 153-64)]

    4.   The person with diabetes must carefully attend to hygiene to prevent infections.

    5.   To assure proper hygiene in their patients, health care professionals must offer education on hygiene. This is in compliance with the National Standards for Diabetes Patient Education Programs.[7]

F.   Dental Care

1.   Dental care and good glycemic control will contribute to the prevention of dental caries and periodontal disease.

   a)   Hyperglycemia may contribute to elevated salivary glucose levels.

   b)   Other pathology may include an alteration in oral microbial flora with a shift from gram-positive aerobic microbiota to gram-negative anaerobic flora.[8]

2.   Periodontal disease, an inflammatory process affecting the supporting tissues of the teeth, may be accelerated in patients with diabetes that is poorly controlled or of long duration.[9,10]

3.   Good dental care practices are mandatory for patients with diabetes.

   a)   Patients should have a dental examination several times a year.

   b)   Bacterial plaque must be kept at a minimum.

      (1)   Brushing and flossing should be done routinely.

      (2)   Professional removal of plaque should be done periodically in association with regular dental exams.

      (3)   The use of baking soda with hydrogen peroxide has been identified as useful in the eradication of subgingival microflora.

   c)   Maintaining good glycemic control will help reduce periodontal disease.[11]

   d)   Efforts should be made to allay apprehension associated with dental examinations and treatment; this will help reduce the patient's stress level.

   e)   Patients with diabetes should schedule dental appointments about an hour after breakfast to allow time for food to be absorbed, thus reducing the chances of hypoglycemia.[12]

G. Infections and Skin Care

1. Patients with uncontrolled diabetes are more prone to infections.

   a) Skin infections may result from staphylococci, beta-hemolytic streptococci, and fungus.

   b) Women with diabetes commonly have the vaginal infection candidiasis.

      (1) Hyperglycemia, and consequent increased glucose in the vaginal mucosa and urine, will cause *Candida* organisms in the mucosa to multiply rapidly, causing vulvovaginitis and pruritus with a cheesy white discharge.

      (2) Also susceptible to *Candida* organisms are axillary areas; under skin folds and breasts; and oral mucosa.

   c) Treatment may include the application of topical powder, vaginal suppositories, and/or oral medication.

2. Infections and carbuncles usually increase the blood glucose level and, consequently, the patient's insulin requirements.

3. Good control of blood glucose levels is important both as a preventative and a treatment.

4. Cleanliness is an important component of good skin care and helps prevent infection. Patients should use mild soap, warm (not hot) water, moisturizing lotion (not oil based), and sunscreen when in the sun.

H. Foot Care

1. Because of vascular insufficiency and neuropathic changes, foot care is one of the most important hygienic considerations for the patient with diabetes.

2. For specific recommendations on foot care, see Chapter XXV: Lower Extremity Problems.

I. Alcohol Consumption

1. Alcohol intake is permitted in moderation for people with diabetes. This is in line with recommendations for the general population.

2. Patients with diabetes should be cautioned about possible problems, however.

   a) Excessive alcohol consumption may cause problems such as hypoglycemia, neuropathy, altered glycemic control, obesity and/or hyperlipidemia.[13] Alcohol may also raise triglyceride levels.

   b) Patients taking oral hypoglycemic agents may experience a disulfiram (Antabuse) reaction if they drink alcohol.

   c) The hypoglycemic effect of alcohol may persist for from 8 to 12 hours after alcohol intake.

   d) Decreased availability of glucose through gluconeogenesis and diminished glycogenolysis may occur with alcohol consumption.[6]

   e) Symptoms of excessive alcohol intake may appear similar to ketoacidosis, including fruity-smelling breath, flushed face, irritability, staggering gait, drowsiness, and coma. Excessive alcohol intake may also mimic hypoglycemia.

3. Diabetes educators need to provide specific information to patients who choose to drink alcoholic beverages.

   a) Food should be eaten with alcoholic beverages. It is vital that patients not skip meals or snacks.

   b) Even if blood glucose levels are high at bedtime, patients who have been drinking alcohol should be advised to eat their bedtime snack because alcohol may lower the blood glucose level during sleep due to the inhibition of gluconeogenesis and diminished glycogenolysis. If a patient's gluconeogenesis or glycogen-releasing mechanisms are inhibited, prolonged hypoglycemia may occur.

c)   Patients should be advised to drink alcohol in moderation. For both insulin-dependent and non-insulin-dependent patients, two alcohol equivalents once or twice a week are all that are recommended.[13]

d)   Because of alcohol's slow absorption, some dietitians recommend substituting alcohol for fat exchanges in the diet.

e)   Cultural considerations concerning alcohol use, blood glucose levels, blood lipid levels, weight, and frequency of hypoglycemic reactions should be considered when advising patients about alcohol consumption.

J.   Other Social Drug Use

1.   Patients with diabetes who are abusing drugs may have symptoms that resemble diabetic ketoacidosis (DKA) or hypoglycemia.

2.   Outward signs that point to drug use may include bloodshot eyes, constricted or dilated pupil size, drowsiness, confusion, inappropriate behavior with emotional swings, and poor physical condition.

3.   Social drugs are categorized as depressants, stimulants, and hallucinogens. All of these have direct or indirect effects on diabetes.

a)   Stimulants include amphetamines, and cocaine and crack. The use of syringes with these drugs is a concern and access to insulin syringes is potentially an enabling factor.

(1)   Amphetamines (speed, uppers, bennies, whites) can be taken orally (pills and capsules), injected intravenously, or smoked (ice).

(2)   Cocaine (snow, coke, toot) is taken orally, sniffed, smoked, or injected. Cocaine causes loss of appetite.

(3)   Crack is made by heating cocaine powder with soda bicarbonate.

(a) The drug stimulates receptors of the pleasure center, producing an immediate high, followed by a desire for more. Addiction often results.

(b) Addiction is marked by loss of appetite and forgetfulness. These conditions have a direct effect on the patient's ability to perform self-care behaviors.[6]

(4) Stimulants affect the central nervous system, increasing blood pressure, pulse, and metabolic rates. Increased metabolism leads to faster glucose utilization and, potentially, to a lower blood glucose level. Speech is also affected.

(5) Persons who take stimulants are sometimes confused and can behave violently.

b) Depressants include heroin and barbiturates.

(1) Known as downers or goofballs, these drugs are taken orally or by injection.

(2) The body builds a tolerance to depressants, requiring more to give the same effect.

(3) Depression of the central nervous system may occur.

(4) Because depressants cause increased metabolism of drugs, the efficacy of oral hypoglycemic agents may be impaired.

(5) Memory impairment and reduced motivation may cause the patient to miss meals and to forget to take medication, to monitor blood glucose levels, and to perform other self-care skills.

(6) A mixture of alcohol and drugs may be fatal.

c) Hallucinogens include lysergic acid diethylamide (LSD), phencyclidine (PCP), and marijuana.

(1) Hallucinogens may be taken orally, injected, or smoked.

(2) These drugs cause flashbacks, "freaking out," and other negative and frightening experiences.

(3) Hallucinogens stimulate the appetite, leading to extra caloric intake and consequent higher blood glucose levels.

K. Smoking

1. The complications of diabetes are devastating enough without adding the health hazards of cigarette smoking.

   a) Smoking is associated not only with cancer but also with coronary artery disease through an increase in triglycerides and a decrease in plasma high-density lipoprotein cholesterol concentration. Studies show that smokers are insulin resistant and hyperinsulinemic.[14]

   b) The person with overt diabetes who smokes may have the additional pathology of peripheral microvascular circulation vasoconstriction from the effect of the nicotine.[15]

   c) An already compromised microvascular system may lead to a number of other complications if the person with diabetes smokes.

   d) Smoking is a risk factor in many disease states, all of which are complicated by diabetes.

      (1) Albuminuria is increased in individuals with IDDM who smoke.[16]

      (2) Studies suggest a connection between cigarette smoking and neuropathy.[17]

2. Not smoking is an imperative for persons with diabetes.

   a) Smoking cessation must be initiated and supported by the diabetes health care team.[18]

   b) Prescription nicotine gum and nicotine patches are available to help the smoker quit smoking.

L. Unusual Schedules

1. One of the most difficult challenges for the patient with diabetes in today's hectic world is to maintain a standard routine. This is especially difficult for people whose careers demand unusual work hours. Farmers, police officers, shift workers, college students, and fire fighters constantly struggle

to attain good blood glucose control while continuing to perform optimally at all hours of the day and night.

2. With few exceptions, persons are not expected to leave or change careers because they have diabetes. However, they are expected to make good self-care practices a part of their lifestyle.

    a) Patients should work with their diabetes health care team to fit their diabetes management protocol into their lives.

    b) Patients who are sophisticated consumers can develop a great deal of expertise in diabetes self-management skills. For example, frequent monitoring of blood glucose values will provide valuable information and increase confidence in making adjustments in the diabetes routine.

3. For the patient who requires insulin, the key to increasing flexibility is for the patient to understand how insulins work.

4. Various options are available to fit different lifestyles and career demands.

    a) The person who is willing to convert to multiple injections of rapid-acting regular insulin can deal with fluctuating meal times.

    b) The insulin pump (CSII therapy) can provide the flexibility needed with unusual schedules. The person who works a swing shift, for instance, may have lunch at noon during one week and at 3 A.M. the next week. The insulin pump will allow the person to take prelunch regular insulin whenever mealtime occurs.

    c) Conceptually, the Ultralente protocol gives the same flexibility. Ultralente administered once or twice a day with the remaining amount taken as a bolus of regular insulin distributed as needed for meal coverage, provides great flexibility.

    d) Another option involves injections of regular insulin before meals, with NPH or Lente insulin taken before sleeping. This regimen provides insulin coverage for food intake and longer-term coverage for hours of sleep.

e)   During harvest, farmers may work 18 to 20 hours a day. Frequent monitoring of blood glucose levels may show that not only must the dose of insulin be adjusted, but extra calories should be consumed to cover the extra activity.

f)   In contrast, a college student studying 18 to 20 hours a day for final exams may find through careful monitoring that few if any additional calories are needed. Stress may actually spike the blood glucose level, making frequent monitoring critically important.

5.   Many combinations of insulin therapies, coupled with frequent glucose monitoring, have empowered health care providers and patients with diabetes to experiment safely until they get the best combination based on the needs of the patient.

REFERENCES

1.   Stephenson JM, Schernthaner G. Dawn phenomenon and somogyi effect in IDDM. Diabetes Care 1989;12:245-51.

2.   Hirsch IB, Smith LJ, Havlin CE, Shah SD, Clutter WE, Cryer PE. Failure of nocturnal hypoglycemia to cause daytime hyperglycemia in patients with IDDM. Diabetes Care 1990;13(2):133-42.

3.   Tomky D, Weinrauch S. Insulin pumps. Diabetes Forecast 1987;40(10):43-45.

4.   Burr RE. Continuous subcutaneous insulin infusion therapy associated with pregnancy. Diabetes Educ 1983;9(2):30-46s.

5.   Strowig SM. Initiation and management of insulin pump therapy. Diabetes Educ 1993;19:50-60.

6.   Guthrie DW, Guthrie RA, eds. Nursing management of diabetes mellitus. 3rd ed. New York: Springer Publishing Co, 1991.

7.   National Diabetes Advisory Board. National standards for diabetes patient education and American Diabetes Association review criteria. Clinical practice recommendations. Diabetes Care 1991-92;15(suppl 2):75-80.

8.   Savitt ED, Socransky SS. Distribution of certain subgingival microbial species in selected periodontal conditions. J Clin Periodont Res 1984;19:111-23.

9.   Sznajder N, Carraro JJ, Rugna S, Sereday M. Periodontal findings in diabetic and non-diabetic patients. J Clin Periodontal 1989;16:215-23.

10. Hugoson A, Thorstenson H, Falk H, Kuyenstierna J. Periodontal conditions in insulin-dependent diabetes. J Clin Periodontal 1989;16:215-23.

11. Hallmon W, Mealey B. Implications of diabetes mellitus and periodontal disease. Diabetes Educ 1992;18:310-15.

12. Villeneuve ME, Treitel L, D'Eramo G. Dental care for the person with diabetes mellitus. Diabetes Educ 1985;11(3):44-47.

13. ADA nutritional recommendations and principles for individuals with diabetes mellitus. Clinical practice recommendations. Diabetes Care 1991-92;15(suppl 2):21-28.

14. Facchini FS, Hollenbook CB, Jeppesen J, Chen YD, Reaven GM. Insulin resistance and cigarette smoking. Lancet 1992;339(8802):1128-30.

15. Parving HH, Noer I, Deckert T, et al. The effect of metabolic regulation on microvascular permeability to small and large molecules in short-term juvenile diabetics. Diabetologia 1976;12:161-66.

16. Chase HP, Garg SK, Marshall G, Berg CL, Harris S, Jackson WE, Hamman RE. Cigarette smoking increases the risk of albuminuria among subjects with type I diabetes. JAMA 1991;265:614-17.

17. Mitchell BD, Hawthorne VM, Vinek AI. Cigarette smoking and neuropathy in diabetic patients. Diabetes Care 1990;13:434-37.

18. Haire-Joshu D. Smoking, cessation, and the diabetes health care team. Diabetes Educ 1991;17:54-64.

KEY EDUCATIONAL CONSIDERATIONS

1. Teaching a patient about basic hygiene can be very challenging. If a patient who has obviously not bathed for a long time presents to your facility, it is important to assess the reason for the person's poor hygiene. If the patient does not have access to bathing facilities, then a social worker may be needed. If the patient does have access but doesn't value cleanliness, then it is important to explore possible cultural or familial values that may explain the patient's attitude. Establish a trusting relationship with the patient before gently discussing your concerns about infection.

2. Many people have misconceptions about continuous subcutaneous insulin infusion (insulin pump) therapy. It may be helpful to show an introductory videotape and/or have a demonstration model of an insulin pump available.

3. Guidelines for safe travel may be taught to patients as part of the diabetes curriculum. Unless a patient plans to take a trip immediately, however, this information is likely to be forgotten, as learning is reinforced and retained when it is applied immediately. To strengthen the learning of travel guidelines, use written instructions and provide a telephone number where a patient can find specific information about crossing time zones and other travel guidelines.

4. The "honeymoon" or remission period can create a potential psychological barrier to diabetes self-management. Initial diabetes education should include information about the potential for a remission period.

SELF-REVIEW QUESTIONS

If you are unsure of the answers to the following questions, please review the materials.

1. Describe the characteristics of the remission period.

2. Discuss the impact of smoking, alcohol, and drugs on diabetes.

3. List special considerations for travel for the person with diabetes.

4. List characteristics of possible candidates for insulin pump therapy.

5. Discuss two issues in hygiene that are important in diabetes management.

6. Describe alternative insulin protocols for patients with unusual schedules.

CASE EXAMPLE

ME is an executive of a national organization, and her work often involves travel between the US mainland and Hawaii. Although ME has had NIDDM for 15 years, she has only recently made the transition to insulin therapy. She called the diabetes educator from her hometown to discuss travel issues.

QUESTIONS

1. What would be important to include in a teaching session concerning travel?

SUGGESTED SOLUTIONS

ME's primary concern was to learn how to adjust her insulin dose for travel. ME and the diabetes educator reviewed ME's carefully recorded blood glucose records and determined some guidelines for ME's insulin and meal adjustments based on the action of insulins. The diabetes educator also inquired about the frequency and usual patterns of hypoglycemia. ME reported that she often experienced hypoglycemia before lunch if lunch is delayed. This became an important consideration, as airline travel frequently involves delays. ME decided to carry a sandwich and piece of fruit in her carry-on luggage in anticipation of flight delays.

ME and the diabetes educator reviewed the importance of ME's wearing diabetic identification when away from home. The diabetes educator also verified that ME's blood glucose meter could be safely scanned by the airport detection systems. ME was given telephone numbers of diabetes educators in different states. She reported feeling more confident about her work-related travel and decided that she would apply her Frequent Flyer mileage toward a European vacation.

OTHER SUGGESTED READINGS

Brink S, Stewart C. Insulin pump treatment in insulin-dependent diabetes mellitus. JAMA 1986;255:616-20.

Brown LS. Clinical aspects of drug abuse in diabetes. Diabetes Spectrum 1991;4:45-47.

Dinwiddie SH. Psychiatric aspects of drug abuse in diabetes. Diabetes Spectrum 1990;3:353-56.

Marcus AO. Patient selection for insulin pump therapy. Prac Diabetol 1992;11(4):12-18.

Reichard P, et al. Intensive treatment and progression of microvascular complications. J Int Med 1991;230:101-8.

Rosenbaum MC, ed. Mastering air travel. Diabetes Trav 1991;5(2):1-6.

MANAGEMENT

XI. HYPERGLYCEMIA

INTRODUCTION

Hyperglycemia stemming from uncontrolled diabetes mellitus can lead to two types of metabolic crises that may result in an altered mental state or even loss of consciousness. These crises are *diabetic ketoacidosis* (DKA) and *hyperglycemic hyperosmolar nonketotic syndrome* (HHNS).

DKA is a complication that results from uncontrolled insulin-dependent diabetes mellitus (IDDM), also called type I diabetes; or, very rarely, from decompensated non-insulin-dependent diabetes mellitus (NIDDM), also called type II diabetes. Persons with IDDM do not progress to the extreme hyperglycemia and dehydration characteristic of HHNS because the nausea, vomiting, and acidosis brought on by severe ketosis usually leads the patient to seek medical help before there is time for major volume depletion to develop.

HHNS is a life-threatening emergency with a high mortality rate. Usually seen in the elderly or undiagnosed person with diabetes, HHNS is characterized by four main clinical features: severe hyperglycemia (blood glucose >800 mg/dL [33.3 mmol/L]); absence of ketoacidosis; profound dehydration; and neurologic signs ranging from depressed sensorium to frank coma.

Although the morbidity and mortality caused by these acute complications have decreased, DKA and HHNS still remain a significant problem. Prevention, early recognition of symptoms, and prompt efficacious treatment must be emphasized.

OBJECTIVES

Upon completion of this chapter, the learner will be able to:

- discuss precipitating factors in DKA;
- discuss the pathophysiology of DKA;
- describe presenting signs and symptoms of DKA;
- discuss possible variations in initial laboratory values;
- state three goals in the treatment of DKA;
- discuss precipitating factors in HHNS;
- discuss pathophysiology of HHNS;
- describe presenting signs and symptoms of HHNS;
- state the major or primary component of treatment for HHNS;

explain major differences between laboratory values found in DKA and HHNS.

A. Diabetic Ketoacidosis (DKA)

1. The characteristics of DKA are hyperglycemia, ketosis, dehydration, and electrolyte imbalance.

2. Precipitating factors of DKA vary from individual to individual.

   a) Illness/infection are the precipitating factors in approximately 25% to 30% of cases. Illness and infection increase production of glucocorticoids by the adrenal gland, promoting gluconeogenesis. Production of epinephrine and norepinephrine are also increased, which in turn increases glycogenolysis.

   b) Inadequate insulin dosage (either physician or patient directed) may lead to DKA and is a major factor in approximately one half of the cases. Patients with gastrointestinal (GI) symptoms often decrease or omit their insulin doses in the mistaken belief that less insulin is needed when food intake is decreased. Because GI signs and symptoms are prominent features of DKA itself, decreasing insulin dosages can be dangerous.

   c) The initial manifestation of IDDM may be DKA. This is the situation in approximately 25% to 30% of patients presenting with DKA.

   d) Emotional stress is a precipitating factor in a small number of cases, particularly among adolescents. In these patients, neglect or mismanagement may be a deliberate "call for help."

B. Pathophysiology of DKA

1. DKA is caused by profound insulin deficiency. Although small amounts of insulin may be circulating, the presence of large amounts of stress hormones, (glucagon, catecholamines [eg, epinephrine and norepinephrine], cortisol, and growth

hormone), render the insulin less effective. All aspects of metabolism (carbohydrate, protein, and fat) are markedly affected (see Fig. XI.1).

FIGURE XI.1: DKA - HHNS Pathways

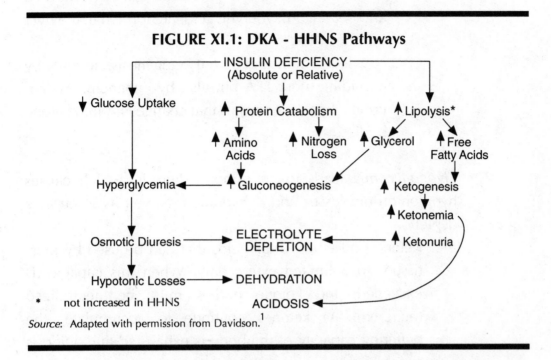

*   not increased in HHNS

Source: Adapted with permission from Davidson.[1]

a) Following a meal, insulin deficiency impairs glucose uptake in the peripheral tissues (mainly muscle) and liver, leading to hyperglycemia. During fasting, insulin deficiency results in excess hepatic glucose production which can also lead to hyperglycemia.

b) Insulin deficiency causes impaired protein synthesis and an excessive protein degradation. The resulting increase in the gluconeogenic amino acids leads to increased hepatic glucose production (by means of gluconeogenesis) and finally hyperglycemia. The failure to build new protein and the increased breakdown of already formed protein are the reasons for the loss of lean body mass in uncontrolled diabetes.

c) Severe insulin deficiency causes excessive hydrolysis of triglycerides, the storage form of fat, yielding increased amounts of glycerol and free fatty acids (FFA). This metabolic pathway is called lipolysis.

(1) Glycerol is an important gluconeogenic precursor leading to increasing hepatic glucose production and more hyperglycemia.

(2) Excessive amounts of *ketone bodies* (acetoacetic acid and beta-hydroxybutyric acid) are formed in the liver from the FFA.

(3) Low levels of insulin permit ketogenesis, not only by providing more FFA but also by enhancing certain critical hepatic enzymes that change FFA into ketone bodies.

2. *Hyperglycemia* leads to an osmotic diuresis, which causes hypotonic fluid losses and dehydration as well as electrolyte depletion.

   a) Ketone bodies are weak acids that can be used by most tissues to a limited extent only. When this capacity is exceeded, the ketone bodies must be neutralized (buffered). As ketones continue to accumulate, the buffering capacity of the body is exhausted and acidosis supervenes.

   b) The excretion of ketone bodies in the urine (*ketonuria*) leads to more electrolyte depletion, because cations must be eliminated along with the anionic ketone bodies to maintain electrical neutrality.

   c) Twelve to 24 hours of insulin deficiency in patients with IDDM (depending on the hyperglycemic state) causes profound fluid and electrolyte losses. Fluids, sodium, potassium, and chloride must be vigorously replaced in the initial hours of treatment. There is controversy concerning the need for magnesium and phosphate replacement.[1,2]

C. Signs and Symptoms

1. Symptoms may mimic other diseases or conditions.

a) Manifestations of hyperglycemia are polyuria, polydipsia, blurred vision and, if insulin deficiency is present long enough (days to weeks), polyphagia.

b) Nonspecific symptoms include weakness, lethargy, malaise, and headache.

c) Gastrointestinal symptoms are nausea, vomiting, and abdominal pain. The cause of these symptoms is unclear, but they are probably related to the ketosis and/or acidotic state.

d) Respiratory symptoms may include an inability to "catch one's breath," and a very deep, sometimes rapid, breathing unrelated to exertion termed *Kussmaul's respiration*. This hyperventilation produces a respiratory alkalosis in a partial, but not completely successful, attempt to correct the metabolic acidosis.

2. There are no specific signs of DKA; rather a constellation of evidence should alert the clinician to the possibility of DKA.

a) Hypothermia is often found; therefore, the presence of fever suggests associated infection.

b) Hyperpnea (deep respirations) is always present in DKA and reflects pulmonary response to acidosis.

c) Acetone breath may be present. Acetoacetate, one of the ketone bodies, is converted to *acetone*, which is excreted by the lungs. It has a fruity odor that can sometimes be detected on the breath of the patient.

d) Dehydration (intravascular volume depletion) is a common sign.

(1) Dehydration can be assessed by observing for decreased neck vein filling from below when the patient is lying absolutely flat.

(2) Orthostatic hypotension (a fall of systolic blood pressure of 20 mm Hg after 1 minute of standing) may occur as a result of decreased intravascular volume from dehydration.

(3) Poor skin turgor and "soft eyeballs" are late signs of profound dehydration in adults. Poor skin turgor is seen earlier in children.

e) "Acute abdomen" is common. Tenderness to palpation, diminished bowel sounds, and some muscle guarding are usual signs, especially in children. A few patients may have more severe signs (absent bowel sounds, rebound tenderness, boardlike abdomen) that suggest a surgical emergency. However, in virtually every case, these signs are due to profound DKA and disappear after treatment.

f) Mentation changes may be present. Patients may be alert, obtunded, stuporous, or in frank coma. Mentation seems to correlate best with serum osmolality, less well with glucose concentrations, and least with pH changes.

g) Hyporeflexia, or decreased reflexes, if not present initially may occur during treatment as the potassium level falls.

h) Hypotonia, uncoordinated ocular movements, and fixed dilated pupils are all late signs that suggest a poor prognosis.

D. Initial Laboratory Values

1. After the diagnosis of DKA is made by clinical impression and bedside testing (a fingerstick blood glucose and blood/urine test for ketone bodies), initial laboratory tests should be obtained before therapy is begun (see Table XI.1).

2. Normal values may vary in relation to the methodology of the test procedure used in an institution.

a) Glucose concentrations are usually >300 mg/dL (>16.5 mmol/L). This value is not a good index of the severity of DKA. Lower levels are not uncommon, especially in children, pregnant women, and patients who have been vomiting frequently.

b) The test for ketone bodies is semiquantitative and involves the development of a purple color when serum or plasma is added to the reagent, nitroprusside.

TABLE XI.1:
Initial Laboratory Values for Patients Experiencing DKA

Test	Result	Remarks
Glucose level	Usually <600 mg/dL (<33.3 mmol/L)	Concentration not related to severity of DKA
Ketone bodies	Strong at least in undiluted plasma	Measures only acetoacetate, not beta-hydroxybutyrate
Bicarbonate concentration	0-15 mEq/L (0-15 mmol/L)	
pH	6.8-7.3	
Sodium concentration	Low, normal, or high	Total body depletion
Potassium concentration	Low, normal, or high	Total body depletion; heart responsive to extracellular concentration
Phosphate level	Usually normal or slightly elevated; occasionally slightly low	Associated with phosphaturia; marked decrease in levels of both serum and urine phosphates following treatment
Creatinine, BUN* concentrations	Usually mildly increased	May be prerenal: spurious increases in creatinine level by acetoacetate in some automated methods
White blood cell count	Usually increased	Possibility of leukemoid reaction (even in absence of infection): >10% band forms usually signify severe infection
Amylase value	Often increased	Predominant form is of salivary gland origin
Hemoglobin, hematocrit, total protein values	Often increased	Secondary to contracted plasma volume
AST (SGOT),† ALT (SGPT),‡ alkaline phosphatase values	Can be elevated	Nonspecific and reversible

* BUN = blood urea nitrogen.
† AST = aspartate aminotransferase (previously SGOT, serum glutamic oxaloacetic transaminase).
‡ ALT = alanine aminotransferase (previously SGPT, serum glutamic pyruvic transaminase).

Source: Adapted with permission from Davidson.[1]

(1) Typically, the serum is serially diluted until a dilution is found in which no purple color is seen. The result is usually expressed as the last dilution that produces a 1+ reaction (eg, 1:8).

(2) Nitroprusside reacts only with acetoacetate, not with beta-hydroxybutyrate. These two ketones exist in equilibrium, with the latter in excess by three- to fivefold in DKA.

(3) This test for ketones can only be used to diagnose DKA; it is not useful in monitoring response to therapy because the excess beta-hydroxybutyrate is converted back to acetoacetate as the patient improves biochemically.

c) The serum bicarbonate (HCO_3) concentration will be low, usually less than 15 mEq/L (15 mmol/L), reflecting acidosis.

d) The pH is obtained on an arterial blood gas determination and will be low (6.80 to 7.30), reflecting acidosis.

e) The carbon dioxide pressure (PCO_2) is obtained by an arterial gas determination and will be low (10 to 35 mm Hg [1.33 to 4.66 kPa]), reflecting the hyperventilatory response to the metabolic acidosis.

f) Even though loss of total body sodium (Na) is profound, the serum sodium level can be low, normal, or high because the sodium level depends on the amount of total body water (H_2O). The sodium concentration at a particular time will reflect the relative amounts of H_2O and sodium lost and replaced up to that point. If the deficit of H_2O is greater than that of sodium, the sodium level will be high; if the deficit of sodium is greater than that of H_2O, the sodium level will be low; if the deficits are approximately equal, the sodium level will be normal.

g) The serum potassium (K) level can also be low, normal, or high despite a profound loss of potassium. The potassium level does not reflect the relative amounts of H_2O lost but depends on the balance between the amount of potassium lost in the urine and other factors that raise the potassium level, such as the lack of insulin, which allows potassium to remain in the circulation rather than enter cells. If potassium entrance from the cells into the circulation exceeds excretion, serum potassium level may be high. Nonetheless, total body depletion of potassium always occurs regardless of the initial serum level.

h) Phosphate concentrations are usually high or high-normal initially, and decrease, sometimes markedly, to very low levels over the next day or two.

i) Creatinine and blood urea nitrogen (BUN) concentrations are usually mildly increased because of the dehydration and prerenal azotemia. After rehydration, raised creatinine and BUN levels indicate renal insufficiency present before DKA.

j) Hemoglobin, hematocrit, and total protein values are often mildly elevated, reflecting the decreased plasma volume (dehydration).

k) White blood cell (WBC) counts are usually increased, occasionally to very high levels. This does not necessarily reflect an ongoing infection, since DKA itself often causes a rise in white count. However, if a differential count is performed, >10% band forms (immature WBC) almost always denotes a severe infection, whereas <10% band forms usually does not.

l) Amylase values are usually increased. This does not reflect pancreatitis because in DKA, salivary glands, not the pancreas, release most of the amylase.

m) Liver function tests often produce mildly elevated values. This does not necessarily reflect acute or chronic liver damage because the values usually return to normal in several weeks (see Table XI.1).

E. Treatment of DKA

1. The goals of treatment are to correct fluid and electrolyte disturbances, provide adequate insulin to restore and maintain normal glucose metabolism and correct acidosis, prevent

complications resulting from the treatment of DKA, and provide patient and family education and follow-up.

2. The treatment of mild DKA (ie, patients who can ingest and retain oral fluids without difficulty) should focus on rehydration, euglycemia, and education. If the patient or family can provide accurate blood glucose values and results of urine ketone tests, therapy directed over the phone by a knowledgeable health care professional may take place at home.

    a) Oral hydration is employed (by definition, the patient is not vomiting). Small sips of sodium-containing fluids should be given at frequent intervals. Although sugar-free fluids may be offered if the blood glucose levels are above 250 to 300 mg/dL (13.9 to 16.7 mmol/L), some programs advocate the use of sugar-containing liquids regardless of the blood glucose level. It is more important to prevent or treat the dehydration than the hyperglycemia (although the latter will maintain an osmotic diuresis leading to continued loss of fluid.)

    b) Patients in mild DKA require some supplemental insulin. If the hyperglycemia is unaccompanied by ketosis, a proportionately smaller amount of insulin is required. Insulin doses in children should be supplemented with regular insulin in the range of 0.25 to 0.5 units/kg of body weight every 4 to 6 hours, as needed. In adults, the dose of subcutaneous regular insulin at 3- to 6-hour intervals will vary (usually between 4 to 10 units or 10 to 20 percent of the usual total daily dose), depending on the patient's known sensitivity to insulin.

    c) Education regarding self-management during illness and stress management is essential (see Chapter XII: Managing Diabetes During Intercurrent Illness).

3. Moderate (ie, patients who cannot retain oral fluids) and severe DKA (ie, patients with altered mentation) require immediate emergency treatment.

a) In the rare situation in which a cardiac or respiratory arrest has occurred, the first step is to ensure an adequate airway and to assess and maintain respiratory function (and oxygen delivery). In all cases, circulation should be maintained by ensuring appropriate fluid volume replacement.[1,2]

b) Diagnosis is established by testing for one or a combination of the following: the presence of urine ketones, serum ketones, lowered serum bicarbonate level, and/or a lowered arterial pH. Hyperglycemia can be established by bedside measuring of the capillary blood glucose level.

c) A preliminary history and rapid physical examination (vital signs, weight, blood pressure in the supine and upright positions, and pulse rate) may be obtained to confirm clinical findings and to identify other emergency measures that may be needed.

d) Baseline laboratory data should be obtained without delay. These should include serum electrolyte values; BUN and creatinine levels; calcium, phosphorus, and serum ketone body concentrations; an arterial blood gas determination; and a complete blood cell (CBC) count.

e) After the initial evaluation has been made and therapy started, a more thorough examination should be performed and may help identify precipitating causes.

4. General principles of treatment apply to almost all patients in a compromised hyperglycemic state.

a) Bladder catheterization is generally not desirable. A patient who is alert will usually cooperate with voiding as required. If patients cannot produce urine initially, they are often successful after several hours of rehydration. If there is no urine flow after 4 hours of appropriate rehydration, bladder catheterization is usually warranted. In small infants and children, urine may be obtained through the use of urine-collection bags.

b) In most patients, hypovolemia is the most acute and critical problem. The largest practical intravenous line for the rapid administration of saline must be started and its patency maintained.

c) An electrocardiogram (ECG), especially leads II, V_1 or V_2, is important. The T-wave configuration (see Fig. XI.2) aids in the determination of serum potassium status on admission and usually allows for earlier decisions regarding potassium therapy. Hypokalemia causes low or flattened T- or U-waves. Hyperkalemia causes peaked T-waves and, if markedly elevated, a widened QRS interval. Serial ECG tracings will reflect changes in potassium levels as therapy proceeds. This information is available immediately before values are returned from the laboratory.

FIGURE XI.2:
T-Wave Configuration

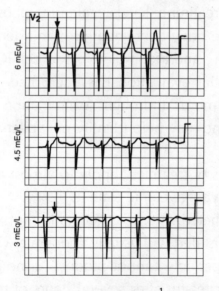

Relation between serum concentration of potassium [K] and T-wave configurations.

Source: Reproduced with permission from Davidson.[1]

d) Placement of a nasogastric tube should be considered in a patient who is stuporous or comatose or who has signs of gastric dilatation, to prevent aspiration should the patient vomit.

e) A flowsheet is an absolute necessity to provide parameters that can be followed sequentially and in an organized fashion by different observers.

5. Fluid and electrolyte replacement is based on specific needs.

a) Adequate fluid replacement is critical for lowering glucose concentrations. Hyperglycemia will persist (even with appropriate insulin therapy) if fluid replacement is inadequate.

b) Considerations should include maintenance needs, replacement requirements, and ongoing losses.

c) Initial fluid replacement should be made with one-half normal (0.45%) or normal (0.9%) saline.

(1) For adults, the initial fluid replacement level depends on the degree of dehydration and the patient's cardiovascular status. In general, 1 to 2 liters should be delivered in the first 1 to 2 hours, then the patient's status should be reassessed.[1,2]

(2) The above quantities are not appropriate for children. Many specialists prefer to state all values for children on the basis of kilograms of body weight. The usual calculation for fluid replacement in children is 20 mL/kg of body weight in the first hour. If no urination occurs, 20 mL/kg of body weight of fluid is given during the second and third hours as well. This is followed by routine fluid replacement calculated on maintenance plus deficit.

d) As soon as the serum glucose level is decreased to approximately 250 mg/dL (13.7 mmol/L), intravenous fluids should be changed to contain glucose. *Remember that the acidosis almost always persists longer than marked hyperglycemia during treatment.* Therefore, adequate amounts of insulin must continue to be given (and glucose concentrations supported) until the acidosis is treated appropriately (see below).

e) Hypokalemia, if not treated properly, can lead to death.

    (1) Potassium should be given immediately if hypokalemia is present as determined by ECG changes or initial laboratory findings. Because of the total body potassium depletion associated with DKA, all patients with urine flow eventually need potassium repletion.

    (2) Potassium may be added in the second to fourth hour of treatment or sooner, depending on T-wave changes confirmed by laboratory values.

    (3) Potassium is usually replaced at concentrations of 20 to 40 mEq/L (20 to 40 mmol/L), depending on the serum potassium level. Half is sometimes given as potassium chloride and the other half as potassium phosphate. Some treatment regimens use only potassium chloride for potassium replacement, especially if the initial phosphate (PO_4) is high or high-normal on admission, as is most often the case.

    (4) As therapy is begun, potassium concentrations can decline rapidly from those initially obtained because of the expansion of the intravascular volume and increased renal excretion due to improved perfusion of the kidneys, both secondary to rehydration. Increased potassium entry into cells also occurs secondary to insulin administration. When the serum potassium level is <3.0 mEq/L (<3.0 mmol/L), potassium replacement using a solution of potassium >40 mEq/L (>40 mmol/L) may be used, but only with the patient on a cardiac monitor. Patients must be carefully observed.

    (5) Clinically significant signs of hypokalemia include skeletal weakness progressing to paralysis, rapid diminution or absence of deep tendon reflexes, and usually arrhythmias. The development of shallow, gasping respirations (in contrast to Kussmaul's deep ventilation) may also be observed.

(6) Continuous, frequent monitoring of ECG status and serum potassium concentration is essential to guide therapy.

f) Phosphate levels should be measured. Some physicians replace phosphate when PO_4 is low or low-normal by using potassium phosphate. Doses exceeding 1.5 mEq/L/kg (1.5 mmol/L/kg) of body weight/24 hours may cause hypocalcemia.

g) Treatment with sodium bicarbonate ($NaHCO_3$) is controversial and is not recommended by most diabetologists.

(1) Some physicians use $NaHCO_3$ in severe metabolic acidosis, as indicated by an arterial pH of 7.0 or less or a serum bicarbonate level of less than 5 mEq/L (5 mmol/L). Even in this situation, a clinical benefit has not been shown with $NaHCO_3$ therapy,[3] and potassium levels will drop faster and must be monitored closely.

(2) Rapid infusions, or large amounts of $NaHCO_3$ over a short time span, should never be routinely ordered (even if potassium levels are elevated) and should be used only in acute cardiorespiratory arrest situations or to treat hyperkalemia-induced cardiac arrhythmias. Potassium values may drop quickly and to low levels, resulting in dangerous hypokalemic-induced arrhythmias.

(3) If used, $NaHCO_3$ should be given by slow intravenous infusion over several hours. It should never be given as a bolus injection except in a cardiac arrest.

6. Insulin treatment protocols may be varied based on physician preference.

a) All patients with diabetic ketoacidosis need insulin.

b) It takes longer to reverse the acidosis than to treat the hyperglycemia with insulin. Regular (crystalline) insulin should always be used. This produces relatively quick results in glycemic adjustments.

c) Intravenous low-dose continuous infusion of insulin is the most popular method to use.

(1) The benefits of low-dose infusions include the reduced risk of hypoglycemia and hypokalemia because decreases in glucose and potassium levels are more predictable. Additionally, the theoretical risk of cerebral edema is decreased, and the need to "guess" doses and administer repeated intramuscular injections is eliminated.

(2) A disadvantage is the increased nursing care required.

(3) The following is a suggested approach for low-dose infusion.

(a) The insulin is administered through a piggyback system into the existing intravenous (IV) line; use a special pump or pediatric drip set.

(b) Attach IV tubing and preflush with at least 50 mL of infusion to allow insulin to bind to the plastic tubing if larger volume containers are used. This ensures that the infusion entering the circulation contains the correct amount of insulin. It is not necessary to use albumin.

(c) Some physicians give 0.1 to 0.2 units/kg of body weight of regular insulin intravenously as a bolus. However, no benefit has been documented.[4]

(d) In children, give 0.1 to 0.2 units/kg of body weight of regular insulin per hour as a continuous infusion. In adults, the rate should be 3 to 10 units per hour as a continuous infusion.

(e) Expect the glucose level to drop approximately 75 to 100 mg/dL/hr (4.2 to 5.5 mmol/L/hr) with proper rehydration and insulin therapy. In the absence of appropriate fluid replacement, insulin will not be very effective in lowering glucose concentrations.

(f) Monitor blood glucose levels after 1 hour and then every 1 to 2 hours. Double the insulin infusion rate if the glucose level has not dropped by 10% over 2 hours *and* the patient is being adequately hydrated. Check electrolyte values every 2 to 4 hours as needed. Urinary ketone bodies may take several days to clear and their presence is not useful for management decisions.

(g) Subcutaneous insulin may be given when the patient is able to eat.

d) Low-dose intramuscular (not subcutaneous) insulin injections are an alternative treatment for DKA.

(1) Benefits of this method over low-dose continuous infusion therapy include a protocol that is easier for staff to comprehend, no complex apparatus needed to deliver the insulin, and no complicated calculations required for mixing the insulin solution.

(2) Potential problems include patient discomfort from frequent injections and minimal numbers of injection sites for repeated injections.

(3) Dosage calculations are determined the same way as they would be for continuous low-dose infusion but the amount per hour is administered intramuscularly instead of intravenously.

7. Response to therapy can, in most instances, be predicted. Glucose levels should fall at the rate of approximately 75 to 100 mg/dL/hr (4.2 to 5.5 mmol/L/hr). Ketosis should be reversed in 12 to 24 hours, although occasionally urinary ketone bodies may be present for several days.

a) The time-course for the reversal of acidosis has not been well studied because serial pH measurements are not carried out. However, as most patients recover from DKA, they go through a transient state of *hyperchloremic acidosis.*[1] This is manifested by bicarbonate levels plateauing at approximately 15 to 20 mEq/L (15 to 20 mmol/L), usually between 12 to 24 hours after treatment is started. Chloride levels are elevated, pH has returned to normal, and serum ketone bodies are low or absent. Patients do not require additional insulin as this is temporary and recovery to a normal acid-base status occurs naturally.

b)   Mortality is less than 10%, with most deaths occurring in older patients primarily because of medical complications other than DKA.[2] Older age and depth of coma are the best prognostic indicators. Death is usually due to infection, arterial thrombosis, or unrelenting shock.

(1)   Even in the most controlled environment, complications in the treatment of DKA can occur. These might include aspiration, unrecognized renal tubular necrosis, pulmonary edema, and unsuccessfully treated precipitating causes.

(2)   Cerebral edema occurs rarely, but is the primary cause of death in children who succumb to DKA. When the patient's mental function begins to improve and then deteriorates while the metabolic condition continues to return to normal, cerebral edema should be suspected. One factor contributing to the development of cerebral edema may be the rate of fall of the blood glucose level. Too rapid a decline may predispose to cerebral edema. Other unknown factors are undoubtedly involved as well.

(3)   Addition of intravenous glucose to the regimen is important once the serum glucose level reaches 250 mg/dL (13.9 mmol/L).

(4)   Treatment of cerebral edema, if it occurs, should include IV osmotic diuretics (Mannitol) and possibly high-dose glucocorticoids (dexamethasone). The earlier the treatment, the better the prognosis.

8. Frequent errors made in the management of DKA include delay in diagnosis or misdiagnosis, delay in instituting therapy, and inadequate fluid replacement. Patients may be misdiagnosed as having gastroenteritis or appendicitis.

   a) Hypokalemia and cerebral edema may also go unrecognized, causing critical delays in the institution of appropriate therapy for these conditions.

   b) It is essential for nurses to assess mental status frequently (every 1 or 2 hours), especially in children, who are more susceptible to cerebral edema than adults. Treatment of cerebral edema at early stages may be beneficial but is usually ineffective at later stages.

9. Prevention of DKA is the best therapy.

   a) Refer to Chapter XII: Managing Diabetes During Intercurrent Illness for more detail on self-management guidelines for patients.

   b) The patient's knowledge and actual use of sick-day management skills should be evaluated following an episode of DKA. Frequent errors include omitting insulin when unable to eat, not monitoring glucose levels frequently enough, and failing to test urine for ketone bodies. The patient and family should understand the specifics of "what to do differently next time."

   c) A multidisciplinary team approach, including psychological intervention, is critical in caring for patients with recurrent episodes of DKA.

F. Hyperglycemic Hyperosmolar Nonketotic Syndrome (HHNS)

1. HHNS is sometimes overlooked and oftentimes confused with other illnesses or conditions.

   a) Unlike DKA, which only occurs in IDDM patients (young or old), HHNS is more commonly found in elderly patients with mild or previously undiagnosed NIDDM.

   b) HHNS often occurs in elderly patients who are taking oral hypoglycemic agents and who may be inadequately monitored; eg, nursing home residents, those who live alone, and elderly hospitalized patients who are not receiving adequate fluid intake and are often unable to communicate their needs. HHNS is often precipitated by illness or other stresses.

c) The symptoms that normally signal the onset of HHNS may go unrecognized for several weeks in the elderly. The absence of significant ketosis (<2+ in a nitroprusside test in a 1:1 dilution of plasma) differentiates HHNS from DKA.

d) The mortality rate in HHNS is greater than in DKA because of misdiagnosis, delay in diagnosis, or other complications in elderly patients.

2. Precipitating factors may include massive fluid loss from prolonged osmotic diuresis secondary to hyperglycemia, severe burns, severe diarrhea, hemodialysis, peritoneal dialysis, and the use of thiazide or other diuretics.

a) Other causes are infections, myocardial infarction, gastrointestinal hemorrhage, uremia, and arterial thrombosis.

b) Hypertonic feeding (prolonged parenteral nutrition via IV infusion, high-protein or gastric tube feeding) and pharmacologic agents (thiazides, propranolol, Dilantin, steroids, Lasix, Hygroton) may precipitate the onset of HHNS.

G. The Pathophysiology of HHNS

1. HHNS is considered to be a syndrome with four primary features: severe hyperglycemia, absence of ketosis, profound dehydration, and neurologic manifestations.

a) HHNS is similar to DKA except that insulin deficiency is probably not so profound, so increased lipolysis does not occur (see Fig. XI.1).[4]

b) The lack of ketosis and acidosis lessens the gastrointestinal symptoms so that patients do not seek medical care as quickly. Consequently, the prolonged osmotic diuresis and dehydration secondary to hyperglycemia lead to decreased renal blood flow and allow glucose concentrations to reach a very high level.

c) Impaired thirst mechanism or impaired ability to replace fluids, especially in the elderly, will exacerbate the tendency towards HHNS. Patients have longer to lose fluids, so may be more dehydrated than in DKA. Thus, BUN and creatinine levels may be higher.

d) Because HHNS patients are more dehydrated, mentation changes are more commonly seen than in DKA.

H. Signs and Symptoms of HHNS

1. The signs and symptoms of HHNS are similar to DKA, with several important exceptions. The gastrointestinal symptoms are usually milder than those found in DKA.

2. Kussmaul's respiration is seldom observed because of a lack of severe acidosis.

3. Decreased mentation (eg, lethargy, mild confusion) is common in HHNS. Frank coma is unusual. As in DKA, mentation correlates best with serum osmolality.

4. Patients with HHNS may also have focal neurological signs (hemisensory deficits, hemiparesis, aphasia, and seizures) that mimic a cerebrovascular accident. These signs will clear as biochemical status is restored to normal. (Comparisons between DKA and HHNS are noted in Table XI.2).

I. Initial Laboratory Values

1. Appropriate laboratory tests such as a complete blood cell (CBC) count, roentgenogram, and cultures (blood, urine, and sputum) may help identify the precipitating cause of HHNS.

TABLE XI.2:
Diabetic Ketoacidosis (DKA) and Hyperglycemic Hyperosmolar Nonketotic Syndrome (HHNS): Comparison of Some Salient Features

	Conditions	
Feature	**DKA**	**HHNS**
Age of patients	Usually <40 years	Usually >60 years
Duration of symptoms	Usually <2 days	Usually >5 days
Glucose level	Usually <600 mg/dL (<33.3 mmol/L)	Usually >800 mg/dL (>44.4 mmol/L)
Sodium concentration	More likely to be normal or low	More likely to be normal or high
Potassium concentration	High, normal, or low	High, normal, or low
Bicarbonate concentration	Low	Normal
Ketone bodies	At least 4+ in 1:1 dilution	<2+ in 1:1 dilution
pH	Low	Normal
Serum osmolality	Usually <350 mOsm/kg (<350 mmol/kg)	Usually >350 mOsm/kg (>350 mmol/kg)
Cerebral edema	Often subclinical; occasionally clinical	Subclinical has not been evaluated; rarely clinical
Prognosis	3% to 10% mortality	10% to 20% mortality
Subsequent course	Insulin therapy required in virtually all cases	Insulin therapy not required in many cases

Source: Adapted with permission from Davidson.[1]

2. Glucose level is usually >800 mg/dL (44.4 mmol/L).

3. Ketone bodies are not present in the blood or urine except in small amounts.

4. Osmolality is markedly elevated.

J. Treatment of HHNS

1. The primary treatment goal is rehydration to restore circulating plasma volume and correct electrolyte deficits. Additional

treatment goals are similar to those for DKA: to provide adequate insulin to restore and maintain normal glucose metabolism; to prevent complications due to treatment of HHNS; to treat any underlying medical condition; and to provide patient/family education and follow-up.

2. Treatment is based on fluid and electrolyte replacement and administration of insulin.[1,4,5]

3. As in DKA, fluid replacement depends on the patient's state of hydration and cardiovascular status. Hydrate elderly patients with caution.

   a) Because older patients are more likely to have a compromised cardiovascular status, fluid replacement with saline should be done cautiously.

   b) Patients need to be examined frequently to ensure that they are not developing congestive heart failure.

   c) Patients with a previous history of cardiovascular disease should be monitored by central venous pressure (CVP) or Swan-Ganz catheter.

4. Although glucose levels will not decrease appreciably without adequate rehydration, insulin administration is also an important treatment of HHNS. In general, follow the same guidelines as in DKA. Glucose and electrolyte levels should be followed every 2 to 4 hours until stable. Because treatment of acidosis is not part of HHNS, insulin can be decreased when glucose values reach acceptable levels.

5. To prevent HHNS from occurring, identify high-risk patients, keep elderly patients well hydrated, and educate patients and family on warning signs and symptoms.

   a) See Chapter XII: Managing Diabetes During Intercurrent Illness for more detail on self-management guidelines for patients/families.

   b) Professional education regarding HHNS and its management will prepare the clinician for this situation.

REFERENCES

1. Davidson MB. Diabetic ketoacidosis and hyperosmolar non-ketotic coma. In: Davidson MB, ed. Diabetes mellitus: diagnosis and treatment. 3rd ed. New York: Churchill Livingstone, 1991:175-212.

2. Walker M, Marshall SM, Alberti KGMM. Clinical aspects of diabetic ketoacidosis. Diabetes/Metab Rev 1989;5:651-63.

3. Morris LR, Murphy MB, Kitabchi AG. Bicarbonate therapy in severe diabetic ketoacidosis. Ann Intern Med 1986;105:836-40.

4. Carroll P, Matz R. Uncontrolled diabetes mellitus in adults: experience in treating diabetic ketoacidosis and hyperosmolar non-ketotic coma with low dose insulin and a uniform treatment regimen. Diabetes Care 1983;6:579-85.

5. Matz R. Hyperosmolar nonacidotic uncontrolled diabetes: not a rare event. Clin Diabetes 1988;6:25.

KEY EDUCATIONAL CONSIDERATIONS

1. Recognition of the signs and symptoms of hyperglycemia and the importance of not omitting insulin and encouraging fluids should be emphasized at diagnosis and reinforced regularly. Instructions should also be given to both patient and significant others as to when, whom, and how to call for help. This should also be repeated frequently.

2. Teaching methods should include the use of analogy (in explaining the physiology behind signs and symptoms) and the use of practice through simulation and role-playing (because patients are usually healthy when sick-day guidelines are taught and they may not be required to use them for some time).

3. Patients who are adept at diabetes management should also be instructed about the proper use of fluids (sugared and sugar-free) and supplemental insulin when experiencing hyperglycemia and/or ketonemia.

4. After an acute episode of DKA or HHNS, the patient and family's use of sick-day guidelines should be assessed. Precipitating factors should be reviewed and specific and individualized guidelines developed to prevent reoccurrence. For children and adolescents who experience repeated episodes of DKA, supervision of insulin injections may be necessary.

5. Elderly patients (especially those living alone) should be checked frequently for signs of hyperglycemia or change in mentation to ensure prompt medical care if symptoms develop. In addition, special attention should be given when patients are started on new medications that may exacerbate hyperglycemia.

If you are unsure of the answers to the following questions, please review the materials.

1. What are the precipitating factors in the development of DKA?
2. What is the pathophysiology of DKA?
3. List three presenting signs and symptoms of DKA.
4. What laboratory values indicate DKA?
5. What are the three major goals for the treatment of DKA?
6. What are the two precipitating factors of HHNS?
7. What is the pathophysiology of HHNS?
8. What are the signs and symptoms of HHNS?
9. What is the primary treatment for HHNS?
10. What are two differences in laboratory values between DKA and HHNS?

CASE EXAMPLE

ML is a 72-year-old woman who lives alone. On the day of hospital admission, she was brought to her physician's office by a daughter. At that time, she had a chief complaint of confusion and weakness. She was oriented to person, time, and place but was obviously mentally slow. ML's daughter reported that her mother had had hypertension for many years and been treated with medication. According to her daughter, ML was on a thiazide diuretic and the dosage was recently increased to twice daily. ML had noted increasing thirst and urination over the past month and had been weak and shaky. A fingerstick blood glucose test, obtained in the physician's office, was extremely high. ML was sent to the hospital emergency room for further evaluation.

In the emergency room, ML was awake but lethargic and fell asleep during the physical examination. Her skin and mucous membranes appeared quite dry. A sinus tachycardia was present. Physical examination was otherwise unremarkable. Laboratory studies disclosed the following values: blood glucose level, 1630 mg/dL (90.5 mmol/L); sodium, 144 mEq/L (144 mmol/L); potassium, 5.5 mEq/L (5.5 mmol/L); BUN, 79 mg/dL (28 mmol/L); creatinine, 2.8 mg/dL (247 μmol/L); serum osmolality, 361 mOsm/kg (361 mmol/kg); pH, 7.33; and bicarbonate, 18 mEq/L (18 mmol/L). Urine was 5% for glucose and negative to trace for ketone bodies.

QUESTIONS

1. What diagnosis do you think will be made?
2. How do you think this patient will probably be treated?

SUGGESTED SOLUTIONS

A diagnosis of HHNS was established. An IV was started and ML was given an infusion of 0.45% normal saline solution with 20 mEq/L (20 mmol/L) potassium chloride. An insulin infusion was begun at a rate of 10 units/hr. Blood glucose levels and electrolyte levels were checked hourly and the insulin drip was adjusted accordingly. On the day following admission, ML's blood glucose level normalized. She was much more alert and was started on oral fluids. The insulin drip was continued until adequate hydration and oral intake were established. ML was then started on a 1500-calorie ADA diet. Subcutaneous insulin administration was initiated and the dose was adjusted over the next several days. A cardiologist who was consulted about ML's hypertension changed her medications.

During her hospital stay, ML and her daughter were seen by the diabetes nurse educator and the dietitian. ML and her daughter were taught to fill the syringe and administer the insulin. Based on an assessment of ML's needs, the dietitian assisted ML in devising a 1500-calorie meal plan consisting of three meals and a bedtime snack. Blood glucose monitoring equipment was obtained with the assistance of the social worker. Mother and daughter were instructed to check blood glucose levels prior to meals and the bedtime snack. Targets were set for blood glucose control, and ML was asked to call daily for further insulin dose adjustment. Because ML was feeling overwhelmed and frightened by the prospect of being on her own at home, a referral was made for a home health nurse to visit daily to provide more extensive diabetes education and to monitor control.

ML's saga is a typical one. Many elderly patients are on medications that can precipitate the onset of diabetes. Classic symptoms may go unnoticed for a period of time because of solitary life styles typical of this age group. ML was fortunate to have received treatment leading to recovery because the mortality rate from this complication is high. She needs lots of support on an ongoing basis to prevent further episodes of HHNS.

OTHER SUGGESTED READINGS

Davidson MB. Diabetes mellitus: diagnosis and treatment. 3rd ed. New York: Churchill Livingstone, 1991.

Matz R. Hyperosmolor nonacidotic diabetes. In: Rifkin H, Porte Jr D, eds. Ellenberg and Rifkin's diabetes mellitus: theory and practice. 4th ed. New York: Elsevier Science Publishing, 1990:617-25.

Sabo CE, Michael SR. Diabetic ketoacidosis: pathophysiology, nursing diagnosis and nursing interventions. Focus Crit Care 1989;16:21-28.

Sperling MA. Diabetic ketoacidosis in children. In: Lebovitz HE, ed. Therapy for diabetes mellitus and related disorders. Alexandria, Va: American Diabetes Association, 1991:36-43.

Walker M, Marshall SM, Alberti KGMM. Clinical aspects of diabetic ketoacidosis. Diabetes/Metab Rev 1989;5:651-63.

White NH, Henry DN. Special issues in diabetes management. In: Haire-Joshu D, ed. Management of diabetes mellitus: perspectives of care across the life span. St Louis: Mosby Year Book, 1992.

MANAGEMENT

XII. MANAGING DIABETES DURING INTERCURRENT ILLNESS

INTRODUCTION

Illness can cause special problems in managing diabetes. During times of illness, the body releases stress hormones that oppose the action of insulin, contributing to hyperglycemia and the formation and accumulation of ketones. If appropriate action is not taken, dehydration and ketosis can result, requiring hospitalization. This chapter will address the knowledge and skills needed by health care professionals and patients to manage diabetes during illness, minimizing the risk of hospitalization.

OBJECTIVES

On completion of this chapter, the learner will be able to:
- describe the physiological effects of illness on blood glucose levels, ketone levels, and fluid and electrolyte balance;
- identify specific guidelines that health care professionals can follow when managing patients with intercurrent illnesses;
- identify situations that require examination and possible treatment in an office, emergency room, or hospital setting.

A. **Physiologic Effects of Illness on Blood Glucose Levels, Ketone Levels, and Fluid and Electrolyte Balance**

1. Physiological stress can be caused by injury, emotional trauma, surgery, drugs, infection, or intercurrent illnesses.

2. During illness (and with other forms of physiological stress), there is an increase in the secretion of *counterregulatory hormones* including cortisol, epinephrine, growth hormone, and glucagon.[1,2]

3. In insulin-dependent diabetes mellitus (IDDM), also called type I diabetes, counterregulatory hormones cause these metabolic changes: glycogenolysis, lipolysis, gluconeogenesis, and ketogenesis.[3,4]
   a) Counterregulatory hormones contribute to the release of glucose from the liver.
   b) Counterregulatory hormones oppose the action of insulin.

4. Clinical manifestations become evident.
   a) Blood glucose levels increase due to glycogenolysis and gluconeogenesis.
   b) Ketones are present due to lipolysis and ketogenesis.

5. With hyperglycemia, urine flow is increased due to osmotic diuresis; fluid requirements increase.
   a) Signs and symptoms resulting from increased urine flow can include muscle weakness and fatigue related to sodium, potassium, and phosphorus loss.
   b) Signs and symptoms related to increased fluid requirements include polydipsia and dry mouth.

6. With ketosis, signs and symptoms include nausea and anorexia.

7. If hyperglycemia persists, dehydration can occur. Vomiting and diarrhea can be warning signs of dehydration.

8. If ketosis goes untreated, acidosis can result, requiring hospitalization. Warning signals include fruity acidic breath, abdominal pain, and/or rapid, labored breathing/Kussmaul respirations.

9. In non-insulin-dependent diabetes mellitus (NIDDM), also called type II diabetes, hyperglycemic hyperosmolar nonketotic syndrome (HHNS) can occur.
   a) HHNS, a manifestation of severe metabolic decompensation, often is not considered a distinct disorder.[5]
   b) HHNS is seen most often in the elderly, who have poor fluid intake or lack a normal thirst mechanism.[6]
   c) Recommendations for prevention and early treatment are similar to those for diabetic ketoacidosis.
   d) Severe hyperglycemia occurs with glucose levels greater than 600 mg/dL (33.3 mmol/L).
   e) In NIDDM, volume depletion results but ketogenesis usually is suppressed secondary to some residual insulin secretion.

f) If undetected, lethargy, impaired mental status, or coma may result.[7]

g) Individuals must be hospitalized for treatment.

B. Guidelines for the Health Care Professional Managing Persons with Diabetes on Sick Days

1. Increase the frequency of monitoring during illness.

   a) The signs and symptoms of a developing acute illness can be signaled by higher than usual blood glucose levels, ketone levels, and, for some, urine glucose levels.

   b) More frequent monitoring is indicated when the person experiences unusual physical symptoms, such as malaise, anorexia, and nausea, or when blood glucose levels are rising. These symptoms may disappear or may develop into an identifiable illness.

   c) The frequency of blood or urine glucose monitoring may need to be increased to every 4 to 6 hours while levels are elevated and/or until symptoms subside. Urine ketone levels also should be tested every 4 to 6 hours.

   d) Monitoring is performed at times when decisions must be made regarding the insulin dose. Preferred times to check the blood glucose and urine ketones on sick days are before usual breakfast time, before usual lunch time, before usual dinner time, and at usual bedtime.

   e) Patients should be instructed to record the monitoring results to read over the telephone to the health care professional if needed.

2. Continue and possibly increase medication during illness.

   a) Insulin or oral hypoglycemic agents are still needed during illness even when the patient is unable to eat. Omission of insulin is a common cause of ketosis. The routine dose of intermediate- or long-acting insulin (NPH, Lente, Ultralente) should be continued. Usually, the full dose of daily insulin is required.

   b) Supplemental doses of short-acting insulin (regular) also may be required for continuously rising or persistent high blood glucose levels, large ketones, or persistent ketones. The patient should call the health care professional for instructions on taking extra insulin.

    (1)   Regular insulin may be given every 4 to 6 hours.

    (2)   The doses of regular insulin depend on the severity of the illness. Ten percent of the total daily dose as a supplemental dose of regular insulin is safe during most illnesses. If the blood glucose is higher than 300 mg/dL (16.7 mmol/L) with large ketones, 20% of the routine dose may be given.

    (3)   In the rare event that hypoglycemia exists, the short-acting insulin should be decreased, but the intermediate- or long-acting insulin should be maintained.

    c)   Over-the-counter and prescribed medications may contribute to hyperglycemia or hypoglycemia (see Chapter VIII: Pharmacologic Therapies).

    d)   Labels on over-the-counter products used to treat cold symptoms often advise against use by persons with diabetes. There are two approaches regarding the use of over-the-counter medications to treat cold symptoms in persons with diabetes.

    (1)   Use of antihistamines/decongestants and cough medicines is acceptable if the patient is performing blood glucose monitoring every 4 to 6 hours and calling the health care professional when levels are elevated. Insulin dose adjustments can be made for hyperglycemia.

    (2)   Use sugar-free antihistamines/decongestants and cough medicines to avoid adding simple sugars that could elevate blood glucose levels.[8]

3.   To maintain adequate hydration, patients should be encouraged to drink at least 8 ounces (240 mL) of calorie-free fluid every hour while they are awake. Decreased fluid intake, polyuria, and evaporative losses from fever, vomiting, and diarrhea all can contribute to dehydration. Examples of calorie-free liquids include diet colas or sodas, water, broth, and sugar-free Kool-Aid®.

Because caffeine acts as a diuretic, the fluids consumed should be non-caffeinated. Bouillon, consomme, and canned clear soups provide sodium as well as fluids.

4. If the patient is unable to tolerate fluids by mouth, antiemetics may be prescribed or intravenous fluids may be required.

5. If nausea or anorexia makes patients unable to tolerate solid foods at meal times, clear liquids should be encouraged.

    a) If the blood glucose level is higher than 250 to 300 mg/dL (13.9 to 16.7 mmol/L) or urine glucose is 2%, the patient should continue to drink calorie-free liquids at that mealtime.

    b) If the blood glucose is 180 to 250 mmol/L (10 to 13.9 mmol/L) the patient should drink or eat the equivalent of 15 grams of carbohydrate at that mealtime.

    c) With intestinal viruses, if the patient's blood glucose level is less than 180 mg/dL (10 mmol/L) or urine glucose is 1% or less prior to a meal, the patient should consume more easily tolerated foods or beverages equivalent to the usual meal plan in carbohydrate content. Note that many people regain their appetite when blood glucose levels return to less than 180 mg/dL (10 mmol/L).

    d) The following information can be used as a guide by the health care professional to calculate sample sick-day meal plans for patients using ADA exchanges:

        (1) Each *Starch/Bread* exchange contains 15 grams of carbohydrate.

        (2) Each *Fruit* exchange contains 15 grams of carbohydrate.

        (3) Each *Milk* exchange contains 12 grams of carbohydrate.

e) The following foods and beverages contain approximately 15 grams of carbohydrate and may be substituted for either one fruit or one starch/bread exchange:

$\frac{1}{2}$ cup apple juice

$\frac{1}{2}$ - $\frac{3}{4}$ cup *regular* carbonated beverage (not diet)

$\frac{3}{4}$ of a double-stick Popsicle®

5 Lifesavers®

1 slice dry toast

$\frac{1}{2}$ cup cooked cereal

6 saltines

1 cup broth-based soup

$\frac{1}{3}$ cup frozen yogurt

1 cup Gatorade®

3 teaspoons honey

$\frac{1}{2}$ cup regular vanilla ice cream

$\frac{1}{4}$ cup sherbet

$\frac{1}{4}$ cup regular pudding

$\frac{1}{3}$ cup *sweetened* gelatin/Jell-O®

f) The following foods contain approximately 12 grams of carbohydrate and may be substituted for one milk exchange:

Milkshake ($\frac{1}{3}$ cup milk and $\frac{1}{4}$ cup vanilla ice cream)

1 cup nonfat, sugar-free yogurt (*not* frozen)

g) EXAMPLE:

(1) If an ADA exchange meal plan is followed and one meal includes:

1 milk exchange (12 g/exchange)	= 12	g
2 starch exchanges (15 g/exchange)	= 30	g
1 fruit exchange (15 g/exchange)	= 15	g
Total	= 57	g

To replace this meal, 57 g of carbohydrate are needed. Note: It is not necessary to replace meat and fat exchanges during a brief illness.

(2) The sample meal plan in (1) contained 57 g carbohydrate that needed to be replaced. A substitute meal could include:

1 cup carbonated beverage	= 20 g
3 saltines	= 7.5 g
$^2/_3$ cup Jell-O®	= 30 g
Total Carbohydrate Replaced	= 57.5 g

Note: For those who are nauseated, vomiting, or unable to tolerate a large volume of fluids, taking in approximately 15 grams of carbohydrate over 1 to 2 hours can be recommended as a "sipping diet."

6. The patient should know which conditions necessitate an immediate telephone call to their health care provider.

a) Some patients hesitate to telephone the health care professional, concerned that their call might be a bother. Patients should be encouraged to call when questions and problems arise.

b) The patient should be instructed to call a health care professional immediately in the following situations:

(1) Vomiting occurs more than once.

(2) Diarrhea occurs more than five times or longer than 24 hours.

(3) Breathing is difficult.

(4) Blood glucose levels are higher than 300 mg/dL (16.7 mmol/L) on two consecutive measurements.

(5) Urine ketones measure moderate or large.

C. Situations that Require Examination and Possible Treatment in an Office, Emergency Room, or Hospital Setting

1. The health care professional should determine if telephone management is possible or if an assessment and evaluation in the clinic or emergency room is indicated.

2. The following signs and symptoms indicate a need for examination, treatment, and possible hospital admission:

a) Persistent vomiting or an inability to tolerate fluids by mouth.
b) Persistent diarrhea and progressive weakness.
c) Difficulty breathing, rapid and labored respirations.
d) Moderate or large ketones which do not improve after 12 to 24 hours of treatment.
e) Change in mental status.

REFERENCES

1. Schade DS, Eaton RP. The controversy concerning counterregulatory hormone secretion: a hypothesis for the prevention of diabetic ketoacidosis? Diabetes 1977;26(6):596-99.

2. Schade DS, Eaton RP. Pathogenesis of diabetic ketoacidosis: a reappraisal. Diabetes Care 1979;2(3):296-306.

3. Alberti KGMM, Christensen NJ, Iversen J, Orskov H. Role of glucagon and other hormones in development of diabetic ketoacidosis. Lancet 1975;1:1307-11.

4. Keller U, Schnell H, Girard J, Stauffacher W. Effect of physiological elevation of plasma growth hormone levels on ketone body kinetics and lipolysis in normal and acutely insulin-deficient man. Diabetologia 1984;26:103-8.

5. Genuth S. Diabetic ketoacidosis and hyperglycemic hyperosmolar coma in adults. In: Lebovitz HE, ed. Therapy for diabetes mellitus and related disorders. Alexandria, Va: American Diabetes Association, 1991:63-75.

6. Carroll P, Matz R. Uncontrolled diabetes mellitus in adults: experience in treating diabetic ketoacidosis and hyperosmolar nonketotic coma with low-dose insulin and a uniform treatment regimen. Diabetes Care 1983;6(6):579-85.

7. Minaker KL. What diabetologists should know about elderly patients. Diabetes Care 1990;13(suppl 2):34-46.

8. Campbell RK. Treating the common cold without sugar. Diabetes Professional 1988;(summer):15-19.

KEY EDUCATIONAL CONSIDERATIONS

1. Sick-day management is a basic survival skill and should be taught at an appropriate level to all patients.

2. Sick-day instruction and reinforcement should be considered a priority before a hospital discharge; before starting day care, school, or college; before the flu season; when administering the flu vaccine; and before overnight travel away from home. Learning is reinforced and retained when it is applied immediately. Because sick-day guidelines usually are taught when patients are healthy, and the guidelines are not applied immediately, evaluation should include assessing the patient's immediate and long-term recall of gained knowledge. Actual use of the skills should be evaluated during and following an intercurrent illness.

3. Use props and simulations for reinforcement and to assist the patient in recalling the sick-day guidelines at a later date. For example, show ketone testing materials, regular insulin, and an 8-ounce plastic glass, and use a telephone call role-play to emphasize sick-day guidelines as you provide instruction.

4. Give patients written instructions as reinforcement, keeping sick-day guidelines as simple as possible. If appropriate, ask the patient to copy the guidelines or take notes on the provided handout to enhance retention. Assist the patient in determining where the guidelines will be posted or placed for easy access when needed.

5. Ask the patient to pack a sick-day box with supplies and nonperishable items that can be stored for use during illness. Acknowledge that the patient may not be accustomed to keeping glucose-containing products such as regular Jell-O®, regular cola, or regular Gatorade® at home. Review the rationale for keeping these items on hand for sick days and assist the patient in determining a site for storage or placement.

6. During an illness, many patients experience malaise, fatigue, and sleepiness, making self-care more difficult. Therefore, family members or significant others should be familiar with sick-day guidelines and

should know where sick-day supplies and instructions are kept. A plan for their role and participation should be negotiated.

SELF-REVIEW QUESTIONS

If you are unsure of the answers to the following questions, please review the materials.

1. What are the physiologic effects of illness on blood glucose levels, ketone levels, and fluid and electrolyte balance?
2. Discuss specific guidelines that health care professionals may use when managing patients with intercurrent illnesses.
3. List situations that require examination and possible treatment in an office, emergency room, or hospital setting during an illness.

CASE EXAMPLE

RS is a 32-year-old sales representative who was diagnosed with insulin-dependent diabetes mellitus (IDDM) one year ago. He manages his diabetes with a split-mixed regimen of insulin consisting of intermediate- and short-acting insulin before breakfast and before dinner. He monitors his blood glucose twice a day, follows a meal plan, and has been instructed on the recognition and treatment of hypoglycemia, ketone testing, and sick-day management. RS returns to the clinic for follow-up once every 3 to 4 months.

This morning he telephones to report that he is feeling nauseated. He states that his blood glucose level before breakfast was 233 mg/dL, he administered his usual dose of insulin, and then was only able to drink one fruit-juice-sized glass of apple juice before becoming nauseated. It is now noon and he is still nauseated and does not feel like eating lunch or going to the office. He reports that he vaguely recalls being instructed on sick-day management, but he is unsure what he should do because this is his first episode of being sick since diagnosis.

QUESTIONS

1. What additional assessment data should you obtain at this point?
2. What instruction and/or advice might be given?

SUGGESTED SOLUTIONS

Information to determine if the patient's condition is stable should include whether the patient has been vomiting or experiencing diarrhea, how often, and for how many hours. The health care professional should be listening for symptoms of respiratory distress and ask whether the patient has had difficulty breathing. Although diabetic ketoacidosis develops over hours, the possibility exists that the patient may not have performed the SBGM procedure properly, thereby skewing the result. RS reported no vomiting, diarrhea, or respiratory distress.

Once acute distress is ruled out, recent blood glucose and urine ketone results would be needed. RS had not tested his blood glucose since before breakfast and had not checked for ketones. He was given positive reinforcement for calling for advice and was asked to obtain blood glucose and urine ketone measurements. Depending on the circumstances, the health care professional may wait for the patient to report the testing results or ask the patient to call back immediately with the results. RS reported a blood glucose value of 363 mg/dL and a small amount of ketones. Morning fluid intake was assessed and RS reported that he had been sipping on a diet soft drink during the morning because of thirst. However, because of nausea he had consumed only a total of approximately 8 ounces. He reported eating no solid foods.

Reinforcing the rationale, RS was given reassurance that administering his morning dose of insulin was appropriate. He then was instructed to administer a supplemental dose of regular insulin immediately after the telephone conversation. Because his blood glucose was 363 mg/dL he was instructed to have bouillon (a source of sodium and fluid) and a diet soft drink for lunch — both items were on hand and were choices he liked. He also was told to drink 8 ounces of fluid every hour during the afternoon and evening hours, drinking in sips if necessary. Avoiding dehydration by consuming plenty of fluids was explained.

RS was instructed to retest his blood glucose and urine ketone levels in 3 hours, pre-supper (7 P.M.), and at bedtime. He was told to call if his blood glucose values were higher than 300 mg/dL and if he had moderate or large ketones. RS was encouraged to telephone the clinic immediately if vomiting occurred more than once, if he experienced more than five episodes of diarrhea, or he had difficulty breathing.

OTHER SUGGESTED READINGS

Ley B, Goldman D. Sick-day management: preparing for the unexpected. Diabetes Spectrum 1991;4:173-76.

Spencer ML. Immediate complications: the ups and downs of blood glucose. In: Franz MJ, Etzwiler DD, Joynes JO, Hollander PM, eds. Learning to live well with diabetes. Minneapolis: DCI Publishing, 1991:185-88.

MANAGEMENT

XIII.   HYPOGLYCEMIA

INTRODUCTION

Hypoglycemia is the most frequently encountered acute complication of therapy in insulin-treated patients with diabetes mellitus. The risk of severe hypoglycemia is greatly increased among patients with insulin-dependent diabetes mellitus (IDDM), also called type I diabetes, using intensive regimens designed to achieve near-normal levels of glycemia.[1,2] Hypoglycemia is also a complication of treatment with oral hyperglycemic agents.

An understanding of the clinical settings and physiologic alterations that result in or increase the risk of hypoglycemia, as well as its treatment and prevention, is an essential component of comprehensive diabetes education.

OBJECTIVES

Upon completion of this chapter, the learner will be able to:

- define three clinical levels of hypoglycemia with associated signs and symptoms;
- describe the physiologic alterations associated with hypoglycemia;
- identify the primary causes of hypoglycemia in insulin-treated patients;
- describe appropriate treatment for each level of hypoglycemia;
- list three major concepts related to the prevention of hypoglycemia that patients should understand;
- state the major approaches to counter hypoglycemia unawareness.

A. Clinical Levels of Hypoglycemia

1. It is generally accepted that a blood glucose level below 70 mg/dL (3.9 mmol/L) should alert the patient of impending hypoglycemia. *Biochemical hypoglycemia* can be defined as a blood glucose level below 50 mg/dL (2.8 mmol/L)[3] (whole blood) with or without the presence of symptoms known to be associated with hypoglycemia. This biochemical definition,

which does not require the presence of subjective interpretation of symptoms, may not be clinically useful.

2. *Clinical severity of hypoglycemia* is poorly correlated with biochemical measures. The blood glucose level that elicits symptoms and the magnitude of the symptoms depend on various modifying variables that may differ from individual to individual and within the same individual from episode to episode.[4] For example, some patients remain alert with few symptoms at blood glucose levels of 40 mg/dL (2.2 mmol/L), while others may develop coma at this same glucose concentration. Also, an individual patient may tolerate a blood glucose level of 40 mg/dL (2.2 mmol/L) on one occasion but be incapacitated at the same blood glucose level on another occasion. The following definitions of three levels of hypoglycemia, based on clinical rather than biochemical criteria, are useful in caring for and educating patients with diabetes.

   a) *Mild hypoglycemia* can be defined as an episode of hypoglycemia associated with adrenergic or cholinergic symptoms such as pallor, diaphoresis, tachycardia, palpitations, hunger, paresthesias, and shakiness. The patient remains totally alert during these episodes.

      (1) Mild hypoglycemia is easily recognized and self-treated with ingestion of any source of rapidly absorbed carbohydrate.

      (2) In both nondiabetic and diabetic individuals, adrenergic symptoms of hypoglycemia sometimes can be elicited by a rapid decline in blood glucose concentrations even in the absence of biochemical hypoglycemia (eg, a decline in blood glucose level from 200 to 100 mg/dL [11 to 5.5 mmol/L] over a period of less than 1 hour).[5]

      (3) Patients should be instructed to measure their blood glucose level when experiencing symptoms associated with mild hypoglycemia. If this is not possible or practical, patients should treat

symptomatic hypoglycemia, regardless of actual blood glucose level, assuming that biochemical hypoglycemia is present or imminent.

b) *Moderate hypoglycemia* can be defined as an episode of hypoglycemia that is associated with neuroglycopenia, which is defined as impaired function of the central nervous system due to cellular deprivation of glucose.

(1) Common symptoms or signs associated with moderate hypoglycemia include inability to concentrate, confusion, slurred speech, irrational or uncontrolled behavior, slowed reaction time, blurred vision, somnolence, or extreme fatigue.

(2) By definition, this level of hypoglycemia is not severe enough to preclude the patient from seeking food or assistance.

c) *Severe hypoglycemia* can be defined as any episode of hypoglycemia in which the neuroglycopenia is so severe that the patient's neurologic function is impaired and the assistance of another person is required for treatment (eg, to administer oral carbohydrate, glucagon, or IV glucose). Symptoms of severe hypoglycemia may include totally automatic, disoriented behavior, loss of consciousness, inability to arouse from sleep, or seizures.

3. The three definitions of hypoglycemia are intended to help educators and patients understand the spectrum of clinical presentations of hypoglycemia. However, it is extremely important to understand that hypoglycemia does not necessarily progress in the linear order presented.[3] Neuroglycopenic symptoms are not necessarily preceded by adrenergic or cholinergic manifestations such as diaphoresis or tremor. Some patients may miss or ignore adrenergic or cholinergic symptoms that would prompt early treatment of hypoglycemia and progress to frank neuroglycopenia. Others may develop neuroglycopenic symptoms first, followed by adrenergic or cholinergic manifestations.

B. Physiological Alterations and Recovery Associated with Hypoglycemia

1. Recovery from acute insulin-induced hypoglycemia occurs if the release of glucose *counterregulatory hormones*, primarily glucagon and epinephrine, are sufficient to cause an increase in blood glucose.[6,7] During prolonged hypoglycemia, secretion of growth hormone and cortisol also may contribute to the recovery from hypoglycemia. In all cases, the circulating insulin level influences recovery from hypoglycemia. High insulin levels blunt, and lower insulin levels enhance, recovery from hypoglycemia.

    a) In response to hypoglycemia, glucagon secretion results in enhanced hepatic glucose release, which subsequently raises the blood glucose level. Glucagon secretion in response to insulin-induced hypoglycemia frequently is impaired early in the course of IDDM (after 2 to 5 years).

    b) In patients with adequate glucagon secretion, epinephrine serves a secondary role to glucagon in recovery from hypoglycemia.

        (1) Epinephrine assumes a primary role when glucagon secretion is impaired. Epinephrine not only increases hepatic glucose production, it also decreases glucose utilization, thus enhancing recovery from hypoglycemia by two distinct mechanisms.

        (2) Diminished epinephrine secretion, presumably the result of autonomic (sympathetic) neuropathy, or hypoglycemia-associated autonomic failure,[1] usually occurs later in the course of diabetes than does glucagon deficiency.

    c) Diaphoresis that occurs during hypoglycemia is due to activation of cholinergic reflexes and not due to epinephrine.[8]

        (1) Sweating can be seen in some patients even in the absence of increased epinephrine levels during hypoglycemia.

(2) The presence of diaphoresis is not necessarily indicative of sufficient epinephrine secretion to defend against hypoglycemia.

2. Recovery from insulin-induced hypoglycemia is markedly impaired when both glucagon and epinephrine deficiencies are present. This condition is referred to as defective glucose counterregulation.[6,7,9,10] Patients with this condition are at a markedly increased risk for recurrent, severe hypoglycemia, particularly during intensive therapy. Thus, the presence of defective glucose counterregulation or hypoglycemia-associated autonomic failure are limiting factors in attempts at achieving near-normoglycemia in patients with IDDM.

a) Patients should be advised that their symptoms of hypoglycemia may change over time (eg, diminished adrenergic symptoms), resulting in *hypoglycemia unawareness*. Such individuals will need to monitor blood glucose levels more frequently in anticipation of any situation that increases the risk of hypoglycemia.

b) Patients and family often need to be taught to recognize subtle symptoms and signs of hypoglycemia. Glucose treatment targets may need to be adjusted in individuals with repeated episodes of severe hypoglycemia as a result of hypoglycemia unawareness, or in those who are unable or unwilling to follow dietary or glucose-monitoring instructions.

C. Primary Causes of Hypoglycemia

1. Insulin excess, either accidental or deliberate, produces hypoglycemia if not compensated for by increased carbohydrate intake or activation of normal glucose counterregulatory mechanisms.

a) Insulin excess predictably occurs at certain times of the day, depending on the type of insulin replacement regimen used. Overinsulinization is likely during attempts to maintain blood glucose at near normal levels with any form of subcutaneous insulin administration.

  b) Oral hypoglycemic medications also have the potential for causing hypoglycemia, especially if the medication is taken and meals are skipped, or with heavy or prolonged exercise.

2. Inadequate or poorly timed nutrient absorption can cause hypoglycemia.

  a) Obvious causes include delayed or skipped meals, as well as meals with low-carbohydrate content.

  b) Less obvious, sometimes unpredictable, causes include delayed or impaired absorption of carbohydrates due to gastrointestinal neuropathy, delayed gastric emptying, or impaired nutrient absorption.

3. Exercise has both an immediate and a prolonged glucose-lowering effect.[11,12]

  a) Exercise has an immediate glucose-lowering effect.

    (1) Exercise increases glucose utilization by muscle.

    (2) Short-term exercise can accelerate insulin absorption from subcutaneous tissue because of enhanced blood flow at the site of injection. The increase in plasma insulin can inhibit the increase in glucose release by the liver that normally occurs during exercise.

    (3) The combination of decreased glucose production by the liver and increased glucose utilization by muscle predisposes persons with IDDM to hypoglycemia during and shortly after exercise.

  b) Exercise has a prolonged glucose-lowering effect.

    (1) Prolonged strenuous exercise depletes glycogen stores in muscle and the liver, resulting in a subsequent need to replenish these depleted stores with glucose.

    (2) It is possible that the increased movement of glucose into muscle after exercise is mediated through an increase in glucose carrier molecules on the surface

of muscle cells. The key point is that exercise can have long-term glucose-lowering effects.

(3) Prolonged, strenuous exercise can result in lower blood glucose levels for as long as 12 to 24 hours. Thus, an untrained individual who exercises strenuously for a long period during the day may be predisposed to hypoglycemia during sleep.

c) Physical conditioning programs can increase insulin sensitivity and reduce insulin requirements. Thus, lean, well-conditioned patients are much more sensitive to insulin than unconditioned persons of similar weight (see Chapter VII: Exercise).

d) In patients with marked hyperglycemia (glucose levels over 240 mg/dL [13.2 mmol/L]), exercise can cause a paradoxical increase in both blood glucose and urine ketones.[11,12] This increase is due to the unopposed glucose-raising effects of glucagon and epinephrine when insulin levels are low.

4. Ingestion of ethanol, especially in a fasted person, may lead to hypoglycemia due to inhibition of hepatic glucose production (gluconeogenesis).[13] This effect can be seen with as little as 2 or 3 ounces of alcohol. Other drugs, such as propranolol, may mask the early adrenergic warning symptoms commonly associated with hypoglycemia and thus predispose individuals to severe hypoglycemia.

5. Hypoglycemia sometimes also is associated with other conditions.

a) At the onset of menses, a rapid decline in blood progesterone level and other physiologic changes can cause a decline in insulin requirements, thus increasing the risk of hypoglycemia. Women using intensive treatment regimens frequently report higher blood glucose levels just prior to menses followed by a lowering of blood glucose levels immediately after the start of menstrual flow. Treatment of the hyperglycemia with insulin supplements may add to the risk of subsequent hypoglycemia.

b) The immediate postpartum period is associated with an increased risk of hypoglycemia. This risk has been attributed to a rapid reduction in the level of placental hormones, such as placental lactogen, that antagonize insulin action.

c) Autonomic neuropathy, with diminished or absent epinephrine release in response to hypoglycemia, may contribute to hypoglycemia.

   (1) Some patients lose premonitory warning symptoms of hypoglycemia. These individuals with hypoglycemia unawareness have a significantly greater risk of developing severe hypoglycemia.

   (2) Autonomic neuropathy also may cause delayed gastric emptying and increase the risk of hypoglycemia after meals.

d) Substantial lowering of mean blood glucose values using intensive regimens can diminish recognition of hypoglycemic symptoms at blood glucose levels of 40 to 50 mg/dL (2.2 to 2.8 mmol/L).[1,6]

   (1) Patients may become more tolerant (less symptomatic) of blood glucose levels in the 40 to 60 mg/dL (2.2 to 3.3 mmol/L) range after prolonged periods (4 to 8 months) of near-normalization of blood glucose levels. This tolerance may be due to the more frequent occurrence of mild or moderate hypoglycemia.

   (2) Some patients may become mentally and physically more tolerant of hypoglycemia, especially patients who believe that very tight blood glucose control will prevent long-term complications. These patients may engage in risk-taking behaviors that predispose them to more hypoglycemia. They view hypoglycemia as a "necessary evil" and, unless it results in seizure or coma, are willing to accept it as

an inconvenient consequence of their diabetes regimen.

(3) Lowering the threshold for developing hypoglycemic symptoms and hormonal counterregulation may decrease the clinical safety of intensive regimens in patients with IDDM.

D. Treatment of Hypoglycemia

1. The appropriate management of hypoglycemia depends on the type of diabetes treatment; the patient's individual history, occupation, and resources; and the severity and individual symptoms associated with hypoglycemia.

2. Immediate treatment should be given for mild, moderate, and severe hypoglycemia.

   a) Mild hypoglycemia is best treated using 10 to 15 grams of carbohydrate (see Table XIII.1).

      (1) Treatment may need to be repeated in 15 minutes if the symptoms do not abate.

      (2) In most instances, normal activity can be resumed almost immediately following treatment.

      (3) Some health professionals will treat at this stage by administering a small amount of food, such as $1/4$ to $1/2$ glass of milk.

TABLE XIII.1: Carbohydrate Sources (15g) for Treatment of Hypoglycemia

3 glucose tablets (5 g each)	$1/2$ cup fruit juice
2 tablespoons raisins	5 Lifesavers® candy
$1/2$ to $3/4$ cup regular soda (not diet)	1 cup milk

---

b) Moderate hypoglycemia may require larger amounts of rapidly absorbed carbohydrate (15 to 30 g) to reverse symptoms and assure prevention of severe hypoglycemia.

   (1) Patients commonly are asked to follow the carbohydrate, in 10 to 15 minutes, with additional food (eg, lowfat milk, cheese, crackers) after initial symptoms subside. Following treatment, the individual may need to wait 10 to 30 minutes or more before resuming prehypoglycemia activity.

   (2) Blood glucose measurements often are helpful during and after initial treatment to ascertain the actual glucose level and to determine whether treatment has been effective. Neuroglycopenic symptoms (fatigue, somnolence, slurred speech, slowed reaction time, agitated behavior, or transitory hemiparesis) may persist in some cases for an hour or more, even after elevation of blood glucose to values above 100 mg/dL (5.5 mmol/L).

c) Severe hypoglycemia is treated most rapidly by administration of intravenous dextrose (25% or 50%). However, since IV access is rarely available outside of the hospital, severe hypoglycemia is best treated at home by administering glucagon (1 mg for adults and older children, 0.5 mg for children under 5 years of age, and 0.25 mg for infants).

   (1) If the individual experiencing severe hypoglycemia is able to swallow without risk of aspiration, glucose gel, honey, syrup, or jelly can be placed on the inside of the cheek.

   (2) Once the person responds, it is advisable to follow glucose gel, IV glucose, or glucagon administration with some rapid-acting carbohydrate-containing liquid until nausea subsides, then give a small snack or meal.

   (3) Monitoring blood glucose levels frequently for several hours after a severe hypoglycemic episode helps to ensure that the blood glucose level does not

fall again, as well as to prevent overtreatment with resultant hyperglycemia.

(4) The patient is advised to notify a health professional and consult with the primary treatment team following most episodes of severe hypoglycemia.

3. Over 50% of all episodes of severe hypoglycemia occur during the night. Nocturnal hypoglycemia occurs for several reasons. First, many patients are not awakened by early warning symptoms of hypoglycemia. Second, insulin requirements are lower between the hours of midnight and 3 AM (the predawn period) than at dawn. Lastly, intermediate-acting insulins (NPH, Lente) given before dinner may cause a relative hyperinsulinemia in the predawn period.

a) Nocturnal hypoglycemia may be prevented or the frequency may be reduced by employing the following measures.

(1) Monitor 3 AM blood glucose levels at least once a week; monitor more frequently in patients with a history of recurrent nocturnal hypoglycemia.

(2) Monitor 3 AM blood glucose levels following a day of unusual or atypical activity or food consumption, or when insulin doses are being adjusted.

(3) Measure bedtime (presleep snack) glucose levels regularly. A larger snack may be needed if the blood glucose level is less than 120 mg/dL (6.7 mmol/L), especially when daytime activity has been increased. This snack should consist of protein and carbohydrate. The ingested carbohydrate has an immediate effect on blood glucose levels, while the protein helps to maintain glucose levels by stimulating glucagon secretion (even in patients who no longer secrete glucagon in response to hypoglycemia).

(4) Decreasing the predinner NPH or Lente insulin to prevent nocturnal hypoglycemia often results in fasting hyperglycemia. In this case, moving the NPH

or Lente dose to presleep may prevent relative hyperinsulinemia in the predawn period without compromising fasting glucose levels. Using Ultralente insulin, instead of NPH, at supper also may be effective.

4. Overtreatment of hypoglycemia is relatively common. Patients often report consuming excessive amounts of carbohydrate when treating a hypoglycemic episode. Overtreatment can be attributed to both physiological and psychological factors. Some patients will eat until hypoglycemic (primary adrenergic) symptoms abate completely, rather than consuming a more reasonable amount of carbohydrate and waiting to see if symptoms subside or blood glucose levels increase. For other patients, the fear of losing control (primarily neuroglycopenic symptoms) compels them to overtreat hypoglycemic reactions. This fear is especially common in patients who live alone, patients who care for small children, or patients who have experienced severe hypoglycemia in the past that resulted in cognitive impairment. Using rapid-acting, commercially available, portion-controlled glucose products may help some patients avoid overtreating physiologic hypoglycemia. Specific therapeutic interventions that address the fear of hypoglycemia and its effect on metabolic control may be required for patients who overtreat hypoglycemia for psychological reasons.

E. **Psychosocial Variables**

1. In addition to unpleasant physical symptoms, hypoglycemia can lead to socially and occupationally compromising situations secondary to associated cognitive and/or motor dysfunction. Personal or vicarious experiences with hypoglycemia may cause some patients to engage in behaviors specifically intended to avoid low blood glucose values. An excessive "fear of hypoglycemia" can be clinically significant, causing poor adherence to prescribed treatment regimens (eg, patients may avoid hypoglycemia by keeping blood glucose levels elevated

or overtreating early symptoms of hypoglycemia). If these behaviors contribute to poor metabolic control, the following specific therapeutic interventions may be indicated.[14]

   a)   Recognize that fear of hypoglycemia may limit efforts to achieve adequate blood glucose control.

   b)   Utilize behavioral therapy designed to reduce avoidance behaviors.

   c)   Clinicians should routinely look for psychological sequelae to hypoglycemia and its behavioral metabolic consequences, using such tools as the Hypoglycemia Fear Survey.[15]

2.   Symptom detection and interpretation can be confusing for some patients. Not all symptoms of hypoglycemia are unique to this clinical condition. In fact, even if symptoms are detected, competing explanations for these may exist which impair the patient's ability to recognize the symptoms as those of hypoglycemia. For example, sweating may be misattributed to the activity at hand rather than to hypoglycemia. Conversely, patients may attribute hunger or nervousness to a declining blood glucose level, then treat as if hypoglycemia was imminent, and subsequently experience hyperglycemia.

3.   Some people may deny symptoms of hypoglycemia because these symptoms represent failure in their self-management, interference with pleasurable activities, incompetence as a professional or caretaker, or admission to having a chronic illness.[4]

F.   Prevention of Hypoglycemia

1.   Educating patients regarding the signs, symptoms, causes, and treatment of hypoglycemia is the mainstay of prevention. For example, patients and family members must know that delaying a meal more than 30 to 60 minutes, or skipping an afternoon snack increases the likelihood of hypoglycemia. For this reason,

patients should be instructed to carry a source of carbohydrate (at least 10 to 15 grams) at all times.

2. Instruct patients to measure their blood glucose level or treat themselves at the first indication of possible hypoglycemia. Initially, frequent blood glucose monitoring may be necessary to help differentiate between symptoms due to mild hypoglycemia and similar symptoms due to other causes. Teach patients that after oral carbohydrate administration for mild or moderate hypoglycemia, it may take 10 to 20 minutes for blood glucose levels to rise and for symptoms to resolve. Teach patients how to measure blood glucose while traveling or at work or school.

3. Hypoglycemia that occurs on a daily basis requires some adjustment in the treatment plan. Adults trying to lose weight or maintain their current weight may need to have their total insulin or oral agent dosage decreased. Children or thin adults may be able to increase daily caloric intake.

4. Educate household or family members and close friends about hypoglycemia, and when and how to measure blood glucose levels. Teach family members and friends how and when to administer glucagon, and to make sure glucagon is available to all insulin-treated patients.

5. Institute an individual program of blood glucose monitoring that is acceptable to the patient. Additional monitoring should be recommended during times of changing the insulin or oral agent dose, activity levels, or dietary intake. Additional monitoring is especially important when trying to lose weight.

6. Teach patients to monitor blood glucose levels before, during, and after strenuous or irregular exercise. When appropriate, teach patients algorithms for altering insulin dose and/or caloric intake prior to, during, or after exercise. The person initiating an exercise program or successfully losing weight will need to

be aware of signs that suggest a need to reduce oral agents and/or insulin.

7. Institute a program of nocturnal (3 AM) monitoring of blood glucose levels on a periodic basis. The patient should do nocturnal monitoring regularly when making adjustments in the evening insulin, when unusually strenuous physical activity has occurred the previous day, and during periods of erratic glucose control or irregular eating schedules.

8. Instruct patients to carry an identification card or medical identification bracelet to advise police, bystanders, or emergency medical personnel of the fact that they have diabetes and take insulin.

9. Initial education at the onset of insulin or oral agent treatment is essential, as is ongoing education. Repeated reviews and updates are needed. Review the causes, signs, symptoms, treatment, and prevention of hypoglycemia regularly. These reviews should include family members and close friends and should be focused on recent or anticipated events in the patient's life (eg, after a hypoglycemic episode, before a trip, etc). Provide written instructions and reading material as part of these reviews.

10. Remember to give patients positive feedback when they demonstrate good judgment in preventing or treating hypoglycemia.

REFERENCES

1. Cryer PE. Iatrogenic hypoglycemia as a cause of hypoglycemia-associated autonomic failure in IDDM. Diabetes 1992;41:255-60.

2. Diabetes Control and Complications Trial Research Group. Epidemiology of severe hypoglycemia in the Diabetes Control and Complications Trial. Am J Med 1991;90:450-59.

3. Widmann FK. Gooddale's clinical interpretation of laboratory tests. Philadelphia: FA Davis, 1973:425.

4. Cox DJ, Gonder-Frederick L, Antoun B, Cryer PE, Clarke WE. Perceived symptoms in the recognition of hypoglycemia. Diabetes Care 1993;16:519-27.

5. Santiago JV, Clarke WL, Shah SD, Cryer PE. Epinephrine, norepinephrine, glucagon and growth hormone release in association with physiological decrements in the plasma glucose concentration in normal and diabetic man. J Clin Endocrinol Metab 1980;51:877-83.

6. Amiel SA, Sherwin RS, Simonson DC, Tamborlane WV. Effect of intensive insulin therapy on glycemic thresholds for counterregulatory hormone release. Diabetes 1988;37:901-7.

7. Cryer PE, Gerich JE. Hypoglycemia in insulin-dependent diabetes mellitus: insulin excess and defective glucose counterregulation. In: Rifkin H, Porte Jr D, eds. Ellenberg and Rifkin's diabetes mellitus: theory and practice. New York: Elsevier, 1990:526-46.

8. Corrall RJM, Frier BM, Davidson NM, Hopkins WM, French EB. Cholinergic manifestations of the acute autonomic reaction to hypoglycemia in man. Clin Sci 1983;64(1):49-53.

9. Cryer PE, White NH, Santiago JV. The relevance of glucose counterregulatory systems to patients with insulin-dependent diabetes mellitus. Endocr Rev 1986;7:131-39.

10. White NH, Skor DA, Cryer PE, Levandoski LA, Bier DM, Santiago JV. Identification of type I diabetic patients at increased risk for hypoglycemia during intensive therapy. N Engl J Med 1983;308:485-91.

11. Smith L, Casso MB. Exercise and the intensively treated IDDM patient. Diabetes Educ 1988;14:510-15.

12. MacDonald MJ. Postexercise late-onset hypoglycemia in insulin-dependent diabetic patients. Diabetes Care 1987;10:584-88.

13. Gaudiani L, Feingold KR. Alcohol and diabetes: mix with caution. Clin Diabetes 1984;2:121-32.

14. Cox DJ, Irvine A, Gonder-Frederick L, Nowacek G, Butterfield J. Fear of hypoglycemia: quantification, validation and utilization. Diabetes Care 1987;10:617-21.

15. Cox DJ, Gonder-Frederick L, Antoun B, Clarke W, Cryer PE. Psychobehavioral metabolic parameters of severe hypoglycemic episodes. Diabetes Care 1990;13:458-59.

KEY EDUCATIONAL CONSIDERATIONS

1. Patients are provided with information about hypoglycemia when they are diagnosed with diabetes. This information needs to be reviewed and updated at subsequent visits for several reasons. First, patients and their families are only able to assimilate and process a fraction of the information provided at the initial diagnosis. Second, patients tend to become less vigilant about hypoglycemia if they have not had any significant or serious episodes in the recent past. Third, as lifestyles and schedules change, so does the risk of hypoglycemia.

    a) Routinely ask patients if they have had any episodes of hypoglycemia since the last visit. Use the patient's experiences with hypoglycemia as a starting point for review and further education.

    b) Provide written material about hypoglycemia, such as articles or handouts.

2. Patients' symptoms of hypoglycemia can change over time. Help patients learn to recognize the more subtle symptoms of hypoglycemia by using a symptom checklist.

3. Even the best-intentioned, well-meaning patients can make judgment errors that predispose them to hypoglycemia.

    a) Regularly review with patients the situations that increase the risk of hypoglycemia (eg, alcohol consumption, increased exercise/activity, changes in diet).

    b) Remind patients to keep rapid-acting carbohydrate with them at all times.

4. Glucagon, often purchased or provided at diagnosis, may never have been used. Family members frequently don't remember how to administer it or where it is kept. Include at every visit questions about glucagon and medical identification cards/bracelets in the discussion of hypoglycemia. Ask patients to check the expiration date on their glucagon and to replace it if necessary.

5. The lifestyle changes and attitudes of adolescents with diabetes put them at increased risk of hypoglycemia. School, work, and social situations can make adherence to a rigid schedule unrealistic and impractical. It is best to assume that most adolescents will try alcohol and will skip meals or eat "forbidden foods." Educational priorities should include helping adolescents adjust the diabetes regimen to meet their personal needs, with prevention of hypoglycemia as an important goal. Adolescents need to be reminded frequently about the effects of alcohol, dietary indiscretion, and other risk-taking behaviors, preferably at every visit. They also need to be reminded about the dangers of operating a motor vehicle while hypoglycemic.

SELF-REVIEW QUESTIONS

If you are unsure of the answers to the following questions, please review the materials.

1. Explain the three clinical levels of hypoglycemia, giving several symptoms/signs of each level.
2. Describe appropriate treatment for each level of hypoglycemia.
3. Which two hormones are primarily responsible for recovery from hypoglycemia?
4. Define hypoglycemia unawareness and explain its role in managing patients with insulin-dependent diabetes.
5. List the three most common causes of hypoglycemia.
6. Describe the effect of prolonged, strenuous exercise on blood glucose levels and insulin requirements.
7. State two behaviors associated with fear of hypoglycemia.

CASE EXAMPLE

LB is a 23-year-old female who has had insulin-dependent diabetes mellitus (IDDM) for 15 years. Her metabolic control had been fair during adolescence and while at college. She now is out of school, working full-time, and living in an apartment with a roommate. She now wants to improve her metabolic control. Her regimen consists of regular insulin and NPH before breakfast and before dinner. She measures her blood glucose levels before each injection. She jogs 3 miles after dinner several evenings per week, and has a bedtime snack only if she is hungry. Recently she has been increasing her predinner NPH due to fasting hyperglycemia. At a routine office visit, she relates that she is having two or three episodes of nocturnal hypoglycemia per week. She has had many blood glucose measurements less than 50 mg/dL (2.8 mmol/L) during which she has had no symptoms of hypoglycemia. She also reports that she had an episode of hypoglycemia that her roommate had to treat by forcing jelly into her mouth.

QUESTIONS

1. What are the principle factors contributing to this patient's hypoglycemia?
2. What steps can be taken to help improve LB's metabolic control while reducing the frequency of nocturnal hypoglycemia?

SUGGESTED SOLUTIONS

This patient should be commended for her desire to improve her metabolic control. However, she also needs education and specific guidelines to follow regarding dose adjustments, blood glucose monitoring, and treatment of hypoglycemia.

At least three factors predispose this patient to frequent episodes of nocturnal hypoglycemia. Treating the nocturnal hypoglycemia with carbohydrate raises the blood glucose level. In an attempt to improve fasting glucose levels, LB increases her predinner NPH dose. She is not checking her blood glucose levels at bedtime and is not having a bedtime snack on a regular basis. This problem is further complicated because LB is exercising in the evening, which has the effect of lowering her blood glucose during the night. Additionally, she appears to have either become more tolerant of lower blood glucose levels due to improved metabolic control or has experienced a change in the early warning symptoms of hypoglycemia. She also may be developing hypoglycemia unawareness.

Several steps can be initiated to help LB achieve her goal of improved metabolic control without risking hypoglycemia. First, she needs to check blood glucose levels at bedtime every night. She should be instructed to consistently have a bedtime snack that consists of carbohydrate and protein. This snack may need to be adjusted based on her blood glucose levels and physical activity. Another option is to move her NPH insulin to bedtime and adjust the amount of predinner regular insulin to eliminate nocturnal hypoglycemia. Other possibilities include switching LB to a regimen of Ultralente twice a day, with preprandial regular insulin. Although practices vary, the usual recommendation is making just one change in the insulin dose at a given time. The effect of that dose change is assessed after a few days, and additional dose changes are implemented as necessary. Frequent contact with the health care practitioner is critical during this time.

Glucagon should be purchased and kept in the apartment. LB's roommate should know where it is kept and how to use it. If LB is developing hypoglycemia unawareness, more frequent blood glucose monitoring may be required to detect episodes of asymptomatic hypoglycemia. She also should be instructed to monitor blood glucose levels before driving.

OTHER SUGGESTED READINGS

Cox DJ, Gonder-Frederick LA, Lee JH, Julian DM, Carter WR, Clarke WL. Effects and correlates of blood glucose awareness training among patients with IDDM. Diabetes Care 1989;12:313-18.

Cryer PE. Hypoglycemia and insulin-dependent diabetes mellitus. In: Alberti KGMM, Krall LP, eds. The diabetes annuals/4. Amsterdam: Elsevier Science Publishing, 1988:272-310.

Horton ES. Role and management of exercise in diabetes mellitus. Diabetes Care 1988;11:201-11.

Santiago JV, Levandoski LA, Bubb J. Definitions, causes, and risk factors for hypoglycemia in insulin-dependent diabetes. In: Bardin CW, ed. Current therapies in endocrinology and metabolism. Philadelphia: BC Decker, 1991:354-59.

Santiago JV, Levandoski LA, Bubb J. Hypoglycemia in patients with type I diabetes. In: Lebovitz H, ed. Therapy for diabetes mellitus and related disorders. Alexandria, Va: American Diabetes Association, 1991:161-69.

MANAGEMENT

XIV.   PERIOPERATIVE ISSUES

INTRODUCTION

The same surgical conditions affect people with and without diabetes. Many people with diabetes, however, also have associated complications, such as coronary artery disease, peripheral vascular disease, neuropathic ulcers, kidney disease, and proliferative retinopathy, that can require surgical interventions. According to Busick[1] and Alberti,[2] the person with diabetes has a 50% chance of requiring surgery during his or her lifetime. Considering the advances in medical and surgical therapies, it is likely that people with diabetes have an even greater chance of undergoing surgery.[3]

An understanding of normal physiology is necessary to provide adequate support to the person with diabetes who is undergoing a surgical procedure. Special care is needed to achieve and maintain euglycemia, maintain fluid and electrolyte balance, provide adequate nutrition, and prevent further complications. The perioperative management of patients with insulin-dependent diabetes mellitus (IDDM), also called type I diabetes, and non-insulin-dependent diabetes mellitus (NIDDM), also called type II diabetes, differs.

Although the patient's physician usually decides the route of insulin administration, the diabetes educator is called upon to educate the staff, patient, and significant other(s) regarding perioperative diabetes-related issues. The key educational considerations focus on patient education concerns.

OBJECTIVES

Upon completion of this chapter, the learner will be able to:
- describe the physiological effect of surgery;
- understand the importance of euglycemia during the preoperative, intraoperative, and postoperative periods;
- describe three components of preoperative care;
- identify three alternative methods of insulin/glucose management for the surgical patient;
- identify special postoperative concerns.

A. Metabolic Effects of Surgery and Anesthesia in Patients With and Without Diabetes

1. Metabolic homeostasis is maintained by the balance of the anabolic hormone insulin, and the major catabolic hormones of glucagon, the catecholamines, cortisol, and growth hormone.

2. The physiological stress of surgery causes the system to release large amounts of catecholamines (epinephrine and norepinephrine). There is an increase in the heart rate, which increases the blood pressure and dilates the bronchi to maximize the amount of oxygen supplied to the body tissues. Blood is shunted from the vulnerable surface of the body to supply the vital organs in the core with essential oxygen. Epinephrine decreases the uptake of glucose by the muscle tissue and inhibits the release of endogenous insulin. Catecholamines cause glycogen that is stored in the liver to break down into glucose (glycogenolysis) and to be released into the bloodstream. The adrenal cortex secretes cortisol, which causes the liver to create additional glucose (gluconeogenesis) from amino acids (alanine), glycerol, and lactate. Uptake of the glucose by the muscle tissue is inhibited by cortisol.

3. During anesthesia and surgery there is an increase in the plasma concentration of counterregulatory hormones. An elevation in the levels of glucagon, catecholamines, cortisol, and growth hormone is observed.[2]

4. The patient with uncontrolled diabetes will already be in a catabolic state. Superimposition of the metabolic stress of surgery will result in a major worsening of this state. In order to minimize the adverse effects on the patient with diabetes, meticulous attention to metabolic control is required.[2]

B. Treatment Goals for the Patient With Diabetes

1. Prevention of hypoglycemia, excessive hyperglycemia, lipolysis, protein catabolism, and electrolyte disturbance are the goals of therapy during the preoperative, intraoperative, and postoperative periods.

    a) Hyperglycemia has been associated with several problems, including decreased effectiveness of leukocytes, increased risk of platelet aggregation, and increased rigidity of the red blood cell, which decreases circulation through the small vessels, depriving them of oxygen and nutrients.

    b) Ketosis and ketoacidosis may ensue with persistent hyperglycemia, leading to a drop in pH concentration. Patients with IDDM undergoing surgery are more prone to developing acidosis even with moderate hyperglycemia.[3]

    c) All patients with glucose intolerance are susceptible to electrolyte abnormalities and volume depletion from osmotic diuresis.

    d) Unrecognized and untreated hypoglycemia may endanger the life of the surgical patient. Because hypoglycemia in the anesthetized patient can be difficult to identify, meticulous perioperative blood glucose monitoring is imperative.

    e) The blood glucose level should be controlled between 125 mg/dL (6.9 mmol/L) and 200 mg/dL (11.1 mmol/L).[2-4]

2. Theoretically, enhanced healing depends on establishing or reestablishing homeostasis. Normal glucose levels are essential for the normal protein synthesis that is required for wound healing.[2,3]

C. General Preoperative Assessment and Preparation for Surgery

1. Preoperative care should include a thorough history and physical examination.

2. The admission history should include the following: date of diabetes diagnosis; medications, including type, manufacturer, and dosage of insulin and/or oral agents and over-the-counter medications; allergies; previous episodes of ketoacidosis and severe hypoglycemia (blood glucose records if available); current weight and maximum weight; previous hospital admissions for surgery and other illnesses; and any current signs and symptoms. For women, the last menstrual period and childbearing history should be obtained if applicable.

3. Diagnostic laboratory data should be reviewed prior to admission for surgery with special consideration being given to the individual's electrolyte balance and blood count. An elevated hemoglobin A_{1c} may indicate that the patient has been in poor control and may have a greater risk for ketoacidosis. A fructosamine (glycosylated albumin) or glycosylated serum protein test may help determine the most recent level of glucose control. Just prior to surgery, a complete blood count and electrolyte profile should be performed.

4. For elective surgery, special considerations should be given to the patient's renal, cardiovascular, peripheral vascular, neurological, respiratory, and cerebrovascular systems.

    a) Cardiovascular considerations:

    (1) The presence of carotid bruits or transient ischemia attacks (TIAs) prior to surgery may indicate cerebrovascular disease. Metabolic and hemodynamic stresses may compromise the cardiovascular system and lead to myocardial infarction, congestive heart failure, cerebral vascular accidents, or acute renal failure. Anesthesia agents can depress heart muscle function and may induce

rhythm disturbances. Several events during surgery place additional stress on the myocardium. For example, bleeding during surgery may result in hypovolemia, hypotension, tachycardia, or bradycardia. Volume overload, fever, and shivering all may put additional stress on the myocardium. A study by Hollenberg[5] found that diabetes mellitus was one of five risk factors for developing postoperative myocardial ischemia.

(2) Preoperative and postoperative electrocardiograms should be obtained as well as measurements of cardiovascular enzyme activity, when indicated.

(3) The blood pressure should be carefully monitored. Antihypertensive medications should be reinstituted promptly after surgery.

(4) A patient with a history of congestive heart failure (CHF) should be assessed for pulmonary and peripheral edema. Caution should be used to prevent overhydration and hypokalemia. The patient with CHF and hypertension may be at risk for developing hypokalemia due to previous diuretic therapy.

b) Neurological considerations:

(1) If the patient has had recent TIAs, a neurological evaluation may be indicated.

(2) The presence of some manifestations of neuropathy may affect recovery from the operation. Orthostatic hypotension, neurogenic bladder, hyperesthesia or hypoesthesia, and gastroparesis are some manifestations of diabetic neuropathies. Physical assessment is necessary to identify these problems and should include lying and standing blood pressure readings, reflex and pinprick assessment of the feet, and determination of residual urine, if indicated.

c) Renal considerations:

(1) The presence of renal disease may alter the types and amounts of fluid infused and the medication

dosages. As part of the general assessment to guide diabetes management, measurement of urine protein and creatinine clearance may be indicated if the patient's diabetes has been diagnosed for more than 5 years and the tests have not been performed recently. If there is inadequate time to collect a 12- or 24-hour collection for a quantitative evaluation, random dipstick for proteinuria may be used as a screen. A serum creatinine should be included in the electrolyte screen.

(2) Arteriography procedures using dye should be undertaken with extreme caution in the patient with renal disease. The use of low osmolar dyes may be indicated. Adequate hydration is essential. A nephrology consult may be warranted.

(3) Amphotericin B and aminoglycosides are extremely nephrotoxic agents. Extreme caution should be used in administering these agents.

d) Respiratory considerations: Obesity in any person increases the risk of developing pneumonia.

5. The preoperative assessment may provide insight into the educational needs of the patient and significant other(s). Assessment of the patient's knowledge will help provide direction for preoperative and postoperative diabetes teaching. Family members or significant others should be included in the preoperative teaching.

D. Perioperative Concerns for the Patient With IDDM

1. *Insulin.* There are a number of alternatives for management of the surgical patient with diabetes. Ideally, a diabetologist or endocrinologist will be consulted for insulin and fluid management. In all of these methods, the usual insulin dosage is altered for the day of surgery. Physician preference will dictate the method used.

a) A glucose-insulin infusion regimen is an option for providing optimal glucose control during surgery and the immediate postoperative period. Rapid-acting insulin (regular) is mixed in a normal saline solution and infused intravenously using an infusion pump. An initial rate of 0.5 to 1.0 unit per hour may be used. This solution is adjusted according to the results of frequent glucose monitoring. According to Alberti,[2] a ratio of between 0.2 and 0.4 units insulin per gram of glucose is suggested. A solution of at least 5% dextrose is given at a variable rate to balance the glucose levels and prevent ketosis.

b) The combined glucose-insulin-potassium infusion (GIK) is a safe, effective method of managing the patient. This method was designed to be simple and reproducible. Thirty-two units of regular insulin plus 20 mmol of potassium chloride are added to one liter of 10% glucose and infused at a rate of 100 ml/h. The GIK infusion has the disadvantage of having a fixed insulin concentration such that the entire bag must be changed each time the plasma glucose is outside the target range.[3] Also, this method is recommended only for patients with normal renal function.

c) Subcutaneous regimens are prescribed for shorter procedures usually when the patient will be able to eat lunch.

   (1) Subcutaneous regular insulin may be given with a 5% or 10% glucose solution plus potassium to maintain the target glucose levels. Numerous methods to calculate the dosage have been used from unit per kilogram to present total daily dose.

   (2) Another subcutaneous method is to withhold the morning rapid-acting insulin and give one-half of the intermediate-acting insulin. This method can lead to unpredictable glycemic exclusions due to the variable absorption times of intermediate-acting insulin and the decreased peripheral perfusion during surgical procedures.

(3) Although the effects of surgery on subcutaneous insulin have not been studied, fluid shifts and hemodynamic changes that occur during and after surgery alter cutaneous blood flow and may result in unpredictable differences in serum insulin concentrations.[3]

2. *Glucose.* Sufficient glucose to prevent hypoglycemia and to provide the basal energy requirement should be administered during surgery in the insulinopenic patient. Most authors recommend the infusion of 5 grams glucose per hour while others suggest that 10 grams per hour may be needed.[3]

3. *Potassium.* According to Hirsch,[3] the patient with diabetes who is normokalemic with normal renal function should have 20 mEq of potassium chloride added to each liter of fluid. Electrolytes should be monitored to verify the patient's status.

4. *Fluids.* If a patient is receiving adequate insulin, glucose, and potassium, any additional fluids given during surgery should be nonglucose-containing. The use of lactated Ringer's solution in patients with diabetes is controversial. Lactate is a gluconeogenic precursor that is rapidly metabolized[3] and may cause hyperglycemia, requiring greater amounts of insulin.

5. *Scheduling.* Surgery or tests that require the patient to have nothing by mouth should be scheduled early in the morning to prevent long periods of fasting. If the test or procedure is scheduled mid- to late morning or in the afternoon, then intravenous fluids and intravenous or subcutaneous insulin should be initiated on the morning of the procedure to prevent hyperglycemia.

6. *Monitoring.* Frequent blood glucose and urine ketone monitoring is necessary to evaluate the adequacy of the insulin dosage and calorie replacement.

a) Urine ketone accumulation should be monitored every 4 to 6 hours, or any time the blood glucose level is greater than 240 mg/dL (13.3 mmol/L).

b) At minimum, blood glucose levels should be checked preoperatively and postoperatively and before insulin administration. If the patient is receiving intravenous insulin, it is essential to monitor the blood glucose every 1 to 2 hours.

c) Ideally, intraoperative blood glucose levels should be checked every 30 to 60 minutes.

d) The ease of obtaining and testing capillary samples makes frequent blood glucose testing feasible with less expense. A blood glucose meter, rather than a visual-read glucose method, should be used by nurses or physicians trained in the use of a meter.

E. Perioperative Concerns for the Patient With NIDDM

1. The majority of patients with diabetes who undergo surgery have NIDDM as opposed to IDDM. Many of these NIDDM patients are taking insulin, although they are not insulin-dependent in the traditional sense. Some of these patients, especially the nonobese, respond metabolically like the classic IDDM patient and should be treated with the same medical regimens.[3] The main determinants for therapy in NIDDM patients are the magnitude of the procedure and the metabolic state of the patient on the day of surgery.[2]

2. Patients whose diabetes is well controlled with diet or diet plus oral hypoglycemic agents (OHA) do not require specific therapy. Patients with fasting blood glucose levels lower than 140 mg/dL (7.8 mmol/L) treated with an OHA can be given their medication and started on a glucose infusion in the morning. Some suggest stopping the OHA the evening before surgery. The longer-acting chlorpropamide should be discontinued 48 to 72 hours prior to the surgical procedure.[2]

3. According to Hirsch[3] and Alberti,[2] perioperative insulin therapy should be considered if the fasting or random glucose level exceeds 200 mg/dL (11.1 mmol/L). According to Hirsch,[3] either the GIK method or subcutaneous insulin may be used in this population. Only human insulin should be given to the NIDDM patient who has never received insulin therapy.

4. Hyperglycemic hyperosmolar nonketotic syndrome (HHNS) has been reported as a postoperative complication in patients with NIDDM.

F. Postoperative Care

1. The literature suggests that impaired wound healing occurs when plasma glucose levels exceed 200mg/dL (11.1 mmol/L).[3]
   a) The wound should be observed carefully for any signs of inflammatory changes or drainage, and alterations in the patient's temperature should be noted. Meticulous wound care is essential.
   b) Maintaining and improving circulation is particularly important for the person with diabetes who may have peripheral vascular disease.

2. Monitoring of blood glucose and electrolytes continues in the postoperative period. Hypoglycemia is a particular concern because the blood glucose level and insulin dose may decrease dramatically as the stress of surgery declines or as an infection is treated.

3. There are two phases of nutritional perioperative management. Successful transition through the phases and reinitiation of medication are essential for a successful surgical outcome.
   a) The first phase is the initial catabolic phase that extends from the period just before surgery into the period immediately following the operation. The second phase is a transition in which the patient moves from being NPO to eating a regular diet.

b) During the reintroduction of foods such as clear liquids, it is preferable to continue a low-maintenance dose of intravenous or subcutáneous regular insulin and fluids.

c) Returning to the normal meal plan as soon as possible will promote healing and reestablish homeostasis. Adequate carbohydrate should be given daily to prevent ketosis due to starvation. Solid foods should be started as soon as they can be tolerated.

4. Once food tolerance is established, the infusion is stopped and a new regimen is planned, considering such elements as infection, pain, steroids, or total parenteral nutrition (TPN). For patients treated with OHA, the usual OHA may be prescribed and the patient may be supplemented with regular insulin. For insulin-treated patients, a combination of intermediate- and rapid-acting insulin may be prescribed. If only rapid-acting insulin is prescribed, care must be taken not to leave insulinopenic patients (IDDM) without basal insulin.

5. Subcutaneous insulin should be given at least 30 minutes prior to the discontinuation of any intravenous insulin infusion.

6. Capillary blood glucose monitoring should be done a minimum of four times per day. The times may vary by physician preference and by the medical regimen.

7. Pain can cause the release of counterregulatory hormones and may increase the blood glucose level. Adequate pain management will help relieve this response.

8. Peripheral neuropathy and peripheral vascular disease increase the risk of the patient developing ulcerations. Careful monitoring of pressure areas and ambulation as soon as possible will help reduce the risk of these postoperative complications.

9. Written instructions are mandatory for post-procedure home care, with instructions for insulin, other medications, meal planning and hydration, and wound care, if applicable.

G. Emergency Surgery

1. Management will depend upon the metabolic condition of the patient. Surgical emergencies, particularly if there is underlying infection, can cause rapid metabolic decompensation, with dehydration and hyperglycemia and ultimately ketoacidosis in the patient with IDDM. If the patient is in early or established diabetic ketoacidosis (DKA), the first priority is metabolic management.
2. In the patient without severe metabolic disturbance, initial diabetic management can be with an intravenous insulin infusion. If the patient is dehydrated, normal saline should be used for a fluid replacement.[2]

H. Surgery in Children

1. There are few published guidelines for the management of diabetes in children during surgery. In general, adult regimens have been adapted.[2]
2. Caution will need to be taken in calculating fluid requirements and insulin requirements. A pediatric endocrinologist should be consulted if available.

REFERENCES

1.   Busick EJ. The medical management of diabetic patients during surgery. Diabetes Educ 1982;8(3):24-25.

2.   Alberti KGMM. Diabetes and surgery. In: Rifkin H, Porte Jr D, eds. Ellenberg and Rifkin's diabetes mellitus: theory and practice. 4th ed. New York: Elsevier, 1990:626-33.

3.   Hirsch IB, McGill JB, Cryer PE, White PF. Perioperative management of the surgical patient with diabetes mellitus. Anesthesiology 1991;74:346-59.

4.   Araua-Pacheco C, Raskin P. Surgery and anesthesia. In: Lebovitz H, ed. Therapy for diabetes mellitus and other related disorders. Alexandria, Va: American Diabetes Association, 1991:147-154.

5.   Hollenberg M, Mangano DT, Browner WS, London MJ, Tubau JF, Tateo IM. Predictors of postoperative myocardial ischemia in patients undergoing noncardiac surgery. JAMA 1992;268(2):205-9.

KEY EDUCATIONAL CONSIDERATIONS

1. Explain to the patient how the insulin dose will be administered and adjusted during surgery. Many patients are fearful of giving the decision-making responsibility for insulin adjustment to others.

2. Explain the need for dextrose in the intravenous solution. Many patients know that dextrose raises the blood glucose and they are concerned that an error may have been made.

3. Explain to patients with NIDDM (type II diabetes) treated with oral hypoglycemic agents that they may need insulin before, during, or after surgery. Many patients are concerned that the insulin therapy may permanently replace their previous treatment.

4. Prepare the patient for frequent capillary blood glucose and urine ketone testing. The blood glucose may be checked every 1 to 2 hours.

5. Provide written discharge instructions for any medications, including insulin (if applicable), meals, activity, and surgical and medical follow-up. Ask the significant other(s) to plan menus for the first few days at home. Use this opportunity to provide updated information.

SELF-REVIEW QUESTIONS

If you are unsure of the answers to the following questions, please review the materials.

1. Describe the physiological responses to surgery and the subsequent effect on the blood glucose level.
2. Describe the effects of surgery on the cardiovascular system.
3. Why is the prevention of hyperglycemia important to the surgical patient with diabetes?
4. List the methods to prevent hypoglycemia in the surgical patient.
5. What should be included in preoperative management?

6. List three alternatives for insulin therapy intraoperatively and immediately postoperatively.
7. Discuss any advantages and disadvantages of these alternatives.
8. List four potential postoperative problems that may be more common in the person with diabetes.
9. What oral agent should be discontinued at least 48 hours prior to surgery?

CASE EXAMPLE

CB is a 42-year-old female diagnosed with IDDM at age 17 years. She will be admitted for an elective cholecystectomy with general anesthesia. CB is hypertensive and being treated with ACE inhibitors. She also has background diabetic retinopathy and proteinuria.

CB manages her diabetes in conjunction with a diabetes care team. She monitors her blood glucose three to four times per day and injects 38 units of NPH, and 6 units of regular insulin every AM, plus 6 units of regular insulin prior to her evening meal, and 8 units of NPH at 10 PM.

In a team meeting the day before CB's admission for surgery, the resident suggests the following insulin regimen. Advise CB to take her usual NPH dose on the morning of surgery. Order capillary blood glucose readings every 4 hours and give regular insulin on a sliding scale.

< 150 mg/dL (8.3 mmol/L) — no insulin
151-200 mg/dL (8.4-11.1 mmol/L) — 4 units
201-250 mg/dL (11.2-13.9 mmol/L) — 6 units
251-350 mg/dL (14.0-19.4 mmol/L) — 8 units

The endocrinologist strongly disagrees.

QUESTIONS

1. What is wrong with the resident's plan?
2. What other insulin option should the physician consider?
3. What teaching needs could be identified for CB?

SUGGESTED SOLUTIONS

Giving no insulin with a blood glucose of less than 150 mg/dL (8.3 mmol/L) would leave an IDDM patient who is insulinopenic at risk for developing ketosis and ultimately ketoacidosis. The resident also recommended advising the patient to take her usual dose of NPH insulin, which could lead to difficulties with hypoglycemia or hyperglycemia because subcutaneous insulin, particularly NPH, has a variable absorption in the surgical patient.

An insulin/glucose infusion would be optimal. The GIK method and any addition of potassium should be avoided due to CB's kidney status.

Preoperative teaching should include information about the frequency of glucose monitoring, the surgical procedure, and postoperative care. Written instructions should be provided on discharge, concerning medication, meal planning, care of the incision, and medical and surgical follow-up.

OTHER SUGGESTED READINGS

Davidson JK. Clinical diabetes mellitus: a problem oriented approach. 2nd ed. New York: Thieme, 1991:648-55.

Guthrie DW, Guthrie RA. Nursing management of diabetes mellitus. 3rd ed. New York: Springer, 1991:251-61.

Hernandez C. Surgery and diabetes: minimizing the risks. Am J Nurs 1987;87(6):788-92.

Saltiel-Berzin R. Managing a surgical patient who has diabetes. Nursing 92;22(4):34-41.

Shuman C. Controlling diabetes during surgery. Diabetes Spectrum 1989;2(4):263-69.

Special Populations

SPECIAL POPULATIONS

XV. PREGNANCY: PRECONCEPTION TO POSTPARTUM

INTRODUCTION

The outlook for pregnant women with diabetes has improved dramatically over the past several years. In centers specializing in the management of diabetes during pregnancy, the perinatal mortality figures for offspring of women with insulin-dependent diabetes approach the 1.6% to 2% found in the general population.[1,2] This success rate is largely the result of more concerted efforts at normalizing maternal metabolism throughout gestation; an emphasis on team care; improved obstetric techniques to assess fetal well-being and maturation in utero; and, pediatric advances in neonatal care. As a result, major system anomalies, which are a first-trimester complication of maternal diabetes, have emerged as the major cause of infant mortality and morbidity in diabetic pregnancies. Preventing these anomalies is highly dependent upon initiating care in the preconception period.

In this chapter, the metabolic abnormalities that occur in maternal diabetes will be described, and the problems that appear to develop from these abnormalities will be reviewed. A preconception counseling and management program will be outlined to offer the best possible chance for a healthy baby. Diabetes management for pregestational and gestational diabetes also will be reviewed.

OBJECTIVES

On completion of this chapter, the learner will be able to:
- identify two types of diabetes in pregnancy, eg, pregestational (overt) diabetes and gestational diabetes;
- describe normal maternal metabolism in pregnancy;
- identify potential maternal complications for the patient with pregestational diabetes;
- list neonatal complications;
- identify risk factors associated with a poor outcome in a pregnancy complicated by diabetes mellitus;
- review two important topics to discuss with patients seeking preconception counseling;
- state treatment guidelines for pregnancy;
- identify educational guidelines for pregnancy;

- describe three types of monitoring methods utilized in the medical management of diabetes in pregnancy;
- define the screening guidelines for gestational diabetes.

A. Definition of Diabetes in Pregnancy

1. When reviewing the types of diabetes in pregnancy, it is helpful to divide them into two groups.

   a) The first group consists of pregestational diabetes, insulin-dependent diabetes mellitus (IDDM), also called type I diabetes, or non-insulin-dependent diabetes mellitus (NIDDM), also called type II diabetes, including patients with vascular complications.

   b) The second group consists of women who develop gestational diabetes defined as carbohydrate intolerance of variable severity with onset or first recognition during pregnancy.[3-6]

2. Approximately 0.2% to 0.3%[7] of all pregnancies occur in women with pregestational insulin-treated diabetes. An additional 2% to 3%[8] or 3% to 5%[9] of apparently healthy pregnant women are found to have gestational diabetes when they are tested during the second half of gestation. The incidence of gestational diabetes may vary considerably with the ethnic background of the pregnant population.

B. Normal Metabolism

1. Attempts to normalize metabolism for the best possible outcome in a pregnant woman with diabetes require an understanding of the metabolic changes that occur in a nondiabetic pregnancy.

   a) The fetus depends upon the mother for an uninterrupted supply of fuel.

   b) To meet fetal needs, several maternal adaptations occur in early pregnancy.

(1) Increased tissue glycogen storage and peripheral glucose utilization. Decreased hepatic glucose production.

(2) A shift toward production of free fatty acids and ketones.

(3) Pancreatic cell hypertrophy with resultant increased insulin response to glucose.

(4) Decreased maternal alanine (gluconeogenic amino acid) leads to hypoglycemia and lower fasting blood glucose levels.[10]

c) There is a passive diffusion of glucose across the placenta.

d) Hyperemesis and food intolerance may occur.

e) The early months of normal pregnancy can be described as a period of maternal anabolism, a time when maternal fat storage takes place.

2. The metabolic changes related to pregnancy are most pronounced during the latter half of gestation and are seen in both fed and fasted states.

a) The fasted state of pregnancy is characterized by a more rapid diversion to fat metabolism (accelerated starvation).[11]

(1) Whenever food is withheld, concentrations of free fatty acids and ketones reach higher levels in pregnant women than in nongravid women.

(2) Plasma glucose levels and amino acids decrease more markedly in pregnant women during a fasting state.

b) The fed state also is modified in pregnant women. Food ingestion results in higher and more prolonged plasma glucose concentrations in pregnant women compared with nongravid women[12] (see Figure XV.1). This more sustained, postprandial hyperglycemia enhances transplacental delivery of glucose to the fetus and promotes growth of the fetus. (Maternal insulin and glucagon do not cross the placenta.)

3. During late pregnancy, a woman's basal insulin levels are higher than nongravid levels, and food ingestion results in a two to threefold increase in insulin secretion[12] (see Figure XV.1). The cause of this state of insulin resistance is related to the increasing levels of human placental lactogen (HPL), prolactin, and free and bound cortisol. Insulin resistance may be responsible for the diabetogenic effect of pregnancy.

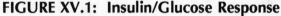

FIGURE XV.1: Insulin/Glucose Response

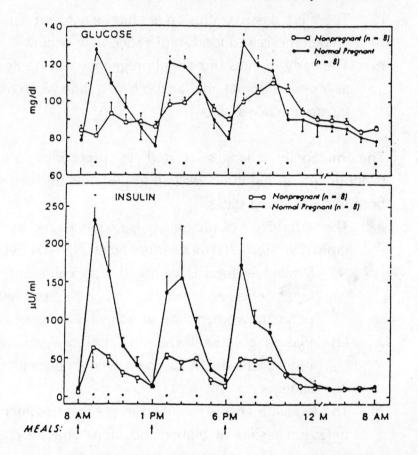

Fig. 1. Mean ± SEM values for plasma glucose and insulin obtained "around the clock" from eight nonpregnant and eight pregnant women in the third trimester. Identical-formula diets were administered in all subjects at the times indicated. Time points where mean values for the two groups are significantly different (p ≤0.05) are shown by asterisks (*). (Adapted from Phelps RL, Metzger BE, Freinkel N: Carbohydrate metabolism in pregnancy: XVII. Diurnal profiles of plasma glucose, insulin, free fatty acids, triglycerides, cholesterol and individual amino acids in late normal pregnancy.[12]

Permission to reprint granted from C.V. Mosby Company.

C. Neonatal Complications

1. Several neonatal complications may occur in pregnancies complicated by diabetes mellitus. Most occur in neonates whose mothers have pregestational diabetes, but some — macrosomia or hypoglycemia can occur in infants of mothers with gestational diabetes as well.

2. Many of the complications can be decreased substantially if good metabolic control is established and maintained prior to and throughout gestation.

   a) In pregestational diabetic pregnancies the incidence of major congenital malformations is 6% to 13%,[13-20] which is two to three times higher than the 2% to 3% incidence found in nondiabetic pregnancies.[13,16,19]

   b) Congenital malformations are formed during the first 5 to 8 weeks of gestation.[21] The types of malformations that occur in infants of diabetic mothers (IDM) affect the central nervous system, the heart and great (major) blood vessels, the kidneys, and the skeleton[21] (see Table XV.1).

   c) There appears to be a relationship between the incidence of birth defects in infants of diabetic mothers (IDM) and maternal glycemic control.

      (1) Studies using maternal glycosylated hemoglobin levels at the end of the first trimester as an index of glycemia during organogenesis generally reveal an anomaly risk of 2% to 5% in diabetic women with normal to moderately elevated glycosylated hemoglobin levels.[15,19,20]

      (2) When glycosylated hemoglobin levels are markedly elevated at the end of the first trimester, the malformation rate rises substantially, reaching as high as 20% to 40% in some studies.[15,20]

      (3) These findings indicate that very poor diabetes control is associated with a very high risk of anomalies, while good to fair control is associated with a much lower risk of anomalies.

TABLE XV.1:
Congenital Malformations
in Infants of Diabetic Mothers (IDM)

Anomaly	Gestational Age After Last Menstrual Period
Sacral Agenesis (Caudal regression)	5 weeks
Spina bifida, hydrocephalus, or other CNS defect	6 weeks
Anencephalus	6 weeks
Heart anomalies	
Transposition of great vessels	7 weeks
Ventricular septal defect	8 weeks
Atrial septal defect	8 weeks
Anal/rectal atresia	8 weeks
Renal anomalies	
Agenesis	7 weeks
Cystic kidney	7 weeks
Ureter duplex	7 weeks
Situs Inversus	6 weeks

Reprinted with permission from Diabetes[21]

  d) The association between poor glycemic control and birth defects has prompted several studies of preconception management in diabetic women. Fuhrmann et al,[22,23] Steel et al,[24] and Kitzmiller et al[25] have reported a virtual elimination of excess anomalies in studies designed to achieve very good glycemic control prior to conception. These studies suggest that it may be possible to eliminate the high rate of congenital malformations in well-managed patients. Therefore, planned pregnancies are extremely important for women with diabetes (see Section E: Preconceptional Counseling).

3. Hypoglycemia in the neonate, the most common metabolic problem, is defined as plasma glucose values less than 35 mg/dL (1.92 mmol/L) in term infants and less than 25 mg/dL (1.37 mmol/L) in preterm infants.[26] In a poorly controlled diabetic pregnancy, the fetus receives larger amounts of

glucose, amino acids, and fatty fuels than are required for normal growth and development. Because insulin does not cross the placenta, the fetus must secrete additional insulin to utilize the larger amounts of glucose and other fuels received from the maternal circulation. At delivery, when the maternal blood supply is eliminated, the fetus continues to produce excess amounts of insulin that may result in neonatal hypoglycemia.

4. There is controversy regarding the definition of fetal macrosomia, another potential complication of a diabetic pregnancy. According to American College of Obstetricians and Gynecologists,[27] any fetus with an estimated weight of more than 4500 grams in utero is considered to be macrosomic. Spellacy et al[28] observed that delivery of an infant weighing greater than 4500 grams occurred 10 times more often in diabetic women than in a control population.

    a) The development of macrosomia in late pregnancy may result from increased secretion of insulin (a growth factor) by the fetal pancreas in response to the excess glucose and other fuels from the diabetic mother. Fetal macrosomia is reflected by increased fetal growth of adipose tissue, muscle, and liver, which are insulin-sensitive structures.

    b) Macrosomia is a risk factor for shoulder dystocia, which can lead to birth trauma such as Erb's palsy. Alternatively, a cesarean section may be required.

5. Stillbirth is a complication of a diabetic pregnancy which can be reduced when excellent diabetes control is maintained and sophisticated fetal monitoring tests are employed.

6. Respiratory distress syndrome now is an infrequent complication of a diabetic pregnancy. Years ago, obstetricians preferred to deliver infants of diabetic mothers several weeks before the due date to prevent a stillbirth and frequently did not document pulmonary maturity prior to delivery. As a result of

a preterm delivery, respiratory distress syndrome sometimes ensued because the infant's lungs were not fully mature. As a result of good diabetes control, sophisticated fetal monitoring, and the ability to document fetal lung maturity, most babies can be delivered close to term (38 to 40 weeks).

7. Hypocalcemia, hyperbilirubinemia, and polycythemia are seen more frequently in infants of diabetic mothers. The pathogenesis of hypocalcemia is not well understood. Polycythemia is related to increased levels of erythropoietin (which correlate directly with maternal insulin levels), and hyperbilirubinemia results when the excess red blood cells are broken down.

D. **Classification Systems Used in Pregnancy Complicated by Diabetes**

1. Classification systems have been developed to identify risk factors in patients who are pregnant and have diabetes.

2. The most widely applied classification system to assess risk factors of a diabetic pregnancy is that of Priscilla White, MD.[29] She observed that the age of onset of maternal diabetes, its duration, and the presence of vascular complications all had an important impact on the outcome of pregnancy.[30] *The White Classification* includes the categories or classes listed in Table XV.2.

3. *Pedersen* et al[31] noted five prognostically bad signs of pregnancy associated with unfavorable outcomes. These signs include ketoacidosis, pyelonephritis, pregnancy-induced hypertension, poor clinic attendance, and self-neglect.

4. Both the White Classification and Pedersen's prognostically bad signs help to identify patients at risk for poor pregnancy outcomes. Probably the most important predictors of perinatal outcome, however, are the degree of achievable metabolic control, the presence of diabetic vascular complications, and

TABLE XV.2: White's Classification[29]

Class	Diabetes Onset Age (y)	Duration (y)	Vascular Disease	Therapy
Gestational diabetes	Abnormal OGTT detected during pregnancy	---	None	Diet alone or Diet and insulin
A	Any	Any	None	Diet alone
True B	>20	<10	None	Diet and insulin
Gestational B	Abnormal OGTT detected during pregnancy	---	None	Diet and insulin
C	10-19 or 10-19		None	Diet and insulin
D	<10 or >20		Background retinopathy or hypertension	Diet and insulin
F	Any	Any	Nephropathy with >500 mg/day proteinuria	Diet and insulin
R	Any	Any	Proliferative retinopathy or vitreous hemorrhage	Diet and insulin
RF	Any	Any	Nephropathy and proliferative retinopathy co-exist	Diet and insulin
H	Any	Any	Arteriosclerotic heart disease	Diet and insulin
T	Any	Any	Prior renal transplantation	Diet and insulin

Pedersen's prognostically bad signs.[32] These factors appear to be more important predictors of perinatal outcome than either the age at onset or the duration of maternal diabetes.

E.   Preconceptional Counseling

1.   Management of pregestational diabetes ideally should begin prior to conception to offer the best outcome for the unborn child.

2.   All women with diabetes of childbearing age should receive counseling about the potential risks of unplanned pregnancy, and appropriate contraception should be emphasized. Women with NIDDM need to make the transition from oral agents to insulin before conception. If excellent diabetes control is not maintained prior to and throughout gestation, and if skilled obstetrical care is not available, neonatal and maternal problems may develop. For this reason, team management by a diabetologist, obstetrician, nurse educator, dietitian, and social worker is highly desirable. In addition, the diabetic woman with vascular complications requires special attention.

3.   The topics of fertility, spontaneous abortion rate, incidence of diabetes mellitus in offspring, incidence of congenital anomalies, and the effects of pregnancy on existing vascular complications are important to discuss with each patient. It is not uncommon for women to experience increased anxiety during this discussion. Psychosocial concerns should be addressed by the team and support offered as an integral part of the treatment plan. The following are some of the findings that relate to diabetes and pregnancy.

   a)   There is no evidence to suggest that diabetic women with well-controlled and uncomplicated diabetes are less fertile than nondiabetic women.

   b)   The risk of spontaneous abortion in women with diabetes appears to be no greater than the risk for nondiabetic women when glycemic control is good to fair.[20,33] In the

Diabetes in Early Pregnancy Project (DIEP)[33] and a study by Greene et al,[20] spontaneous abortions were similar to those expected in nondiabetic pregnancies when first trimester glycosylated hemoglobin levels were in normal to moderately elevated ranges. The spontaneous abortion rates increased dramatically in each of these studies when glycosylated hemoglobin levels were extremely elevated.

c) The risk of transmitting diabetes to offspring does not constitute a specific contraindication to pregnancy. One long-term follow-up study indicated that the net cumulative risk for IDDM (type I diabetes) in children born to insulin-dependent (type I) mothers is 2%.[34] In contrast, the prevalence of IDDM (type I diabetes) in the offspring of insulin-dependent (type I) fathers is reported to be 6%.[34] The risk for offspring of mothers with NIDDM (type II diabetes) is not precisely known but is related to ethnic origin and the presence or absence of obesity. The empiric risk of offspring to develop diabetes or some form of glucose intolerance is 33%.[35]

d) An essential preconception consideration is excellent diabetes control prior to and throughout early pregnancy to reduce the excess risk of congenital anomalies.

(1) Women are counseled that if they achieve excellent blood glucose control and normal or near-normal glycosylated hemoglobin levels in early pregnancy, they may decrease their risk for giving birth to an infant with a birth defect. They are reminded, however, that no one can be guaranteed a perfectly healthy baby, because the risk of birth defects is approximately 2% to 3%[13,16,19,22] even in the general population.

(2) Women with poor glucose control, as reflected by markedly elevated glycosylated hemoglobin levels, are counseled that they may be at higher risk for an infant with a congenital malformation[15,17,20] and that the risk may be as high as 10% to 25%.

(3) When counseling about birth defects, the concepts of maternal serum alpha-fetoprotein screening for neural tube defects and ultrasonographic detection of central nervous system, heart, renal, and skeletal anomalies may be introduced. It should be emphasized that none of these tests is 100% sensitive for detecting fetal malformations.

(4) The following preconception protocol for women with diabetes is recommended prior to discontinuing contraception.

(a) A thorough assessment should be done for any vascular complications.

(b) Oral agent therapy should be discontinued if applicable.

(c) Dietary counseling should be updated because the patient's meal plan may not be appropriate for current needs.

(d) Diabetes self-management skills should be assessed. The patient should be observed obtaining capillary blood glucose levels to assess technique and accuracy, and to make sure that she is not using an outdated meter. She also should be observed while filling the syringe and administering insulin. Additionally, she and her significant other should receive extensive education concerning hypoglycemia, including glucagon administration.

(e) Optimal diabetes control should be achieved as evidenced by glycosylated hemoglobin levels within or close to the normal range and acceptable mean blood glucose levels.

(f) Contraception should be discontinued only when diabetes control is optimal. Basal body temperatures at this time are helpful to accurately date conception.

(g) A serum pregnancy test should be obtained if menses does not occur within 15 to 18 days following ovulation.

e) Women with vascular complications present with additional concerns.

(1) Women who have diabetic retinopathy should be counseled about the effect of pregnancy on their eyes. Preconception fluorescein angiography is indicated since dye studies during pregnancy may be contraindicated.

(a) Worsening of background and untreated proliferative retinopathy has been reported during pregnancy.[36-37] It is not clear whether this worsening reflects the effects of pregnancy, the natural history of diabetic retinopathy, or the rapidly improving glycemic control that frequently is instituted in pregnant women.[36,38-40] In most situations, background retinopathy that occurs during pregnancy regresses after delivery.[41] Although this regression suggests an effect of pregnancy on eye disease, it indicates that background retinopathy should not be considered a contraindication to pregnancy.

(b) Women with proliferative disease who have had photocoagulation prior to pregnancy encounter a low (~5%) risk of significant disease progression during gestation.[41] If their retinopathy does progress, these patients generally can be treated successfully with minimal loss of vision.[39,42,43]

(c) Women with untreated proliferative retinopathy are at greatest risk for progression[41] and pregnancy is contraindicated in these women until they receive laser photocoagulation to stabilize their eye disease.

(2) Women who have diabetic nephropathy (defined as proteinuria >400 mg/24 hours and/or a reduced

glomerular filtration rate [GFR]) should be counseled about the effect of pregnancy on their kidneys and the effect of diabetic nephropathy on the developing baby.

(a) In general, the chances for a successful outcome are good in patients with diabetic nephropathy. Studies[44-47] have shown that the perinatal survival rate in this patient group has been between 89% and 100%. However, the course of pregnancy is not necessarily easy because these women are at risk for a small-for-gestational-age infant, a preterm delivery, and an increased incidence of stillbirth.[44-46] Additionally, pregnancy in women with renal disease frequently is complicated by the development or worsening of hypertension and an increase in proteinuria.[48]

(b) The impact of pregnancy on the natural history of renal disease remains a matter of controversy. In general, pregnancy does not appear to accelerate the rate of deterioration of renal function if the underlying renal disease is mild.[44] However, women with moderate renal disease, defined as a serum creatinine from 1.7 to 2.7 mg/dL;[48] (150.3-238.7 µmol/L) may experience a decline in renal function that is faster than predicted by the natural history of diabetic glomerulopathy. Additionally, since diabetic nephropathy tends to worsen over time, women with this condition must consider the possibility of motherhood complicated by dialysis or renal transplantation.

(3) Other women with diabetes who might experience a problematic pregnancy are those who have symptomatic ischemic heart disease, congestive heart failure, or diabetic neuropathy with severe gastroparesis.

(a) Women with symptomatic or ischemic heart disease and/or congestive heart failure should be counseled not to attempt a pregnancy because these conditions carry a high risk of maternal mortality.[49]

(b) Diabetic neuropathy with severe gastroparesis may lead to significant nausea, vomiting, hypoglycemia, and problems with maternal and, indirectly, fetal nutrition.

F. Conception: Treatment and Education During Pregnancy

1. Normal pregnancy must be used as a reference point when attempting to normalize metabolism in a diabetic pregnancy.

   a) Lower values for fasting and preprandial blood glucose levels are normal during the second and third trimesters of pregnancy (see Figure XV.1).

   b) The heightened tendency for maternal ketosis during fasting and the possible adverse effects of ketones on the fetus suggest that periods of fasting during pregnancy should be avoided to help prevent ketonemia.[50-51]

   c) Increasing doses of rapid-acting insulin with meals often are necessary because of the increased resistance to insulin during the latter half of pregnancy. In addition, larger amounts of long- or intermediate-acting insulin are necessary to maintain basal insulin levels overnight. It is not unusual for a woman's insulin requirement to increase two- to three-fold during the course of pregnancy.

2. No general consensus exists regarding the optimal dietary guidelines for women who have pregnancies complicated by diabetes mellitus. Because no evidence exists to indicate otherwise, it is generally assumed that nutritional guidelines for pregnant women with type I and type II diabetes will be similar to recommendations for women who do not have diabetes.

   a) The goals of nutrition during pregnancy are to provide adequate nutrition throughout pregnancy for the baby and mother; to assist in appropriate gestational weight gain that is neither subnormal nor excessive; and to assist with blood glucose normalization.

b) Weight gain.

(1) The 1990 National Academy of Science[52] recommended total weight gain ranges for pregnant women based on prepregnancy body mass index (BMI):*

Weight-for-height category	Recommended total weight gain
Low (BMI <19.8)	28 - 40 lb (12.5 - 18 kg)
Normal (BMI 19.8 - 26)	25 - 35 lb (11.5 - 16 kg)
High (BMI 26 - 29)	15 - 25 lb (7 - 11.5 kg)
Obese (BMI >29)	~15 lb (6 kg)

*BMI = weight (kg)/height (m)^2 x 100

(2) However, weight gain by women giving birth to healthy infants is highly variable. Obese women have significantly heavier babies independent of weight gain. It is generally recommended that obese women gain a minimum equivalent to the products of conception (6.8 kg, 15 lb), although lower weight gains are often compatible with optimal birth weight.[53]

(3) Women should gain approximately 1 lb/wk (0.3 to 0.7 kg or 0.7 to 1.4 lb) during the second or third trimester; overweight women can gain at half that rate. Gains of less than 2 lb/month (0.9 kg/month) or more than 6.5 lb/month (3 kg/month) for normal weight women should be evaluated.[52]

c) Calories

(1) Adequate calories are needed to provide for weight gain in underweight and normal weight women and for weight maintenance or gain in obese women — weight loss is contraindicated.

(2) There are no universal recommendations for determining calories required during pregnancy (see Chapter VI: Nutrition). One method that can be used is to determine caloric requirements based on prepregnancy weight and add an additional 100 to 300 calories per day for the last two trimesters.[54-55] Another method is to take a diet history, individualize a meal plan, follow up with food records and monitor weight gain.

(3) Every attempt should be made to avoid ketonemia either from ketoacidosis or accelerated starvation ketosis in all pregnant women.[51]

(4) Monitoring blood glucose levels, urine ketones, appetite, and weight gain can guide the counselor in developing an appropriate individualized meal plan, and in making adjustments to the meal plan throughout the pregnancy.[56]

d) Insulin can be matched to food intake, but consistency of times and amounts of food eaten is essential. Smaller frequent meals and snacks are helpful. A snack at bedtime is important.

e) High-intensity sweeteners.

(1) Saccharin can cross the placenta to the fetus although there is no evidence that this is harmful to the fetus. However, avoiding excessive use during pregnancy would seem prudent.[57]

(2) Aspartame is safe for use during pregnancy with the exception of women with phenylketonuria.[57] Reproduction studies in laboratory animals show that consumption of aspartame at intake levels of at least three times the 99th percentile, poses no risk to the mother or fetus.[57]

(3) Although Acesulfame K crosses the placenta, reproduction studies show no adverse effect. It can be concluded that Acesulfame K is safe for use during pregnancy.[57]

f) Morning sickness can present a challenge. The following guidelines may be helpful:

(1) Encourage women to eat dry crackers or toast before rising.

(2) Small frequent meals help some women minimize nausea.

(3) Advise women to avoid caffeine, and foods that are spicy or have a high fat content.

(4) Encourage women to drink fluids between meals rather than with meals.

(5) Some women find it beneficial to take their prenatal vitamins before bedtime.

3. If a woman was previously sedentary, pregnancy generally is not a time to introduce strenuous activity into her lifestyle. A woman who previously was active should continue to include similar activity during her pregnancy, although she should avoid becoming dehydrated, overheated, tachycardic (HR >140 bpm), or dyspneic.

4. There is controversy regarding the goals of glycemia in the preconception period and during the course of pregnancy. Some diabetologists advocate preprandial plasma glucose levels in the range of 100 to 120 mg/dL (5.6 to 6.7 mmol/L) because these levels are associated with a minimum risk to the developing embryo.[58] Kitzmiller et al[25] advocate preprandial blood glucose ranges of 60 to 100 mg/dL (3.3 to 5.6 mmol/L) and 1-hour postprandial blood glucose ranges of 100 to 140 mg/dL (5.6 to 7.8 mmol/L) because the frequency of birth defects in patients who followed these goals in the preconception period and in early pregnancy was comparable to a nondiabetic population (approximately 2%).

a) When stating goals of glycemia, it is important to recognize that not all patients are able to achieve these goals. In Kitzmiller's successful preconception study,[25] 90% of his patient population achieved mean blood glucose levels of 104 to 160 mg/dL (5.8 to 8.9 mmol/L) during organogenesis, substantially higher than the recommended goals of glycemia. Even with these blood glucose ranges, there was no excess of congenital anomalies.

b) Additionally, when determining goals of glycemia, one must look at the individual patient and set realistic goals for her. If a woman has impaired glucose counterregulation or hypoglycemic unawareness, preprandial blood glucose levels under 100 mg/dL (3.3 to 5.6 mmol/L) may not be suitable. Hypoglycemia has not been found to be teratogenic in human studies,[19,24,25] although animal studies suggest otherwise.[59]

5. To achieve the desired ranges of glycemia, many patterns of insulin administration can be utilized. For example, some patients may do well with twice-daily injections of intermediate- and rapid-acting insulin. Others may fare better with rapid-acting insulin prior to meals and intermediate-acting insulin at bedtime. It is important to keep activity and the timing and content of meals constant from day to day so that the insulin dosage can be varied to keep up with the changing insulin requirements of pregnancy. Caution should be exercised in the first trimester because women with IDDM (type I diabetes) may have an increased incidence of hypoglycemia.

a) An estimate of the patient's insulin requirement is based on blood glucose monitoring results, weight, gestational age, and caloric intake.

b) Continuous subcutaneous insulin infusion (CSII) using an infusion pump is another efficient way to achieve normal or near-normal glucose levels in the pregnant woman with diabetes. Pregnant women using insulin pumps require extensive education to avoid complications that could arise from any interruption in insulin delivery.

6. Diabetes control is monitored through blood glucose levels, urinary ketone measurements, and glycosylated hemoglobin concentrations. In addition, some centers have successfully

measured glycosylated serum protein levels to evaluate short-term glycemic control.[60]

a) Blood glucose levels are monitored by the patient before each meal and before the bedtime snack. Additionally, postprandial measurements are necessary to evaluate the effectiveness of rapid-acting insulin and 3 A.M. levels are helpful to evaluate unexplained fasting hyperglycemia.

b) Urine monitoring for ketones is performed daily on the first morning urine specimen, any time the premeal blood glucose level exceeds 150 mg/dL (8.25 mmol/L), during illness, or when unable to eat as a result of nausea and/or vomiting. Urine measurements for ketones are important because of the increased tendency towards fat catabolism during pregnancy. Ketones cross the placenta if the patient has ketonemia and may be potentially harmful to the fetus.

(1) The presence of ketonuria with normal or low blood glucose levels suggests inadequate food intake.

(2) The presence of ketonuria in the face of mildly elevated blood glucose levels may indicate incipient ketoacidosis.

(a) The main cause of ketoacidosis is infection.

(b) Ketoacidosis in pregnancy is associated with a high perinatal mortality rate.

(c) B-sympathomimetic therapy such as Yutopar (ritodrine) to treat premature labor has been reported to cause deterioration of blood glucose control and ketosis in pregnant diabetic women.[61] These agents should be used only during careful monitoring of blood glucose levels.

c) Glycosylated hemoglobin measurements may be obtained monthly during pregnancy. Ideally, patients should achieve normal or near normal values.

d) Food records are helpful to assess actual food intake.

7. Hospitalization may be indicated whenever pregnancy is diagnosed in a patient with diabetes who has not been following an intensive management regimen prior to conception. Other indications for hospitalization include a lack of self-management skills, nausea and vomiting that prevent adequate caloric intake, deterioration of blood glucose control that is unresolved by close telephone contact, hyperglycemia with moderate or large ketonuria, patient nonadherence, and any obstetric complication such as preeclampsia or premature labor.[32]

G. Monitoring of the Fetus During Pregnancy

1. Fetal ultrasonography in the first or early second trimester allows confirmation of gestational age and helps to verify the absence of certain malformations such as neural tube defects. A fetal echocardiogram in mid-pregnancy screens for congenital heart defects. Serial ultrasounds thereafter assess growth of the fetus and amniotic fluid volume.

2. A blood test to screen maternal serum alpha-fetoprotein (MSAFP) levels provides additional information when trying to identify the fetus at risk for a neural tube defect. In women with diabetes, the incidence of neural tube defects is 20 per 1000, 10- to 20-times greater than in the general population.[62] Thus, all diabetic women should be referred for targeted ultrasound regardless of their MSAFP test result.

   a) Neural tube defects develop from defective closure of the neural tube during embryogenesis which results in anencephaly, encephalocele, and all variants of spina bifida.

   b) The MSAFP test should be offered between 14 and 18 weeks of gestation, and if the result is elevated, it provides evidence that the fetus may have a neural tube defect or other abnormality.

FIGURE XV.2: Fetal Movement Record[63]

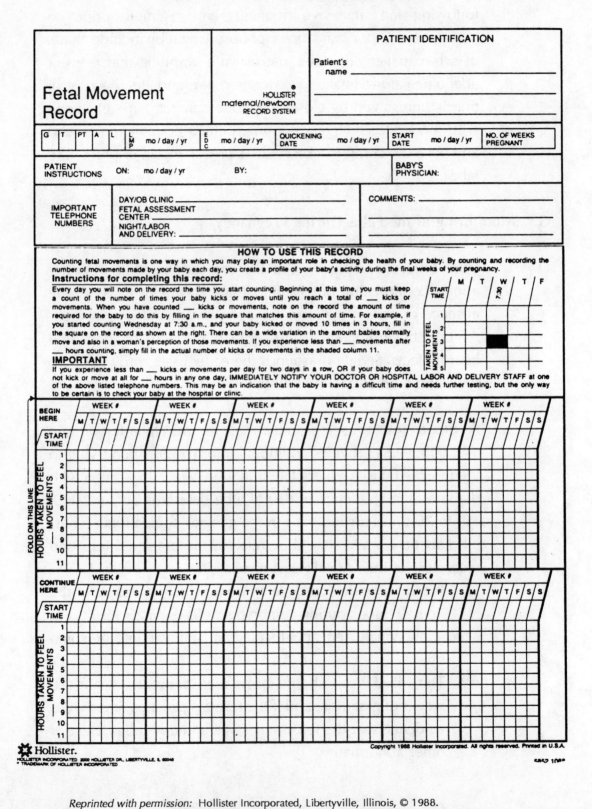

3. Fetal activity can be monitored by all women in the third trimester of pregnancy. One method is to keep track of fetal movements over a 12-hour period. If fewer than 10 movements are observed during the 12-hour period, or if it takes progressively longer before the 10 movements are identified, the woman should notify her obstetrician immediately for further evaluation of fetal status.[63] Another method is to count fetal movement for several 30-minute or 1-hour periods each day. The patient may be asked to keep written records of fetal movement (see Figure XV.2).

4. The nonstress test (NST) helps identify fetuses that are doing well in utero and those that may be at risk for fetal demise. The NST uses ultrasound to monitor the fetal heart rate and a sensor to detect any uterine contractions.

    a) In some centers, nonstress tests are performed weekly from the gestational age of 32 to 34 weeks, then twice weekly from 36 weeks until delivery. If a nonstress test is abnormal or nonreactive, a contraction stress test or a biophysical profile may be ordered.

    b) Earlier and more frequent testing may be necessary for patients who have vascular disease.

5. Weekly contraction stress tests are used by some centers to assess fetal well-being beginning at 32 to 34 weeks. The contraction stress test (CST) is a record of the fetal heart rate response to mild uterine contractions, which are induced by intravenous pitocin or by nipple stimulation.

    a) If late decelerations of the fetal heart rate occur following more than 50% of the uterine contractions, the test is considered positive.

    b) A positive CST may indicate fetal distress and the need for delivery.

6. A biophysical profile is another test to discriminate between fetuses that are well-adapted to their intrauterine environment and those in danger of fetal demise.

a) A biophysical profile involves the evaluation of 5 parameters. Ultrasound is used to assess 4 components: fetal breathing, fetal body movement, fetal tone, and amniotic fluid volume. Fetal heart-rate activity is evaluated by means of a nonstress test. Two points are given for the normal observation of each of these five parameters. The lowest score is 0 and the highest score is 10.

b) A biophysical profile sometimes is performed when a NST is nonreactive or a CST is positive.

7. An amniocentesis generally is performed to assess fetal lung maturity. Amniocentesis may be part of the protocol when an induction of labor or elective caesarean section is planned prior to 39 weeks.

8. Many pregnancies can be allowed to progress to term as long as fetal health does not appear to be compromised and no maternal complication (such as preeclampsia) is present.

H. Monitoring Glycemia During Labor and Delivery

1. The goals of managing maternal diabetes during labor are to provide adequate carbohydrate intake to meet maternal energy requirements and to maintain maternal euglycemia.

a) To accomplish the goal of meeting maternal energy requirements and thus prevent ketosis, glucose is administered 2.0 to 2.5 mg/kg/min by continuous intravenous infusion.[64] This dosage corresponds to approximately 5 to 10 g/hour in lean individuals.

b) To accomplish the goal of maintaining maternal euglycemia, maternal blood glucose values are measured every 1 to 2 hours, and rapid-acting insulin is administered by multiple subcutaneous doses or by continuous intravenous infusion as necessary. Maintaining euglycemia may help prevent undue stimulation of fetal insulin secretion prior to delivery that could result in neonatal hypoglycemia.[63]

(1) Insulin pumps (CSII) have been used successfully during labor and delivery.

(2) Regardless of the method, the key to successful intrapartum management is to monitor blood glucose levels frequently and administer insulin and glucose as necessary.

I. Postpartum Period

1. The postpartum period is characterized by an immediate decrease in insulin requirements lasting for a variable time until prepregnancy requirements are re-established. An occasional patient may require little or no insulin during the first 24 to 48 hours following the delivery of her baby. If no reduction in insulin requirements occurs, an underlying infection, such as endometritis or a urinary tract infection may be present.

2. Many issues surround the patient in the postpartum period. She needs to balance her own self-care needs with the needs of the infant. She requires close follow-up of diabetes control to re-establish her baseline insulin requirement. She may need referral to a registered dietitian concerning weight reduction and/or prevention of hypoglycemia while breast-feeding. As always, the educator's role should be supportive during this period of adjustment.

J. Lactation

1. Patients should be encouraged to breast-feed as long as they are not taking medications that affect breast milk. In some situations, the breast-feeding mother may require less insulin because of the calories expended with nursing. She also may need counseling concerning the risk of hypoglycemia.

2. Patients who decide to breast-feed should remain on a meal plan approximately the same as that of the third trimester of pregnancy. The bedtime snack may need to be adjusted

because of an increased potential for hypoglycemia following the nighttime breast-feeding.

K. **Contraception and Family Planning**

1. There are a number of contraceptive options for the woman who has diabetes.

    a) Barrier methods create mechanical and/or chemical barriers to fertilization. Barrier methods include diaphragms, male condoms, spermicidal foam or jelly, cervical caps, and contraceptive sponges. Although these methods pose no health risks to women with diabetes, they are user-dependent, require correct application or insertion before intercourse, and have a high failure rate of 12% to 28%[65,66] in the first year because people do not use them correctly. With experience and motivation, these failure rates may be reduced to levels of 2% to 6%.[65,66]

    b) Oral contraceptives remain the most popular form of birth control despite controversy over potential side effects. The main reasons for their popularity are their low failure rate of generally less than 1% and the ease with which they are taken. Low-dose formulations are preferred and should be restricted to patients without vascular complications or additional risk factors such as smoking or a strong family history of myocardial disease.[63]

    c) The intrauterine device (IUD) is the most effective nonhormonal device.[65] It should only be offered to women who have a low risk of sexually transmitted diseases because any infection might place the patient with diabetes at risk for sepsis and ketoacidosis. Patients should be educated about the early signs of sexually transmitted diseases, such as increased and abnormal vaginal discharge, dyspareunia, heavy painful menses, lower abdominal pain, and fever.[65] The patient should receive prompt medical attention if any of these symptoms occur.

d) Depoprovera® and Norplant® are long-acting progestins that provide excellent pregnancy protection. Depoprovera® is administered intramuscularly every 3 months and works by inhibiting ovulation. Norplant® is a long-acting, reversible, silicone-rubber covered, hormonal implant that offers 5-year protection and 99% effectiveness.[67] Norplant® works by inhibiting ovulation, thickening cervical mucus, and changing the uterine-lining.[67] The high efficiency and long period of action of Depoprovera® and Norplant® make them attractive options for women with diabetes or previous gestational diabetes mellitus (GDM), especially women with a history of poor medical compliance.[65] Unfortunately, these long-acting progestins have not been studied in this patient population.

e) Permanent sterilization, including tubal ligation and vasectomy, may be offered to the patient or her partner when they have completed childbearing and desire no more children.

L. Gestational Diabetes

1. Gestational diabetes mellitus (GDM) usually is detected during the 24th to 28th week of pregnancy when the insulin resistance of pregnancy becomes marked.

   a) GDM is defined as carbohydrate intolerance of variable severity, with onset or first recognition during pregnancy.[3-6] This definition applies regardless of whether insulin was instituted during pregnancy or the condition persisted following pregnancy.

   b) The definition does not exclude the possibility that unrecognized glucose intolerance may have antedated the pregnancy.

2. Pregnancies complicated by GDM have implications for both the mother and her offspring. Women who develop this condition have an increased risk for perinatal loss when GDM

is undetected or goes untreated, and are at a high risk for developing glucose intolerance in later life.

a) A 6.4% perinatal mortality rate has been observed in pregnancies complicated by untreated GDM in women over 25 years of age compared with a 1.5% rate in pregnant women with normal glucose tolerance.[68]

b) In patients with appropriately treated GDM, the likelihood of intrauterine death is not significantly higher than in the general population.[6]

c) GDM also is associated with many of the same fetal and neonatal morbidities observed in patients with pregestational diabetes, including macrosomia, hypoglycemia, hypocalcemia, polycythemia, and hyperbilirubinemia. Macrosomia is the most important of these perinatal concerns and is observed two to three times more often than expected.[6] GDM, with its onset in late pregnancy, is not associated with an increased incidence of birth defects. However, pre-existing diabetes, which is diagnosed for the first time during pregnancy as GDM, may result in a higher risk of birth defects.[6]

d) Studies suggest that the long-range implications for offspring of women with GDM may include an increased risk of obesity in adolescence[69,70] and impaired glucose tolerance later in life.[71]

e) The maternal implication of gestational diabetes is a high risk for developing overt non-insulin-dependent diabetes mellitus later in life.[72,73] Elevated fasting plasma glucose levels, increased maternal age, and relative insulinopenia during pregnancy appear to be related to an increased risk for abnormal glucose tolerance in the first postpartum year.[74]

3. All pregnant women should be screened for glucose intolerance because clinical risk factors such as previous birth of a large baby, maternal obesity, glycosuria, or family history of diabetes have been shown to be poor predictors of GDM.[75-77] Furthermore, GDM generally is an asymptomatic condition.

a) Screening for GDM should take place between the 24th and 28th week of gestation if a woman has not been identified as having glucose intolerance before the 24th week of gestation.[4,6]

b) Any woman who presents with a history suggestive of prior or current glucose intolerance should be screened immediately. A fasting plasma glucose measurement ≥140 mg/dL (7.8 mmol/L) or a plasma glucose measurement ≥200 mg/dL (11.1 mmol/L) outside the context of a formal glucose challenge suggests a diabetic state and warrants immediate further investigation.[6]

    (1) The screening test involves obtaining a plasma glucose measurement 1 hour after consuming 50 grams of oral glucose without regard to the time of the last meal or the time of day. A value of 140 mg/dL (7.8 mmol/L) or greater is a positive screening test[4,6] and requires further evaluation with an OGTT (see Table XV.3). Test strips and reflectance meters are not sufficiently accurate for screening and diagnosis.[6]

    (2) Women who have a clinical history suspicious of glucose intolerance, but have a normal screening test during the 24th to 28th week of gestation, should be considered for rescreening during the 32nd to 34th week.

    (3) Women with an abnormal screen followed by a normal 3-hour OGTT might be considered candidates to repeat the 3-hour OGTT at 32-34 weeks.

4. Diagnosis of GDM is based on the results of the 100 gram oral glucose tolerance test according to the diagnostic criteria of O'Sullivan and Mahan.[78]

a) The oral glucose tolerance test should be performed in the morning after an overnight fast of at least 8 hours but no greater than 14 hours.

TABLE XV.3: Screening/Testing for GDM

Who	When	Type of Test	Results
All Women	24 to 28 Weeks	BG level 1 hour post 50 g oral glucose	+ Screen if BG result ≥140 mg/dL (7.8 mmol/L)
Women who have a positive screen	24 to 28 weeks	100 g 3-hour OGTT	+ Diagnosis if meets O'Sullivan and Mahan criteria
Women who have a Clinical history/ Normal screen	32 to 34 weeks	Repeat 1-hour post 50 g oral glucose	Repeating the screen is based upon clinical judgement
Women diagnosed with GDM	6 to 8 weeks postpartum	75 g 2-hour OGTT	Classify according to National Diabetes Data Group

Abbreviations: OGTT, oral glucose tolerance test; BG, blood glucose.

b)   At least 3 days of unrestricted diet (≥150 g carbohydrate per day) and unrestricted activity should precede the test.

c)   Subjects should remain seated and not smoke during the test.

d)   A definitive diagnosis of GDM requires that two or more of the venous plasma glucose levels listed in Table XV.4 are met or exceeded.[78]

e)   It may be prudent to notify the physician of the fasting blood glucose level before administration of the glucose load if possible. A high fasting level may be sufficient to make the diagnosis and may make further glucose administration dangerous.

5.   Treatment consists of improving the metabolic abnormalities associated with GDM through meal planning and insulin therapy (if indicated), and providing close obstetric surveillance.

TABLE XV.4:
GDM Diagnostic Criteria of O'Sullivan and Mahan[78]

Time (h)	Venous Plasma Glucose Levels	
	[mg/dL	(mmol/L)]
0	105	5.8
1	190	10.6
2	165	9.2
3	145	8.1

a) The goals and strategies for nutrition care are the same for a GDM pregnancy as for pregestational diabetic pregnancy (see section F.1 above and Chapter VI: Nutrition). Individualization of the meal plan is recommended based on the woman's prepregnancy body weight.[79]

b) Calories

(1) The goal is to provide adequate calories and optimal nutrition needed for pregnancy without hyperglycemia or ketonemia. Frequent small feedings with limited carbohydrates at breakfast often will return blood glucose levels to normal.

(2) The use of caloric restriction in treating obese women with GDM requires further study.[80,81]

c) Macronutrients

(1) The ideal percentage and type of carbohydrate is controversial. A reasonable meal plan will have between 30% and 45% of the carbohydrate at meals and when snacks are included approximately 45% of the calories for the total day are from carbohydrate, 20% from protein, and 35% from fat. However, more important than percentages are the actual grams of carbohydrate. Breakfast meals generally require less

than 30 grams of carbohydrate to prevent excessive elevations of postprandial blood glucose levels. Concentrated sources of carbohydrates should be eliminated.

d) Exercise can also help to lower postprandial glucose elevations.

(1) Women with GDM who have an active lifestyle may continue a program of moderate exercise[6] combined with frequent blood glucose monitoring.[82] Studies are necessary to determine the effects of cardiovascular fitness training on fetal outcome and the effects of such exercise on ketone production.[6] Exercise programs should be individualized and conducted under careful medical scrutiny.

e) Insulin therapy may be beneficial to some patients with GDM. The major benefit derived from this therapy is some reduction in the incidence of macrosomia in the newborn.[83,84]

(1) The initiation of insulin is now widely recommended when standard dietary management does not consistently maintain a fasting plasma glucose level <105 mg/dL (<5.8 mmol/L) and/or a 2-hour postprandial plasma glucose level <120 mg/dL (<6.7 mmol/L).[6]

(2) There appears to be a relationship between the level of glycemia and neonatal weight.[85] Consequently, overtreatment with insulin may result in small-for-gestational-age (SGA) infants. Langer et al[85] have reported that a mean blood glucose level consisting of both preprandial and postprandial values <87 mg/dL (4.8 mmol/L) increased the incidence 2.55-fold for the development of SGA infants.

(3) When insulin is prescribed, non-animal-source (human) preparations should be used.

(4) Oral hypoglycemic agents are not recommended during pregnancy because they cross the placenta and may potentiate fetal hyperinsulinism.

(5) More studies are necessary to determine if the routine use of insulin should be advocated in all pregnancies complicated by GDM.

6. No data are available concerning the optimal approach to metabolic monitoring of GDM. Surveillance of diabetes control should be directed at monitoring for elevations of fasting and postprandial glucose values in capillary blood or venous plasma samples.[4,6] Daily urinary ketone accumulation should be measured in the first voided morning specimen to determine if dietary carbohydrate and caloric intake are adequate.

7. Fetal monitoring tests are an important part of the management of GDM. The tests that are utilized are the same as those described in the section on pregestational diabetes fetal monitoring. The time in pregnancy to initiate these tests depends upon the practice in a given institution and whether the woman with GDM is taking exogenous insulin.

8. Patients generally are permitted to begin labor spontaneously at term unless fetal health appears compromised. The goals of managing the gestational diabetic woman in labor are the same as those previously outlined in the pregestational diabetes section.
    a) The blood glucose is periodically monitored during labor. Normal or near-normal glucose levels frequently are maintained during labor without the need for insulin therapy in gestational diabetic women.
    b) Insulin treatment can be discontinued in the immediate postpartum period. Women who then manifest nongravid diabetes can be managed with meal planning, oral agents, and/or insulin therapy as indicated.

9. The postpartum period demands special education and follow-up because of the high risk of subsequent diabetes in the mother.

a) Following delivery, all women should be re-evaluated for glucose intolerance. The American Diabetes Association[86] and the Second and Third International Workshop — Conferences on Gestational Diabetes[4,6] recommend that all women receive their initial evaluation (a 2-hour oral glucose tolerance test with 75 grams of glucose) at the first 6- to 8-week postpartum visit.

b) Based on the result of this test, a woman then should be categorized as having previous abnormality of glucose tolerance, impaired glucose tolerance, or diabetes mellitus in the nonpregnant adult in accordance with the National Diabetes Data Group (see Chapter V: Pathophysiology).

c) Because the risk of subsequent diabetes is so high, some centers test all patients with an oral glucose tolerance test in the postpartum period and yearly thereafter.

d) Patient education should include the importance of attaining and maintaining a reasonable body weight, receiving annual blood glucose testing, and contacting a member of the medical team if symptoms of hyperglycemia develop. Low-dose oral contraceptives appear to be safe in women with prior GDM who demonstrate normal glucose tolerance in the postpartum period.[6] High-dose synthetic estrogen/progestin contraceptives should be avoided in these patients. Additionally, the use of other medications that may affect glucose metabolism adversely, such as thiazides, steroids, and beta-blockers, requires careful consideration.[6]

e) Patients should be encouraged to breast-feed as long as they are not taking medications that affect breast milk. Patients who elect to breast-feed are maintained on their third trimester diet to meet lactation needs. The postpartum 75 g 2-hour OGTT may be affected by lactation.

REFERENCES

1. Freinkel N, Metzger BE, Potter JM. Pregnancy in diabetes. In: Ellenberg M, Rifkin H, eds. Diabetes mellitus: theory and practice. 3rd ed. New York: Medical Examination Publishing, 1983:689-714.

2. Jovanovic L, Druzin M, Peterson CM. Effect of euglycemia on the outcome of pregnancy in insulin-dependent diabetic women as compared with normal control subjects. Am J Med 1981;71:921-27.

3. National Diabetes Data Group. Classification and diagnosis of diabetes mellitus and other categories of glucose intolerance. Diabetes 1979;28:1039-57.

4. Freinkel N, Gabbe SG, Hadden DR, et al. Summary and recommendations of the second international workshop-conference on gestational diabetes mellitus. Diabetes 1985;34(suppl 2):123-26.

5. Freinkel N, Josimovich J, Conference Planning Committee. American Diabetes Association workshop-conference on gestational diabetes. Summary and recommendations. Diabetes Care 1980;3:499-501.

6. Metzger BE, Organizing Committee. Summary and recommendations of the third international workshop-conference on gestational diabetes mellitus. Diabetes 1991;40(suppl 2):197-201.

7. Connell FA, Vadheim C, Ammenual I. Diabetes in pregnancy: a population-based study of incidence, referral for care and perinatal mortality. Am J Obstet Gynecol 1985;151:598-603.

8. Freinkel N. Gestational diabetes 1979: philosophical and practical aspects of a major public health problem. Diabetes Care 1980;3:399-401.

9. O'Sullivan JB, Harris MI, Mills JL. Maternal diabetes in pregnancy. In: Harris MI, Hammon RF, eds. Diabetes in America. Washington, DC: US Government Printing Office, 1984;XX:1-17.

10. Metzger BE, Hare JW, Freinkel N. Carbohydrate metabolism in pregnancy. IX: Plasma levels of gluconeogenic fuels during fasting in the rat. J Clin Endocrinol Metab 1971;33:869-72.

11. Jovanovic L, Druzin M, Peterson CM. Effects of the conceptus on maternal metabolism during pregnancy. In: Liebel BS, Wrenshall GA, eds. On the nature and treatment of diabetes. Amsterdam: Excerpta Medica, 1965:679-91.

12. Phelps RL, Metzger BE, Freinkel N. Carbohydrate metabolism in pregnancy. XVII. Diurnal profiles of plasma glucose, insulin, free fatty acids, triglycerides, cholesterol and individual amino acids in late normal pregnancy. Am J Obstet Gynecol 1981;140:730-36.

13. Pederson J. The pregnant diabetic and her newborn infant. 2nd edition. Baltimore, Md: Williams and Wilkins, 1977;191-97.

14. Karlsson K, Kjellmer I. The outcome of diabetic pregnancies in relation to the mother's blood sugar level. Am J Obstet Gynecol 1972;112:213-20.

15. Miller E, Hare JW, Cloherty JP, et al. Elevated maternal hemoglobin A_{1c} in early pregnancy and major congenital anomalies in infants of diabetic mothers. N Engl J Med 1981;304:1331-34.

16. Simpson JL, Elias S, Martin AO, et al. Diabetes in pregnancy, Northwestern University series (1977-1981): prospective study of anomalies in offspring of mothers with diabetes mellitus. Am J Obstet Gynecol 1983;146:263-70.

17. Ylinen K, Aula P, Stenman UH, et al. Risk of minor and major fetal malformations in diabetics with high hemoglobin A_{1c} values in early pregnancy. Br Med J 1984;289:345-46.

18. Miodovnik M, Mimouni F, Dignan PS, et al. Major malformations in infants of IDDM women: vasculopathy and early first trimester poor glycemic control. Diabetes Care 1988;11:713-18.

19. Mills JL, Knopp RH, Simpson JL, et al. Lack of relation of increased malformation rates in infants of diabetic mothers to glycemic control during organogenesis. N Engl J Med 1988;318:671-76.

20. Greene MF, Hare JW, Cloherty JP, et al. First trimester hemoglobin A_1 and risk for major malformation and spontaneous abortion in diabetic pregnancy. Teratology 1989;39:225-31.

21. Mills JL, Baker L, Goldman AS. Malformations in infants of diabetic mothers occur before the seventh gestational week: implications for treatment. Diabetes 1979;28:292-93.

22. Fuhrmann K, Reiher H, Semmler K, et al. Prevention of congenital malformations in infants of insulin-dependent diabetic mothers. Diabetes Care 1983;6:219-23.

23. Fuhrmann K, Reiher H, Semmler K, Glockner E. The effect of intensified conventional insulin before and during pregnancy on the malformation rate in offspring of diabetic mothers. Exp Clin Endocrinol 1984;83:173-77.

24. Steel JM, Johnstone FD, Hepburn DA, Smith AF. Can prepregnancy care of diabetic women reduce the risk of abnormal babies? Br Med J 1990;301:1070-74.

25. Kitzmiller JL, Gavin LA, Gin GD, et al. Preconception care of diabetes: glycemic control prevents congenital anomalies. JAMA 1991;265:731-36.

26. Cornblath M, Schwartz R. Disorders of carbohydrate metabolism in infancy. Philadelphia: WB Saunders, 1976.

27. American College of Obstetricians and Gynecologists. Technical Bulletin 159. Fetal macrosomia. ACOG 1991;159:1-5.

28. Spellacy WN, Miller S, Wingos A. Macrosomia-maternal characteristics and infant complications. Obstet Gynecol 1985;66:158.

29. Hare JW, White P. Gestational diabetes and the White classification. Diabetes Care 1980;3:394.

30. White P. Pregnancy complicating diabetes. Am J Med 1949;7:609-16.

31. Pedersen J, Pedersen LM, Anderson B. Assessors of fetal perinatal mortality in diabetic pregnancy: analysis of 1,332 pregnancies in the Copenhagen series 1946-1972. Diabetes 1974;23:302.

32. Buchanan TA, Unterman TG, Metzger BE. The medical management of diabetes in pregnancy. Clin Perinatol 1985;12:625-50.

33. Mills JL, Simpson JL, Driscoll SG, et al. Incidence of spontaneous abortion among normal women and insulin-dependent diabetic women whose pregnancies were identified within 21 days of conception. N Eng J Med 1988;319:1617-23.

34. Warram JH, Krolewski AS, Kahn CR. Determinants of IDDM and perinatal mortality in children of diabetic mothers. Diabetes 1988;37:1328-34.

35. Kobberly J, Tallil H. Empirical risk figures for first degree relatives of non-insulin-dependent diabetics. In: Genetics of Diabetes Mellitus, Proceedings of the Serone Symposia, Vol. 47 London: Academic Press, 1982:201.

36. Phelps RL, Sakol P, Metzger BE, et al. Changes in diabetic retinopathy during pregnancy: correlations with regulation of hyperglycemia. Arch Ophthalmol 1986;104:1806-10.

37. Klein BE, Moss SE, Klein R. Effect of pregnancy on progression of diabetic retinopathy. Diabetes Care 1990;13:35-40.

38. The Kroc Collaborative Study Group. The Kroc study at two years: a report on further retinal changes. N Engl J Med 1984;311:365-72.

39. Chang S, Fuhrmann M. The diabetes in early pregnancy study group. Pregnancy, retinopathy, normoglycemia: a preliminary analysis. Diabetes 1985;34(suppl):3A.

40. Moloney JB, Drury MI. The effect of pregnancy on the natural cause of diabetic retinopathy. Am J Ophthalmol 1982;93:745-56.

41. Kitzmiller JL, Gavin LA, Gin GD, et al. Managing diabetes and pregnancy. Curr Probl Obstet Gynecol Fertil 1988;11:125-26.

42. Dibble CM, Kochenour NK, Worley RJ, et al. Effect of pregnancy on diabetic retinopathy. Obstet Gynecol 1982;59:699-704.

43. Cassar J. Kohner EM, Hamilton AM, et al. Diabetic retinopathy and pregnancy. Practical Diabetol 1978;15:105-11.

44. Kitzmiller JL, Brown ER, Phillipe M, et al. Diabetic nephropathy and perinatal outcome. Am J Obstet Gynecol 1981;141:741-51.

45. Reece EA, Coustan DR, Hayslett JP, et al. Diabetic nephropathy: pregnancy performance and feto-maternal outcome. Am J Obstet Gynecol 1988;159:56-66.

46. Grenfell A, Brudenell JM, Doddridge MC, Watkins PJ. Pregnancy in diabetic women who have proteinuria. Q J Med 1986;59:379-86.

47. Jovanovic R, Jovanovic L. Obstetric management when normoglycemia is maintained in diabetic pregnant women with vascular compromise. Am J Obstet Gynecol 1984;149:617-23.

48. Hou SH, Grossman SD, Madias NE. Pregnancy in women with renal disease and moderate renal insufficiency. Am J Med 1985;78:185-94.

49. Kitzmiller JK, Aiello LM, Kaldany A, Younger MD. Diabetic vascular disease complicating pregnancy. Clin Obstet Gynecol 1981;25:107.

50. Churchill JA, Berendes HW. Intelligence of children whose mothers had acetonuria during pregnancy. In: Perinatal factors affecting human development. Pan American Health Organization Scientific Publication. Washington, DC: Pan American Health Organization, 1969;185:300.

51. Rizzo T, Metzger BE, Burns WJ, Burns K. Correlations between ante partum maternal metabolism and child intelligence. N Engl J Med 1991;325:911-16.

52. National Academy of Science. Nutrition during pregnancy. National Academy Press, Washington DC. 1990.

53. Abrams BF, Laros RK. Prepregnancy weight, weight gain, and birthweight. Am J Obstet Gynecol 1986; 154:503-507.

54. Durnin JVGA. Energy requirements of pregnancy. Diabetes 1991; 40(Suppl 2):152-156.

55. National Research Council. Recommended Dietary Allowances, 10th edition. National Academy Press, Washington DC. 1989.

56. Powers MA, Metzger BE, Freinkel N. Pregnancy and diabetes. In: Powers MA, ed. Handbook of diabetes nutritional management. Rockville, Md: Aspen Publishers, 1987:332-51.

57. Position of The American Dietetic Association. Use of nutritive and non-nutritive sweeteners. J Am Diet Assoc 1993:93(7):816-21.

58. Metzger BE, Buchanan TA. Diabetes and birth defects: conclusions. Diabetes Spectrum 1990;3:181-83.

59. Buchanan TA, Schemmer JK, Freinkel N. Embryotoxic effects of brief maternal insulin-hypoglycemia during organogenesis in the rat. J Clin Invest 1986;78:643-49.

60. Nelson DM, Barrows HJ, Clapp DH, Ortman-Nabi J, Whitehurst RM. Glycosylated serum protein levels in diabetic and nondiabetic pregnant

patients. An indicator of short-term glycemic control in the diabetic patient. Am J Obstet Gynecol 1985;151:1042-47.

61. Mordes D, Kreutner K, Metzger W, Colwell JA. Dangers of intravenous ritodrine in diabetic patients. JAMA 1982;248:973-75.

62. Main DM, Mennuti MT. Neural tube defects: issues in prenatal diagnosis and counseling. Obstet Gynecol 1986;67:1-16.

63. Landon MB. Diabetes mellitus and other endocrine disorders. In: Gabble SG, Niebyl JR, Simpson JL, eds. Obstetrics: normal and problem pregnancies. New York: Churchill Livingstone, 1991:1097-136.

64. Jovanovic L, Peterson CM. Insulin and glucose requirements during the first stage of labor in insulin-dependent diabetic women. Am J Med 1983;75:607-11.

65. Kjos SL. Contraception in women with diabetes mellitus. Diabetes Spectrum 1993;6:80-86.

66. Trussel J, Hatcher RA, Cates W, et al. Contraceptive failure in the United States: an update. Stud Fam Plan 1990;21:51-54.

67. Lipinski KA. Birth control choices. Diabetes Self-Manage 1991;May/June:6-16.

68. O'Sullivan JB, Charles D, Mahan C. Gestational diabetes and perinatal mortality rate. Am J Obstet Gynecol 1973;116:901-4.

69. Pettitt DJ, Baird HR, Aleck KA, Bennet PH, Knowler WC. Excessive obesity in offspring of Pima Indian women with diabetes during pregnancy. N Engl J Med 1983;308:242-45.

70. Pettitt DJ, Knowler WC, Bennett PH, Aleck KA, Baird HR. Obesity in offspring of diabetic Pima Indian women despite normal birth weight. Diabetes Care 1987;10:76-80.

71. Pettitt DJ, Baird HR, Aleck KA, Knowler WC. Diabetes mellitus in children following maternal diabetes during gestation. Diabetes 1982;31(suppl 2):66A.

72. Mestman JH, Anderson GV, Guadalupe V. Follow-up study of 360 subjects with abnormal carbohydrate metabolism during pregnancy. Obstet Gynecol 1972;39:421-25.

73. O'Sullivan JB. Long-term follow-up of gestational diabetes. In: Camerini-Davalos RA, Cole HS, eds. Early diabetes in early life. Third International Symposium. New York: Academic Press, 1975:503-18.

74. Metzger BE, Bybee DE, Freinkel N, et al. Gestational diabetes mellitus: correlations between the phenotypic and genotypic characteristics of the mother and abnormal glucose tolerance during the first year postpartum. Diabetes 1985;34(suppl 2):111-15.

75. Lavin Jr JP. Screening of high-risk and general population for gestational diabetes. Diabetes 1985;34(suppl 2):24-27.

76. O'Sullivan JB, Mahan CM, Charles D, et al. Screening criteria for high risk gestational diabetic patients. Am J Obstet Gynecol 1973;116:895-900.

77. Coustan DR, Nelson C, Carpenter MW, Carr SR, Rotondo L, Widness JA. Maternal age and screening for gestational diabetes: a population-based study. Obstet Gynecol 1989;73:557-61.

78. O'Sullivan JB, Mahan CM. Criteria for the oral glucose tolerance test in pregnancy. Diabetes 1964;13:278-85.

79. King JC. New national academy of sciences guidelines for nutrition during pregnancy. Diabetes 1991;40(suppl 2):164.

80. Algert S, Shragg P, Hollingsworth DR. Moderate caloric restrictions in obese women with gestational diabetes. Obstet Gynecol 1985;65:487.

81.   Knopp RH, Magee S, Vidmantas R, Bendetti T. Metabolic effects of hypocaloric diets in management of gestational diabetes. Diabetes 1991;40(suppl 2):165-71.

82.   Durak EP, Jovanovic-Peterson L, Peterson CM. Physical and glycemic responses of women with gestational diabetes to a moderately intense exercise program. Diabetes Educ 1990; 16:309-12.

83.   Coustan DR, Imarah J. Prophylactic insulin treatment of gestational diabetes reduces the incidence of macrosomia, operative delivery and birth trauma. Am J Obstet Gynecol 1984;150:836-42.

84.   Drexel H, Bichler A, Sailer S, et al. Prevention of perinatal morbidity by tight metabolic control in gestational diabetes mellitus. Diabetes Care 1988;11:761-68.

85.   Langer O, Levy J, Brustman L, et al. Glycemic control in gestational diabetes mellitus — how tight is tight enough: small for gestational age versus large for gestational age. Am J Obstet Gynecol 1989;161:646-53.

86.   American Diabetes Association. Gestational diabetes mellitus. Ann Intern Med 1986;105:461.

KEY EDUCATIONAL CONSIDERATIONS
FOR PREGESTATIONAL DIABETES

1. Many women are referred to the diabetes educator for preconception counseling. They may present with an outmoded blood glucose meter, outdated insulin administration skills, and/or few healthy eating habits related to diabetes self-management. The educator should be sensitive to the needs of the patient. The patient may be defensive of skills practiced over many years or may be open and welcome to change. As always, the educator should focus on the patient's strengths and recognize that it may take working with the patient over several months to achieve optimal diabetes control.

2. When counseling the patient in the pre- and/or early postconception period, help motivate her by describing the effect of maternal diabetes on the fetus. Explain that glucose and ketones cross the placenta, and insulin and glucagon do not.

3. Explain to the patient that it is normal for her insulin dosage to increase during pregnancy and that she may see a two- to threefold increase in her dosage toward the end of pregnancy. Discuss how the placenta is thought to produce hormones that act against insulin action which is why her insulin requirement will increase. Many patients have the misconception that more insulin means that the diabetes is worse.

4. Present the goals of glycemic control for pregnancy that have been established by your individual institution. Explain how difficult it may be to accomplish these goals. Be sure to make adjustments for the patient who has problems with hypoglycemia awareness.

5. Refer all patients to a registered dietitian for nutritional counseling. Comprehension of sick day rules is important because hyperemesis can be a problem in early pregnancy.

6. Assess the patient's technique with her blood glucose meter at least once a month. Send the patient to your laboratory for a venous plasma glucose test and have her simultaneously obtain a capillary

blood glucose reading. Ideally, the capillary value should be within 10% to 15% of the laboratory value.

7. Due to the emphasis on euglycemia in pregnancy, it is important to review the signs, symptoms, causes, treatment, and prevention of hypoglycemia with the patient and a family member. Instruct the family member on glucagon administration. Treatment choices may change from the use of concentrated sources of carbohydrates such as orange juice to the use of milk.

8. Review rotating injection sites with the patient and reassure her that it is fine to rotate to her abdomen.

9. Ask the patient about her daily routine and work out a schedule together with times for meals, testing, and insulin injections. If the patient does not follow a schedule, it is virtually impossible to successfully titrate her insulin dosage to keep up with changing requirements of pregnancy.

10. Provide the patient with written parameters for when to contact you or another member of the team. Suggest that she or a family member notify you if any of the following occurs: a marked change in blood glucose levels; moderate or large ketonuria; vomiting; hypoglycemia requiring a glucagon injection or any severe episode; vaginal bleeding; severe headache; blurred vision; a decrease in fetal movement (in the second half of pregnancy); or, other pregnancy complications.

11. Following the birth of her baby and months of intensive monitoring, it is common for the mother to lose motivation for her own self-management. Remind her that careful diabetes management will help ensure future successful pregnancies and may reduce the possibility of long-term diabetes complications such as retinopathy and/or nephropathy.

12. Work with the mother closely in the postpartum period to avoid maternal hypoglycemia, which can be a safety issue for her infant and/or herself.

KEY EDUCATIONAL CONSIDERATIONS
FOR GESTATIONAL DIABETES

1. When educating women about gestational diabetes, it is important to recognize that they may be casual about following treatment guidelines because they feel well and are approaching the end of pregnancy.

    a) When teaching the pathophysiology of GDM, describe the role of insulin action in the body to keep blood glucose levels in the normal range. Explain that in the second half of pregnancy, the need for insulin increases because the placenta produces hormones that tend to work against the insulin's ability to lower blood glucose levels. Review with the patient that 3% to 5% of all women develop GDM because they are unable to produce enough of the additional insulin needed during pregnancy. Consequently, their blood glucose levels become elevated. Reassure the patient that she did not do anything to cause this condition and that her infant will not have diabetes. Explain that GDM is easily treated with meal planning or a combination of meal planning and insulin injections. Reinforce that oral agents cannot be taken during pregnancy because they cross the placenta to the developing baby.

    b) Review the results of the patient's 3-hour OGTT with her.

2. Emphasize that GDM is important to diagnose and treat because it has implications for both the mother and her baby. The maternal implication is a higher incidence of NIDDM (type II diabetes) later in life. The potential neonatal implications are macrosomia at birth and a greater propensity toward obesity and diabetes later in life.

3. Review the basics of diabetes education, explaining the relationship between diet, endogenous insulin (also exogenous insulin if the patient requires insulin therapy), and activity.

    a) Refer all patients to a registered dietitian. Emphasize the importance of ingesting all of the recommended portions so that the baby receives adequate nutrition. (Some patients may eat less than recommended in an effort to lower their blood glucose levels and thus avoid insulin injections. This eating pattern may lead to starvation ketosis).

4. Discuss your goals of glycemia with the patient and explain that there may be a need for insulin injections if her fasting and/or postprandial blood glucose levels are consistently elevated despite healthy eating. Reassure the patient that if she requires insulin, it will most likely be only for the duration of pregnancy.

5. Teach the patient how to perform capillary blood glucose monitoring. Capillary blood glucose monitoring helps the patient understand the glycemic response of foods and aids in insulin adjustments if she requires insulin.

6. Teach all patients with GDM to test their first morning urine sample for ketones.

7. As always, be alert for patients who present with a second GDM pregnancy and are using an outdated meter or strips.

8. Provide the patient with written guidelines describing when to contact you or another member of the team. Suggest that she notify you if any of the following occurs: elevated blood glucose levels; hypoglycemia (if the patient requires insulin); moderate or large ketonuria; a decrease in fetal movement (in the second half of pregnancy); vaginal bleeding; severe headache; blurred vision; or, other pregnancy complications.

9. Stress the importance of maternal follow-up in the postpartum period for glucose intolerance.

If you are unsure of the answers to the following questions, please review the materials.

1. What are the normal metabolic changes related to pregnancy during the latter half of gestation?
2. Why is it important to achieve optimal diabetes control prior to conception?
3. What are four potential neonatal complications that may occur in pregnancies complicated by diabetes mellitus?
4. Why are nonstress tests routinely ordered in pregnant women with diabetes?
5. What are three maternal complications associated with diabetes and pregnancy?
6. When should pregnant women with diabetes test their urine for ketones?
7. What should preconception counseling include?
8. Define gestational diabetes.
9. Why should all women be screened for gestational diabetes between the 24th and 28th weeks of pregnancy?
10. What are two methods that might be used to assess fetal status?
11. What should be addressed with women who have gestational diabetes in the postpartum period?
12. Discuss contraceptive options for women with diabetes.

CASE EXAMPLE 1
PREGESTATIONAL DIABETES

NC is a 29-year-old newly married woman with insulin-dependent diabetes mellitus (IDDM) who presented to the Diabetes in Pregnancy Center for preconception counseling and care. NC was diagnosed with IDDM at age 10 years, and has maintained good health with the exception of one episode of DKA at age 12 years, when she had the flu. She has never been pregnant and is using a diaphragm with spermicidal cream as her method of contraception. NC denies a history of diabetic nephropathy and claims that she is normotensive. Her history is significant for background retinopathy that was diagnosed 1 year ago.

At this initial visit, a physical was performed in addition to recording NC's history. NC's blood pressure was 110/70 and her urine sample tested 1+ for protein on dipstick. Her blood glucose records during the previous 2 weeks were reviewed. She appeared to be in reasonably good diabetes control with fasting blood glucose values ranging from 80 to 130 mg/dL (4.4 to 7.2 mmol/L) and pre-supper values from 95 to 140 mg/dL (5.3 to 7.8 mmol/L). NC tested blood glucose levels only twice daily. She was on a three-injection regimen with short- and intermediate-acting insulin prior to breakfast, short-acting insulin prior to supper, and intermediate-acting insulin prior to bedtime. NC did not bring her capillary blood glucose meter with her during this initial visit.

QUESTIONS

1. What laboratory tests would be recommended for this patient?
2. What topics would you counsel her about?
3. How would you involve her husband in the education?

SUGGESTED SOLUTIONS

NC would be asked to obtain baseline renal function studies including a 24-hour urine for creatinine clearance and quantitative protein. A urinalysis also would be performed to rule out a urinary tract infection which might cause the 1+ proteinuria. Additionally, a glycosylated hemoglobin would be obtained to assess overall glycemic control, as well as a rubella titer to assess her immune status. If the patient is nonimmune, an inoculation could be administered during this preconception period. In addition to these laboratory tests, NC would be referred to a retinal specialist for a reassessment of her background retinopathy, and to a team dietitian to evaluate her nutritional intake. The dietitian would work with NC to integrate exercise into her management plan.

NC would be counseled about the goals of glycemia and would be asked to check capillary blood glucose levels prior to each meal and her bedtime snack on a daily basis, as well as 1-hour postprandial levels 2 to 3 days a week. She would be asked to call the diabetes educator at least once a week so that any necessary insulin and/or dietary adjustments could be made. NC would be counseled not to discontinue her barrier method of contraception until she, her husband, and the medical team agree it is safe to do so (eg, when blood glucose levels are optimal and the glycosylated hemoglobin level is in the normal or near-normal range).

The topics of fertility, spontaneous abortion rate, incidence of diabetes mellitus in offspring, effects of pregnancy on existing vascular complications, and the incidence of congenital anomalies in IDMs would be discussed, and any questions would be answered. NC would be encouraged to bring her husband to her next appointment in 1 month so that he could learn how to administer glucagon and be educated about diabetes in pregnancy. Additionally, NC would be asked to bring her glucose meter so her technique and accuracy could be assessed.

CASE EXAMPLE 2
GESTATIONAL DIABETES

RG is a 24-year-old G2P1000 (gravida, term, preterm, abortion, live), obese Hispanic woman who presented to the outpatient Diabetes in Pregnancy Center at 30 $^1/_7$ weeks of gestation. RG stated that she was referred to the center by her family practitioner because he thought she had an excessively large baby with this pregnancy.

RG's past obstetric history was significant for GDM in her first pregnancy, 2 years earlier. That pregnancy resulted in the delivery of a 9 lb 12 oz (4.4 kg) stillborn son at 38+ weeks of gestation. RG's family history was positive for NIDDM, which was diagnosed in her mother at 40 years of age.

A 3-hour OGTT was obtained on RG 3 days later. The results were:

Time (h)	Plasma Glucose mg/dL(mmol/L)
FBS	112 (6.2)
1	250 (13.9)
2	224 (12.4)
3	190 (10.6)

RG was diagnosed with GDM and was started on two injections per day of insulin. She was counseled by a dietitian and agreed on a meal plan.

In addition, RG learned how to monitor capillary blood glucose levels and urine ketone levels. Weekly nonstress tests were instituted at 34 weeks of gestation and RG was instructed to call immediately if she experienced any decrease in fetal movement. As a result of intensive diabetes education and management, and careful fetal monitoring, RG successfully delivered a healthy, term, 7 lb (3.2 kg) infant.

QUESTIONS

1. What other information would you like to have received about this patient?
2. How would you have handled this patient if she had come to you at 6 weeks of gestation instead of at 30 $\frac{1}{7}$ weeks?
3. What advice would you give RG about the long-term implications of GDM?

SUGGESTED SOLUTIONS

It would be important to find out if RG had received an OGTT following the delivery of her stillborn son to determine if she still had diabetes, had impaired glucose tolerance, or was normoglycemic when she was not pregnant. In addition, more information surrounding the stillbirth would have been helpful. Was she preeclamptic? Was there a cord accident? Did she have a placental abruption? The absence of these obstetric complications suggests, but does not prove, that the stillbirth was related to maternal diabetes.

If RG had first presented for care at 6 weeks rather than at 30 $\frac{1}{7}$ weeks of gestation, she would have been screened for diabetes immediately because she had several risk factors for GDM (obesity, family history of diabetes, history of a stillborn macrosomic infant). In fact, she may have remained hyperglycemic following her first pregnancy. Screening early in pregnancy helps to identify those women who probably were glucose intolerant prior to conception.

In the postpartum period, RG would be informed that she was at a high risk for developing diabetes later in life. She would be scheduled for an OGTT and would be advised to lose weight after she discontinued breast-feeding. Additionally, she would be encouraged to obtain annual blood glucose testing and would be advised to contact her physician if she developed any signs or symptoms of hyperglycemia. If RG desired any more children, she also would be advised to be tested for diabetes before discontinuing contraception.

OTHER SUGGESTED READINGS

AADE Task Force on Diabetes and Pregnancy. Educational guidelines for pre-existing diabetes complicated by pregnancy. Diabetes Educ 1993;19:15-17.

California Diabetes and Pregnancy Program. Sweet success: guidelines for care. Campbell, Calif: Education Program Associates, 1992.

Franz, M, Cooper N, Mullen L, Birk PS, Hollander P. Gestational diabetes: guidelines for a safe pregnancy and a healthy baby. Minneapolis, Minn: Diabetes Center Inc, 1988.

Kitzmiller JL, Gavin LA, Gin GD, et al. Managing diabetes and pregnancy. Curr Probl Obstet Gynecol Fertil 1988;11:113-67.

Kitzmiller JL, Gavin LA, Gin GD, et al. Preconception care of diabetes: glycemic control prevents congenital anomalies. JAMA 1991;265:731-36.

Metzger BE, Buchanan TA, eds. Diabetes and birth defects. Diabetes Spectrum 1990;3:149-83.

Metzger BE, Organizing Committee. Summary and recommendations of the third international workshop-conference on gestational diabetes mellitus. Diabetes 1991;40(suppl 2):197-201.

Radak JT. Why worry about gestational diabetes? Diabetes Forecast 1991; April:27-29.

Wason CJ, Metzger BE. You can do it: diabetes management for mothers-to-be. Elkhart, Ind: Ames Center for Diabetes Education, 1986.

SPECIAL POPULATIONS

XVI. CHILDHOOD AND ADOLESCENCE

INTRODUCTION

Diabetes can profoundly affect the normal physical, cognitive, and emotional developmental stages of childhood and adolescence. The unrelenting demands of diabetes management affect families and their social network and may disrupt the developmental tasks of the child within the family. Understanding the unique considerations of diabetes management in children and adolescents, the impact of diabetes on normal development, and the dynamic nature of managing diabetes in youth will help health professionals provide support, flexible care, and age appropriate education.

OBJECTIVES

On completion of this chapter, the learner will be able to:
- describe the major developmental concerns of diabetes in the infant and toddler, preschool-age, school-age, preadolescent, and adolescent child;
- describe how the care and education of children and adolescents with diabetes, including meal planning, insulin therapy, blood glucose monitoring, and exercise, are different from that of adults;
- describe the parental burden of managing a child's diabetes and the benefit of social networks and support;
- describe the acute and chronic complications of diabetes in childhood;
- identify age-appropriate educational materials and considerations for each respective age group.

A. Incidence

1. Insulin-dependent diabetes mellitus (IDDM), also called type I diabetes, occurs in children and adolescents at a rate of 1.6 per 1000. Approximately 120,000 children in the United States today have IDDM.[1] Worldwide, the prevalence and incidence varies from one geographic location to another, with the

incidence being highest in the Scandinavian countries of Sweden, Finland, and Norway, and lowest in Japan.[2]

2. Approximately 95% of new cases of early onset diabetes in children and adolescents are classic IDDM. The remaining cases are Maturity Onset Diabetes in Youth (MODY), or non-insulin-dependent diabetes mellitus (NIDDM).

3. The incidence of IDDM increases with age, with the peak incidence occurring in adolescence. Seasonal variations have also been reported, with diabetes being diagnosed more frequently in the winter than in the summer months.[3]

4. Diagnostic criteria for children and adolescents are generally the same as those for adults[4] (see Chapter V: Pathophysiology).

B. **General Therapy**

General goals of therapy for the child or adolescent are to achieve normal growth and development, optimal glycemic control, minimal acute or chronic complications (see Table XVI.1), and a positive psychosocial adjustment to diabetes.

1. *Insulin therapy* for children and adolescents has some unique considerations. Adequate growth and appropriate pubertal development are important indices of insulin sufficiency. When insulin insufficiency occurs during childhood and adolescence, normal growth and development may be delayed.

   a) The Mauriac syndrome, a diabetes-related growth disorder, is characterized by delayed linear growth, delayed sexual maturation, hepatomegaly, and limited joint mobility, among other findings.[5]

   b) Children's height and weight should be carefully plotted at 3- to 4-month intervals on a standard growth chart. If height and weight begin to fall below the child's normal growth percentile, a careful evaluation of glycemic

TABLE XVI.1: POSSIBLE COMPLICATIONS OF DIABETES IN CHILDHOOD AND ADOLESCENCE

Acute
Hypoglycemia — especially unrecognized in young children
Ketoacidosis
Vaginal yeast infections/thrush
Cellulitus — infection/injury

Intermediate
Mauriac syndrome — insulin insufficiency, growth and pubertal delay (rare)
Necrobiosis lipoidica diabeticorum (rare)
Lipodystrophy at injection sites

Chronic (adolescence)
Hypertension
Nephropathy
Retinopathy
Eating disorders
Depression

control, insulin sufficiency, nutritional adequacy, or other endocrine disorders needs to be made.

c) Therapy should be designed to balance the fluctuating food and insulin requirements and exercise levels that are characteristic of the growing and developing child.

d) Most children do well with two to three daily injections of insulin taken 30 minutes before breakfast and the evening meal (two-injection regimen) or before breakfast and evening meal and at bedtime (3-injection regimen). Most frequently, regular insulin is given in combination with NPH or Lente.[6]

(1) Commercially prepared premixed insulins generally do not allow for the flexibility of daily dosage adjustment based on blood glucose values and exercise levels, which are especially variable in children. It is important to be able to adjust insulin to avoid hypoglycemia. However, commercially available premixed insulin may be useful for some

adolescents who are unable or unwilling to learn to regularly adjust their insulin doses.

    (2)   Young children may require dose adjustments in one-half unit increments.

e)   Approximately 70% of children and adolescents with diabetes move into a remission phase, requiring decreased insulin dosages. Sometimes the evening dose can be discontinued for as long as a year following diagnosis. Remission is less common in preschool children, who seem to do best with continued split-dose therapy.[3]

f)   Most children require approximately 1 unit of insulin per kg of body weight.[7] A range of 0.5 to 1.5 units/kg is acceptable and allows for differences based on age, activity, eating habits, and metabolic requirements of the individual child or adolescent.

g)   With supervision, school-age children are frequently capable of giving themselves insulin injections. It is important to identify learning readiness and individual considerations, such as locus of control, maturity, and family factors, rather than to define specific age ranges for task performance when determining the ability of a child to perform self-care skills. Broad differences have been identified between children and adolescents in their ability to master and take responsibility for these tasks. Parental involvement and/or supervision appears to enhance adherence and glycemic control.[8,9]

h)   Usual injection sites for young children are legs, arms, and the upper-outer quadrant of the buttocks. School age children and adolescents can be encouraged to use the abdomen on a regular basis. However, abdominal injections in children with little subcutaneous abdominal fat, or in very young children, may not be advisable. For these children, the abdomen is usually the least-favored site. Rotating sites in a consistent manner, (eg, arms in the morning, legs in the evening) is frequently advisable. It is not yet clear, however, whether adult studies relating to insulin absorption are applicable to children.[10]

2. The principles of *nutrition therapy* in children and adolescents differ from those in adults because children usually do not require weight reduction; children need sufficient calories for growth and pubertal development.

a) The specific goals of nutritional therapy for children are the maintenance of normal growth, weight, and sexual development; prevention of obesity, excessive glycemic excursions, hypoglycemia, and hyperlipidemia; control of blood pressure; and prevention of the future complications of diabetes.

b) It is generally recommended that children receive 55% to 60% of total calories from a carbohydrate source, 30% from fat, and 12% to 15% from protein. This lower protein recommendation is based on a concern for the effect of excess dietary protein on renal plasma flow and the potential for resulting kidney damage.[11]

c) Most children over the age of 6 years require 3 meals a day plus snacks in mid-afternoon and at bedtime. Children under the age of 6 or children who must go more than 4 or 5 hours between breakfast and lunch usually require a midmorning snack. When older children and adolescents dislike having to eat during schooltime, insulin dosages can usually be adjusted to make snacks at school unnecessary.

d) Unless the child or adolescent is over his or her ideal body weight, the usual caloric guidelines for healthy children are followed. For example, it is not uncommon for a normal-weight, very active adolescent boy with diabetes to require between 3500 and 4500 calories per day.

e) Meals and snacks are timed to correspond with the peak action of the injected insulin. For this reason, it is generally recommended that children and teens try not to deviate by more than an hour from their normal schedule.

f) Meal planning, meal timing, and children's normally variable appetites and food preferences can be worrisome and stressful to parents who are trying to balance their child's exercise level and insulin dose with food. When children refuse to eat, the adult present can offer a carbohydrate-containing beverage, such as milk or juice, and monitor blood glucose levels more closely.

3. Although *exercise* may not always result in better glycemic control in every child with diabetes, it is encouraged to promote cardiovascular fitness and long-term weight control and to enhance social interaction and esteem through team play.[10,12] Physically fit adolescents with diabetes have greater insulin sensitivity.[13]

   a) Additional carbohydrate with protein or fat may be eaten before activity. Typical snacks before exercise might be a peanut butter sandwich or cheese crackers and skim milk or juice. Some adolescents prefer to use drinks like Gatorade® or fruit juice before, during, and after sports because of the difficulty of exercising with a full stomach.

   b) School personnel, especially gym teachers and coaches, should be informed that children and adolescents with diabetes require a snack before and/or sometimes during strenuous exercise. They must also be prepared to identify and treat hypoglycemia with a form of readily available glucose.

   c) Parents are frequently concerned about the possibility of their child's developing hypoglycemia during the night because of the prolonged hypoglycemic effect of exercise. To replenish glycogen stores depleted during high-intensity exercise, a child or adolescent with diabetes may require additional food at bedtime. Parents may also want to occasionally monitor their child's blood glucose level during the night if they fear the possibility of nocturnal hypoglycemia (see Chapter VII: Exercise).

4. *Monitoring of blood glucose and urine ketone levels* must be done regularly to enable parents and children to interpret symptoms and make the necessary adjustments in insulin doses.

a) In general, the recommended frequency for blood glucose monitoring for children is before each meal and bedtime snack, with additional tests performed if the child has symptoms of hypoglycemia, hyperglycemia, ketosis, or illness.

b) It may not be necessary to test blood glucose levels daily before lunch when in school if the child is not having problems with glucose control and is feeling well. The decision to test regularly in school is based partially on the individual child's ability to cope with the situation, the perceived disruption to the classroom, and the child's sensitivity to feeling different.

c) It is generally recommended that children and adolescents test their urine for ketones once daily in the morning; when blood glucose levels exceed 240 mg/dL (13.3 mmol/L); and when illness occurs.

d) Ketones may be present in the urine following hypoglycemia. Therefore, persistent small amounts of ketones found in the urine in the morning may be indicative of nocturnal hypoglycemia. To verify nocturnal hypoglycemia, parents may be asked to test their child's blood glucose level between 1 and 3 AM.

e) Target ranges for blood glucose levels of children and adolescents vary, depending on the judgement of the medical provider and the individual goals set for the child. Target levels can range from 80 to 120 mg/dL (4.4 to 6.7 mmol/L) at fasting and from 80 to 180 mg/dL (4.4 to 9.9 mmol/L) at other times of the day. Permissible levels for children under 6 years of age may range from 90 mg/dL (4.9 mmol/L) to as high as 130 mg/dL (7.1 mmol/L) at fasting and from 90 to 200 mg/dL (4.9 to 11.1 mmol/L) at other times[3] because of the fear that undetected hypoglycemia in the early years may cause neurologic impairment in later years.[14]

f) Blood glucose monitoring results can also be used to help parents determine food types and quantities when balancing activities and food intake, or providing a bedtime snack to avoid nocturnal hypoglycemia.

5. *Education and support of the family* is essential.

   a) Optimally, all family members of the child or adolescent with diabetes should be educated regarding diabetes management. This includes grandparents and baby-sitters, when possible.

   b) The educational process must be an open-ended, ongoing experience between the child, family, friends, and the diabetes therapeutic team.[3]

   c) Stress management and the development of effective coping skills should be considered as important to successful therapy as insulin administration, diet, blood glucose monitoring, and exercise[6] (see Chapter III: Stress Management).

C. Impact on the Family

The role of the parent varies greatly, depending upon the child's age and ability to perform self-care activities. Daily manipulation of insulin, food, monitoring, and exercise are required to achieve successful management. These tasks are either assumed by or supervised by a parent or caretaker.

1. This burden can be quite stressful to parents, causing worry, anxiety, and family disruption; in some instances, it can contribute to dysfunctional methods of coping by both the child and the family.[15]

2. Children with diabetes who come from families with few supports, a lower socioeconomic status, or a chaotic home environment may be at greater risk for acute and chronic complications.

3. By educating extended family members, encouraging counseling, closely supervising blood glucose monitoring

results, and enhancing family support networks, the educator can help to provide parents with the guidance and support needed.

D. Issues of Childhood and Adolescent Development

1. A number of developmental factors must be considered in managing the *infant and toddler (birth to 2 years)* with diabetes.

    a) Normal growth and development for infants and toddlers progresses rapidly and predictably, from large muscle developmental tasks to fine motor skills. Infants may require significant amounts of sleep, and toddlers usually need daily naps. Parents and caretakers must try to fit naps into the child's schedule at times when they do not interfere with meals or snacks.

    b) In normal development, differentiation and "hatching" begin at around 4 to 5 months of age. Tentative experimentation with separation-individuation begins at around 6 months; early practicing of crawling begins at around 9 months. Children aged 10 to 12 months practice walking and manual skills. This stage has been described by Mahler as having "a love affair with the world."[16] As infants approach 2 years of age, they begin to separate and individuate, testing their separateness by saying no and behaving in an oppositional manner. Most parents know this as the "terrible twos." Providing choices at this age can give the toddler with diabetes some control, but the choices should be framed in such a way that the child is not allowed to make important decisions. For example, asking "Which finger shall we choose?" works better than asking, "Do you want to do your blood test now?"

    c) Infants usually nurse or eat predictably, but appetite may become erratic in the toddler when rapid growth begins to subside.

        (1) The normal sporadic eating habits of toddlers can be worrisome for parents who try to balance food with insulin and activity.

(2) Normal activity in infants and toddlers is also sporadic and spontaneous, with bursts of whole body movement.

(3) Parents must try to balance activity with extra food, which is quite often challenging if a picky toddler will not eat. Parents may prevent hypoglycemia in their toddler by offering sips of juice or milk if the child will not eat.

d) Infants and young children may dehydrate quickly because a large percentage of their body surface areas is water and they are unable to retain large volumes of fluids taken by mouth. Dehydration can take place rapidly in any young child when illness occurs, and the effect is enhanced in the infant or toddler with diabetes.

(1) The potential for rapid dehydration makes infants and young children especially vulnerable when illness, vomiting, or diarrhea occurs. Parents should notify their diabetes care team or physician whenever a young child is ill, and they should carefully monitor the child's blood glucose and urine ketone levels. If vomiting does not subside and the child shows signs of dehydration, urinary ketones, ketoacidosis, or hypoglycemia, intravenous hydration may be necessary (see Chapter XII: Managing Diabetes During Intercurrent Illness).

e) Infants and toddlers who are developmentally unable to effectively communicate symptoms of hypoglycemia must rely on the observations of caretakers for recognition and treatment of hypoglycemia. Signs of hypoglycemia in an infant may be pallor, listlessness, crying, clammy skin, irritability, sleepiness, hunger, and/or shakiness. In addition, toddlers may have uncoordinated gait, stumbling, or inactivity.

f) Onset of diabetes early in life is associated with impaired cognitive functions, such as abstract and visual reasoning, later in life, possibly due to undetected hypoglycemia.[14]

g) Infants are usually placed on a 3- to 4-hour flexible feeding schedule to maintain a steady blood glucose level; they may be given additional cereal at feedings preceding the peak effect of insulin. Toddlers usually consume three meals and three snacks daily, but additional snacks may be required. Food and feeding can be problematic for parents or caretakers of a picky toddler. To help prevent hypoglycemia, parents can offer favorite foods and substitute alternative choices of carbohydrate-containing beverages if the child will not eat. However, parents should try to avoid becoming a "short order cook" for their demanding child.

h) To provide a steady state of insulin, one successful approach to insulin therapy in the infant is a split dose of NPH insulin given morning and evening.[3]

i) Treatment of hypoglycemia in the infant consists of providing 5 to 10 g of carbohydrate (CHO) in the form of 1 to 2 teaspoons Karo Syrup, 4 oz (15 g CHO) of undiluted baby fruit juice or glucose water, or 1 small tube (15 to 30 g CHO) of cake decorator or commercially prepared glucose gels.

j) Parents of infants and toddlers must rely on frequent blood glucose monitoring to distinguish normal infant and toddler behaviors from those of hypoglycemia because infants and toddlers are often defiant, demanding, sleepy, or cranky as part of their normal development. Test results will help parents to make daily management decisions.

k) Blood for glucose monitoring can be obtained from the child's fingers, big toes, and external, lateral aspect of the heel.

l) The burden of responsibility for constant care can be quite difficult for parents and caretakers of children with diabetes. Supportive extended family, friends, or baby-sitters can offer some relief by sharing the care.

m) Blood glucose readings in young children are frequently erratic at best. Parents may require additional support from the therapeutic team during this difficult period.

2. Developmental considerations of the *preschool-age child (3 to 5 years)* include many of the concerns pertinent to the toddler in addition to specific developmental issues of the preschool child.

   a) Physical growth slows after the toddler stage but is still relatively rapid. Fine motor skills continue to develop in the preschool child, and cognitive language develops rapidly as children learn to play and enjoy stories.

      (1) Children of this age engage in magical thinking; they may believe that if they think or wish something, they can cause it to happen.[17] For example, when Susan was admitted to the hospital with diabetes, her 4-year-old brother, who earlier that day had shouted angrily that he wished she would go away, later revealed that he thought he had caused Susan's diabetes to happen.

      (2) Separation-individuation continues during this stage, as children learn to define themselves as being separate from their parents.

   b) Preschool children are concerned about the intactness of their bodies. Fear of intrusive procedures is characteristic of this age, and children may act out their anxieties at insulin injection and blood testing times. Preschool-age children have a difficult time understanding the need for insulin injection and blood tests, particularly if they are feeling well.

   c) The advantages and use of play therapy have been well-recognized.[18-20] Children establish a balance between their inner life and reality by continual exploration and testing through their play. Guided play, or play therapy, provides a forum and vehicle for children to express their concerns, and provides a mechanism for emotional release by helping the child learn to deal with these issues through creative expression. Giving a child a "safe" syringe, family and health professional dolls, meter supplies, and other diabetes paraphernalia will provide an opportunity for supervised play. Children will frequently assign one of the dolls to have diabetes, and will play out their life and concerns with diabetes through doll or puppet play.

d) Normal eating patterns for preschool age children are often unpredictable. This is not considered harmful and is normal from a developmental point of view. For example, children may want to eat only bananas and peanut butter for days at a time, then they will switch to grilled cheese and apples. Increased appetites tend to precede growth "spurts" and, nutritionally, are usually balanced over a period of weeks. This erratic eating makes diabetes control difficult for this age, as parents worry about hypoglycemia when children will not eat. Parents can allow the child some control by providing reasonable choices without allowing the child to control eating situations. By giving young children limited choices, parents may avoid a battle of wills.

e) Undetected hypoglycemia is still a risk in the preschool years. Therefore, desirable blood glucose goals should still be in the 90 to 200 mg/dL (4.9 to 11.1 mmol/L) range.[3] Frequent blood glucose testing helps parents and caretakers in the decision-making process. Many preschool-age children are able to identify symptoms of hypoglycemia and alert adults.

f) Infants, toddlers, and preschool-age children are especially vulnerable to elevated blood glucose values and ketonuria when acute infections of childhood, such as otitis media, vomiting illnesses, or the common cold, occur. Wide excursions in blood glucose levels are common and can be quite frustrating for parents. Dehydration and diabetic ketoacidosis (DKA) can develop rapidly.

g) Many young children attend preschool or day-care centers. Educating the staff is of paramount importance to prevent, detect, and treat hypoglycemia. Unfortunately, some insurance policies for these centers prohibit the staff from monitoring a pupil's blood glucose level. This lack of monitoring data can complicate the management of a young child's diabetes.

3. The *school-age child (6 to 10 years)* is better coordinated physically, has a vivid fantasy life, speaks fluently, has a conscience, and is able to share and cooperate. This is the age of concrete reasoning, and repetition compulsion is played out in games and skills.

   a) Although the school age child has increasing need for independence, the power and protection of the parent is very important to the child's feeling of well-being. In terms of diabetes management, the parent's role is to perform diabetes care tasks while moving the child toward independence by means of supervision, encouragement, and support.

      (1) At times, the child may be willing and able to perform blood glucose monitoring, prepare his or her own snacks, and administer insulin. At other times, the parent performs the test or administers insulin. Parent-child sharing of these responsibilities is essential during the school-age years.[8]

      (2) Understandably, parents of the school-age child with diabetes may be more protective than other parents. This can make it difficult for the child with diabetes to attain the independence of the nondiabetic child of the same age. Therefore, diabetes management planning for special events and activities is important to promote independence for these children. By planning ahead, they should be able to join almost any activity their friends are doing.

   b) One of the greatest drives of school-age children is to avoid failure. They acquire strategies to keep them from feeling different from their peers. Fear of peers witnessing symptoms of hypoglycemia or hyperglycemia can alter diabetes self-care routines and ultimately affect self-esteem. Helping the child to fit diabetes management into normal routines both at home and at school can minimize differences. One teacher, for example, had all children in her classroom break for a morning snack.

c)   Because school-age children spend a large portion of their day in school, it is reasonable to expect school personnel to become informed about diabetes care. School districts and personnel are obligated by federal law to provide an individualized plan to accommodate a child's special health care needs. A conference with child, parents, and school personnel at the beginning of each school year is desirable.[21] Certain topics, including the importance of communication, are essential to include in such a conference.

   (1)   The administration of glucagon in schools is highly variable, depending on state laws. However, upon receiving a physician's order, most schools will designate a person to administer glucagon in the same way they are required to give epinephrine to an acutely allergic child who sustains a bee sting.

   (2)   Parents should describe the child's usual signs and symptoms of hypoglycemia as well as the causes for hypoglycemia. They should then help school personnel develop a plan of treatment, including location of the treatment supplies.

   (3)   Parents should provide a basic explanation of diabetes and the requirements of the daily management plan. When scheduling changes occur in the daily school routine, such as field trips or parties, parents should be notified by the school prior to the event.

   (4)   Meal plan basics should be reviewed so that school personnel have a general awareness of what the child eats. Providing a plan to enable the child to manage parties and snacks in school is also beneficial.

d)   Children with diabetes can have feelings of sadness, anxiety, friendlessness, and isolation.[15] Support groups, individual counseling, or diabetes camps can be useful in assisting the child to resolve these feelings.

4. There are large differences between the stages of adolescence. The stages include *early adolescence or preadolescence (≤12 years), middle adolescence (13 to 15 years), and late adolescence (16 to 18 years)*.

a) At no other time of life do environment and heredity produce such a variance in individual development. Broad differences normally occur in emotional, social, and physical development.

  (1) Onset of breast budding and the growth of pubic hair occur at an average age of 10 to 11 years in girls, and pubic hair growth and enlargement of the testicles at 12 to 16 years in boys.

  (2) Changes in size, weight, body proportions, muscular development, strength, coordination, and skill are seen at this age. These changes may occur slowly or rapidly.

  (3) The age of onset of pubescent growth is determined by genetic familial determinants but can also be affected by culture, economy, nutrition, health, and habitat. Poor glycemic control can delay the onset of puberty.

b) Puberty is characterized by the onset of hormonal activity, which is under the influence of the central nervous system, especially the hypothalamus and pituitary gland. The major consequences are the increased production of adrenocortical and gonadal hormones and the production of mature ova and spermatozoa.

  (1) In the adolescent with diabetes, metabolic control, as indicated by increasing glycosylated hemoglobin levels, deteriorates during adolescence despite significantly higher insulin doses.[22,23]

  (2) The hormonal changes cause a state of relative insulin resistance as a result of declining peripheral insulin action and changing counter-regulatory hormonal responses.[24]

c) Certain important characteristics mark the normal period of *early adolescence*.

      (1)   The child becomes acutely aware of body image.

      (2)   Dependent versus independent struggles begin between parent and child.

      (3)   There may be great vacillation between childlike and adult behaviors.

      (4)   There is less social involvement with family, more with peers.

      (5)   Parental criticism becomes difficult to accept.

      (6)   Turmoil and conflict within the parent-child relationship may begin.

d) Certain important characteristics are typical of the normal period of *middle adolescence.*

      (1)   Peer group allegiance develops.

      (2)   Greater experimentation and risk taking occurs.

      (3)   Physical and social activity increases.

      (4)   Sexual relationships emerge and are important.

      (5)   Formal operational thinking begins with the beginning of abstract reasoning.

      (6)   Teens and parents struggle.

e) Certain important characteristics are part of the normal period of *late adolescence*:

      (1)   Cognitive abilities and abstract morals develop.

      (2)   The peer group loses its primary importance.

      (3)   There is increasing separation from the family unit.

      (4)   Teens become future oriented.

      (5)   Conscience is able to stand without outside support.

f) Diabetes affects normal adolescent development.

      (1)   Identity and self-image concerns can revolve around diabetes concerns such as injection site appearance or self-identification as "the diabetic."

      (2)   Normal independence issues may be thwarted as a result of parental protectiveness or the teen's failure to assume responsibility for self-care.

      (3)   Physical growth and development have a strong impact on a teen's self-image.[25,26] Although most adolescents with diabetes display normal growth patterns and normal onset and progression of

pubertal development, they can be concerned about their growth and sexual maturation.

(4) Attitudes of experimentation, rebellion, and risk-taking behaviors normally associated with adolescence can revolve around diabetes issues, such as taking insulin regularly, monitoring, and the quality and quantity of food consumption.

g) Poor adherence to health recommendations is widespread, especially among adolescents. Family dynamics, family health beliefs, communication style, and support networks all affect adolescents' ability to do what is requested of them.

5. Several important conditions in children and adolescents may be associated with poor glycemic control and/or health outcomes.

a) Biologically, the adolescent's earlier and greater epinephrine responses to moderate drops in blood glucose concentrations, when added to a heightened insulin resistance, may contribute to some of the lability in metabolic control.

b) Chaotic home environments and chronic family stress can contribute to poorer metabolic control for children and adolescents as a result of increased epinephrine responses to physical or psychological neglect or abuse or to the frank omission of insulin.

c) Knowledge and level of cognitive maturity is instrumental to proper diabetes management. Occasionally, developmental delay or learning disabilities may hamper understanding of diabetes care.

d) Emotional disturbance can cause disequilibrium and precipitate frequent episodes of ketoacidosis. Insulin insufficiency may occur in response to physical or emotional stress, resulting in over-production of counter-regulatory hormones. Early adolescent girls who are extraordinarily sensitive to emotional stress are most likely to demonstrate recurrent DKA.[3] Repeated episodes of DKA warrant investigation, as DKA can be deliberately induced to displace family tensions. Family patterns of interaction may reveal family enmeshment, rigidity, poor communication, and over-protectiveness.[27] Treatment may include family counseling and aggressive insulin therapy when illness, stress, or ketones appear.

e) Adolescents frequently develop DKA because they fail to take their insulin. Insulin doses can be missed when parents are not involved in an adolescent's diabetes management.[28]

f) The diabetes regimen has been described as providing the right conditions for the development of an eating disorder. There has been an increasing number of case reports and general reviews on the subject, but whether the incidence of eating disorders is significantly increased in the diabetic population has not been firmly established. It is important for educators to be aware of an increased tendency toward pathologic eating behaviors, particularly among adolescent and young adult females because of the focus on food and discipline required in the diabetes regimen (see Chapter II: Psychosocial Assessment and Support).

REFERENCES

1. LaPorte RE, Tajima N, Akerblom HR, et al. Geographic differences in the risk of insulin-dependent diabetes mellitus: the importance of registries. Diabetes Care 1985;8(suppl):101-7.

2. Cruickshanks KJ, LaPorte RE, Dorman JS. The epidemiology of insulin-dependent diabetes mellitus: etiology and prognosis. In: Ahmed PI, Ahmed N, eds. Coping with juvenile diabetes. Springfield, Ill: Charles C. Thomas, 1985:332-57.

3. Drash A. Clinical care of the diabetic child. Chicago: Year Book Medical Publishers, 1987:16.

4. Office guide to diagnosis and classification of diabetes mellitus and other categories of glucose intolerance. Position statement of the American Diabetes Association. Diabetes Care 1992;15(suppl 2): 4.

5. Becker D. Complications of insulin-dependent diabetes mellitus in childhood and adolescence. In: Lifshitz F, ed. Pediatric endocrinology, a clinical guide. 2nd ed. New York: Marcel Dekker, 1990:701-18.

6. Drash A, Becker DJ. Behavioral issues in patients with diabetes mellitus with special emphasis on the child and adolescent. In: Rifkin H, Porte Jr D, eds. Ellenberg and Rifkin's diabetes mellitus: theory and practice. 4th ed. New York: Elsevier Science Publishing, 1990:922-33.

7. Drash A. Management of the child with diabetes mellitus: clinical course, therapeutic strategies, and monitoring techniques. In: Lifshitz F, 2nd ed. Pediatric endocrinology, a clinical guide. 2nd ed. New York: Marcel Dekker, 1990:681-700.

8. Follansbee D. Assuming responsibility for diabetes management: what age? what price? Diabetes Educ 1989;15:4:347-52.

9.   Wysocki T, Meinhold P, Abrams K, et al. Parental and professional estimates of self-care independence of children and adolescents with IDDM. Diabetes Care 1992;15:43-52.

10.   Becker D. Management of insulin dependent diabetes mellitus in children and adolescents. Curr Opinion Pediatr, 1991;3:710-23.

11.   Brodsky I, Robbins D, Hiser E, et al. Effects of low-protein diets on protein metabolism in insulin dependent diabetes mellitus patients with early nephropathy. J Clin Endocrinol Metab 1992;75:351-57.

12.   Diabetes mellitus and exercise. Position statement of the American Diabetes Association. Diabetes Care 1992;15(suppl 2):36.

13.   Arslanian S, Nixon P, Becker D, Drash A. Impact of physical fitness and glycemic control on in vivo insulin action in adolescents with IDDM. Diabetes Care 1990;13:9-15.

14.   Ryan C, Vega A, Drash A. Cognitive deficits in adolescents who develop diabetes early in life. Pediatr 1985;75:921-27.

15.   Kovacs M, Feinberg T. Coping with juvenile onset diabetes mellitus. In: Singer JE, Baum A, eds. Handbook of medical psychology. Vol 2. Hillsdale, NJ: Lawrence Erlbaum, 1982:2:165-212.

16.   Mahler M, Pine F, Bergman A. The psychological birth of the human infant. New York: Basic Books, 1975.

17.   Fraiberg S. The magic years: understanding and handling the problems of early childhood. New York: Charles Scribner's Sons, 1959.

18.   Rogerson C. Play therapy in childhood. New York: Oxford University Press, 1939.

19.   Pothier P. Resolving conflict through play fantasy. J Psychiatr Nurs 1967;5:141-47.

20. Marcus S. Therapeutic puppetry. In: Philpott AR, ed. Puppets and therapy. New York: Plays Inc., 1977.

21. Puczynski S, Betschart J. Foundation for the future: understanding the student with diabetes. Chicago: American Association of Diabetes Educators, 1990.

22. Daneman D, Wolfson D, Becker D, Drash A. Factors affecting glycosylated hemoglobin values in children with IDDM. J Pediatr 1981;99:847-53.

23. Blethen S, Sergeant D, Whitlow M, Santiago J. Effect of pubertal stage and recent blood glucose control on plasma somatomedian C in children with insulin-dependent diabetes mellitus. Diabetes 1981;30:868-72.

24. Amiel S, Sherwin R, Simonson D, Lauritoano A, Tamborlane W. Impaired insulin action in puberty: a contributing factor to poor glycemic control in adolescents with diabetes. N Engl J Med 1986;315:215-19.

25. Normal adolescence: its dynamics and impact. Formulated by the Committee on Adolescence/Group for the Advancement of Psychiatry. New York: Charles Scribner's Sons, 1968.

26. Blos P. On adolescence: a psychoanalytic interpretation. New York: Free Press, 1962.

27. Anderson B, Auslander W. Research on diabetes management and the family: a critique. Diabetes Care 1980;3:696-702.

28. Golden M, Herrold A, Orr D. An approach to prevention of recurrent diabetic ketoacidosis in the pediatric population. J Pediatr 1985;107:195-200.

KEY EDUCATIONAL CONSIDERATIONS

1. The old paradigm, You Can't Treat the Child Without Treating the Parents, can be expanded to include education. Parents, friends, neighbors, caretakers, baby-sitters, and any other support persons can help or hinder a child's adjustment to diabetes and the diabetes regimen. When the same information is heard by all involved, a consistent approach is likely to evolve.

2. Materials, content, and expectations obviously must be age appropriate, and education times matched to the age and attention span of the individual child.

    a) Educating the preschool child is often limited to spontaneously occurring opportunities that revolve around diabetes management and questions asked by the child.

    (1) Young children often do well when provided with choices: for example, "Do you want raisins or a banana?" or "Shall we do your fingerstick in your pinky or thumb?"

    (2) Explain insulin injections and fingersticks in terms of "keeping you healthy."

    (3) Preschool and school-age children primarily process what they have learned through play. Doll play or puppet play are valuable learning modes for this age.

    (4) The education of the young child should focus on the identification of symptoms of hypoglycemia, the basic knowledge that juice or food is required, and the need to tell an adult. Discussing how the child felt before each hypoglycemic episode can help a child recognize symptoms the next time. Many young children are able to identify symptoms of hypoglycemia and tell an adult.

    (5) Frequently, parents are concerned that they may not recognize an episode of hypoglycemia. Reading a detailed description of or seeing a video about hypoglycemia can be helpful.

    b) The school-age child needs to be individually assessed for learning readiness, which can be highly variable. However, school-age children are able to learn concrete survival skills quite well, and they learn diabetes content best when the work is interesting and fun for them.

   (1)   Games, puzzles, and videos are important educational tools.

   (2)   The school-age child also learns well through play.

c)   Most health professionals agree that it is not learning educational content that is most difficult for the adolescent with diabetes but rather doing what is recommended. When educational content is pertinent to adolescent issues, learning occurs best. Topics should include diabetes and sexuality (including contraception), alcohol and tobacco use, drugs, medical identification, driving issues, and special concerns such as party advice, managing diabetes and sports, prom night management, career information, and travel. Educational materials can include books and videos, but discussion groups among peers are often the most effective tool. Educators can use a number of strategies for dealing with teens:

   (1)   Enhance self-esteem by promoting feelings of normalcy. A teen's behavior frequently matches self-image.

   (2)   Develop a primary relationship with teens and a collaborative one with parents.

   (3)   Provide honest communication and don't minimize feelings.

   (4)   Listen to what is being said as well as what is not being said. Negative feelings exist before negative acts.

   (5)   Solve problems together and negotiate treatment strategies.

   (6)   Enlist the assistance of a supportive person (boyfriend, girlfriend, sibling).

   (7)   Candidly discuss perceptions of barriers.

   (8)   Provide ongoing positive reinforcement.

   (9)   Convey enjoyment in working with adolescents.

d)   Diabetes camps provide an excellent setting for facilitating formal and informal learning. Children and adolescents learn from each other in an environment where no one feels different because of his or her diabetes.

e)   Support groups also promote learning but are most effective when structured around an activity that is fun.

f) Factors that contribute to nonadherence are family dynamics (including the family's health belief model), communication style, emotional tone, and inappropriate expectations of children and adolescents.

g) It is important for both children and adolescents that blood glucose results be treated as information only and not as "bad" or "good" numbers. Using such expressions as "in range" or "out of range" for blood glucose readings sounds less judgmental. The same is true for the commonly used word *cheating* to describe nonadherence to the prescribed meal plan. The word is judgmental, meaning to defraud or deceive, and may create more anger, guilt, and acting out behaviors.

SELF-REVIEW QUESTIONS

If you are unsure of the answers to the following questions, please review the materials.

1. Describe three characteristics of the following developmental stages: infancy and toddlerhood; preschool; school-age; early, middle, and late adolescence.
2. Explain the potential impact of diabetes on each developmental stage.
3. Describe the burden of care and potential stress that falls on parents and caretakers and list two possible sources of support.
4. List three conditions that may be associated with poor glycemic control or health outcomes.
5. Describe two educational considerations of preschool, school-age, and adolescent learning styles and abilities.

CASE EXAMPLE 1

HP is a 21-year-old single mother whose 11-month-old son (BP) has just been diagnosed with IDDM. The mother is a high school graduate, now employed part-time as a waitress, working a 4 P.M. to midnight shift. Finances are a problem. Her sister, who has four children of her own, has agreed to watch BP on the nights his mother works. BP's doctor has prescribed two injections of NPH per day, which BP receives before breakfast and dinner. Regular insulin was tried and discontinued at this time because of hypoglycemia. BP is still being bottle-fed, and receives a bottle before bedtime. His dietitian has prescribed a 1200-calorie ADA exchange diet with three meals and three snacks per day.

QUESTIONS

1. What are the primary management and social issues?
2. What educational strategies might be employed?
3. What interventions could or should be employed immediately, and which can be planned for a later time?

SUGGESTED SOLUTIONS

One of the main concerns for this single mother will be finding the support and resources needed to adequately care for her child. Exploring relationships with other family members, including the sister, as well as neighbors and friends, and including them in the education process from the beginning might alert those in HP's support network to the severity of her need and provide her with both caretaking and possibly financial help from the beginning. It will need to be determined if the sister is able and willing to learn to give insulin injections, do monitoring, and so forth. Social service workers might be able to assist with community resources and to explore financial considerations such as expansion of Social Security benefits for this mother. This mother will most likely also need close supervision and a positive relationship with her health care providers. The infant should not be weaned from the bottle during the period of diagnosis and hospitalization, although this is a goal to be worked toward after the child is settled at home. Hospitalization is a traumatic enough period for a very young child without the stress of being weaned from an obvious comfort. Home health care nurses might be consulted to look in on and assist this young mother in her efforts to provide a regular schedule and care for her child.

CASE EXAMPLE 2

JJ is a 15-year-old male who has been diagnosed with IDDM for 8 years. As a child, he did reasonably well with glucose control, and had no hospital admissions. Over the past year, JJ has been admitted to the hospital three times for DKA and once for severe hypoglycemia. His glycosylated hemoglobin (HbA$_1$) concentration has risen over the past 2 years from 10.3% to 14.8% (normal 5.5% to 7.4%). He has been frank about admitting that he has not been testing his blood glucose level, and states that he occasionally forgets to take his insulin, especially the second injection of the day. He lives at home with both parents and two younger siblings, does average work in school, and has a girlfriend. He has been very oppositional at home and argues frequently with his parents.

QUESTIONS

1. What concerns described above are typical adolescent behavior from a developmental perspective?
2. What educational approaches might be effective?
3. What are the primary goals of therapy for this young man?

SUGGESTED SOLUTIONS

The main goals of therapy are: (1) to prevent the recurrent DKA, (2) to prevent severe hypoglycemia, and (3) to decrease JJ's HbA$_1$ concentration. Critical to this is for JJ to take his prescribed dose of insulin and eat regularly. Exploring the reasons for not taking insulin might reveal insights that can lead to solutions. If JJ is out with friends and is either too embarrassed to take his insulin or has not had the foresight to bring it, these issues can be addressed. If JJ agrees, his friends, including his girlfriend, can be asked to support these efforts and be invited to attend education classes. Asking parents to observe JJ taking his insulin can reinforce the importance of this request. JJ also probably needs an educational review since he was at a developmentally younger age when he last received education. The educator might contract for small behavior changes that are achievable and mutually agreeable, and maintain frequent contact to monitor progress. JJ can be guided in the problem-solving process, using hypothetical adolescent situations. One strategy might be to remove the parents from the center of the conflict and communicate directly with JJ without eliminating parental involvement. A referral for counseling, peer support groups, or camp might also be beneficial as JJ passes through a very difficult period of development.

OTHER SUGGESTED READINGS

Anthony E, Benedek T, eds. Parenthood: its psychology and psychopathology. Boston: Little, Brown, 1972.

Chase, P. Understanding insulin dependent diabetes. 7th ed. Denver: Children's Diabetes Foundation, 1992.

Daneman D. Childhood, adolescence, and diabetes: a delicate developmental balance. Diabetes Spectrum 1989;2(4):225-43.

Drash A. Clinical care of the diabetic child. Chicago: Year Book Medical Publishers, 1987:16.

Fraiberg S. The magic years: understanding and handling the problems of early childhood. New York: Charles Scribner's Sons, 1959.

Giordano BP, Petrila AT, Mamien CR, et al. Transferring responsibility for diabetes self-care from parent to child. Pediatr Health Care, 1992;6(Sept-Oct):5.

Kleinberg S. Educating the chronically ill child. Rockville, Md: Aspen Publishers, 1982.

Lorenz R, Wysocki T. The family and childhood diabetes. Diabetes Spectrum 1991;4(5):261-92.

Petrillo M. Emotional care of hospitalized children. Philadelphia: JB Lippincott, 1980.

Siminerio L, Betschart J. Children with diabetes. Alexandria, VA: American Diabetes Association, 1986.

Travis L, Richter N, Cavanaugh B, Carpenter G, et al. Curriculum for youth education. Alexandria, Va: American Diabetes Association, 1983.

Vandagriff J, Marrero D, Ingersoll G, Fineberg N. Parents of children with diabetes: what are they worried about? Diabetes Educ 1992;18:299-302.

SOME EDUCATIONAL MATERIALS
FOR CHILDREN AND ADOLESCENTS

Betschart J. It's time to learn about diabetes. Minneapolis: Chronimed, 1991.

Betschart J. It's time to learn about diabetes (Video). Minneapolis: Chronimed, 1993.

Childs B. Caring for children with diabetes. Alexandria, Va: American Diabetes Association, 1990.

Diabetes and you series (children, teens, young adults). Alexandria, Va: American Diabetes Association, 1988.

Diabetes: one part of me. Boston: Joslin Diabetes Center, 1986.

Miller J. Grilled cheese at four o'clock in the morning. Alexandria, Va: American Diabetes Association, 1988.

Moynihan P, Balik B, Eliason S, Haig B. Diabetes youth curriculum: a toolbox for educators. Minneapolis: International Diabetes Center, 1988.

Moynihan P, Haig B. Whole parent whole child. Minneapolis: DCI Publishing, 1989.

Strodtman L, Knopf R, Funnell M. Sexual health and diabetes. Ann Arbor: Michigan Diabetes Research and Training Center, 1988.

SPECIAL POPULATIONS

XVII.   DIABETES IN THE ELDERLY

INTRODUCTION

The incidence of diabetes is highest in the oldest age groups: 18.5% of individuals over age 65 years are thought to have diabetes. If the traditional oral glucose tolerance tests were used for evaluation, nearly half of the elderly population would have diabetes or impaired glucose tolerance.[1] At the same time, older individuals may not have clinical signs or symptoms of hyperglycemia. More often, secondary effects of long-term hyperglycemia lead to diagnosing diabetes in the elderly. As the US population ages, diabetes educators will need to direct more of their attention and skills toward the needs of the elderly with diabetes. An understanding of the atypical manifestations of diabetes in the aged is necessary to educate and appropriately manage this population.

OBJECTIVES

On completion of this chapter, the learner will be able to:
- describe relevant effects of aging;
- identify unique risks of hyperglycemia in the elderly population;
- identify specific treatment adaptations for older individuals with diabetes;
- list potential barriers and strategies for teaching the elderly.

A. Effects of Aging

1. Certain normal changes of aging mimic the long-term complications of diabetes (decreased vision; elevated blood pressure; decreased glomerular filtration; changes in the bone, muscle, and skin of the foot). When these changes coexist with diabetes complications, each effect is compounded, placing the individual at risk for serious medical disorders.

2. Some kinds of organically caused mental deterioration are more common in elderly people. An estimated 15% of dementia in this age group is caused by nutritional disorders, alcoholism, and diabetes, and is reversible. Some studies indicate that people with diabetes over age 65 years have more cognitive

impairment in specific areas than others of the same age group.[2] Systematic evaluation of cognition can identify specific individual limitations. Several instruments are available to assist with cognitive assessment, including Mini Mental State, Short Portable Mental Status, and the Neurobehavioral Cognitive Status Examination.[3]

Effects of Aging and Diseases of the Elderly Related to Diabetes Care

Eyes

Decreased acuity
Slower light/dark adaptation
Less color perception
Increased blinding diseases (senile cataracts, macular degeneration)

Cardiovascular

Conduction defects
Systolic hypertension
Decreased cardiac output
Increased vascular resistance

Gastrointestinal

Decreased secretion, absorption, motility
Changes in appetite

Dental

Tooth loss
Gum/periodontal disease

Musculoskeletal

Arthritis, joint diseases
Decreased muscle strength
Foot deformities

Neurological

Slower learning, processing time
Slower reactions
Decreased taste, smell, and thirst
Increased cerebral vascular accidents
Increased organic brain diseases

Renal

Decreased glomerular filtration rate (GFR)

---

3. Age-related glucose intolerance seems to be caused mainly by defects in insulin action. Impaired glucose tolerance increases the risk of cardiovascular disease. Because treatment itself can be hazardous to older adults, and because research is lacking

on the effects of impaired glucose tolerance among the aged, elderly people should be treated cautiously when fasting glucose results are abnormal. However, undiagnosed diabetes can cause unnecessary suffering and a shortened life span for those with fragile health. The frequency of undiagnosed diabetes in the elderly may be twice that of younger adults, making screening a critical part of routine health care.[4]

B. Management Issues

1. In the later years, the diabetes that is diagnosed almost exclusively is non-insulin-dependent diabetes mellitus (NIDDM), also called type II diabetes. Decreased muscle mass and inactivity, two problems of aging, contribute to impaired glucose utilization. Modest efforts toward weight loss and improved activity can markedly improve glucose control in some people.[5]

2. Weight reduction meal plans should be designed for gradual weight loss, incorporating other modifications such as sodium restrictions when appropriate, adequate protein and calcium intake, and reduced fat. Aging can reduce taste, smell, salivation, and the ability to see foods. Palatable foods of a consistency that allows for dental or swallowing problems and that accommodates lifelong eating habits will be the most acceptable. Food preparation must be discussed to uncover any physical limitations, accessibility problems, or financial concerns.

3. Although exercise recommendations must allow for the high prevalence of cardiovascular diseases in elderly people, improved aerobic power may be accomplished with less effort than in younger people.[5] Functional capacity should be determined before any exercise program is begun. Stationary bicycling, lap swimming, pool aerobics, walking, or chair exercises can accommodate the limitations of arthritis or

neuromuscular problems, and contribute to flexibility and strengthening.

4. Exercise-associated hypoglycemia from hypoglycemic agents can be avoided by careful blood glucose monitoring, adequate food intake, and appropriate timing of exercise. Exercising with others can provide safety as well as an opportunity for socialization (see Chapter VII: Exercise).

5. Elderly people frequently have several coexisting chronic diseases that require multiple medications. At times, these medications are incompatible and duplicative. An age-related decline in renal function can result in increased drug accumulation. Oral hypoglycemic agents should be initiated only when diet and activity changes have failed, and therapy should be started at the lowest possible doses. The patient's medications should be reviewed for those that interfere with or potentiate sulfonylureas. A pharmacy drug profile can be useful. Patients can be instructed on using assistive devices (eg, date/time pill boxes) and other methods to reduce errors while taking multiple medications.

6. When treatment goals have not been met using other methods, insulin is initiated. Many older people have no difficulty giving insulin and appreciate relief from the symptoms of hyperglycemia. Some individuals will need more assistance with learning self-administration of insulin and monitoring of blood glucose levels. Magnification and enhanced lighting may be helpful for reading syringe markings. Supervised practice and coaching generally result in success. Family, friends or visiting nurses may prefill syringes of insulin for administration later (see Chapter VIII: Pharmacologic Therapies).

7. Goals for diabetes control in the elderly must take into account life expectancy, presence of diabetes complications, coexisting medical or neuropsychiatric disorders, and the patient's ability and willingness to follow the treatment program.[6] The elderly

deserve to be asymptomatic from preventable hyperglycemia and to avoid secondary illnesses, hospitalizations, and untreated complications. Treatment methods should be chosen that optimize social functioning and quality of life.

8. Monitoring diabetes control is best accomplished with self-monitoring of blood glucose (SMBG). Urine glucose results are of limited value due to the increased renal threshold for glucose with aging. The frequency and methods of testing used will depend on the stability of the individual's diabetes. Age alone should not prevent offering self-testing to older patients. In addition, periodic evaluation of fructosamine and/or glycosylated hemoglobin values can indicate the effectiveness of treatment methods.

9. Negative attitudes toward the elderly can affect the behaviors of health care professionals. Treatment choices and educational opportunities should not be withheld due to assumptions about mental competence. Elderly people are as varied in their capabilities as young people. Cultural or social barriers may exist between the older person and the educator. Any differences can be reduced by offering only meaningful, practical information, avoiding jargon, and creating a comfortable, accepting environment. The educator must know the social and financial supports available to the patient and the expectations patients have about the relationship between themselves and their providers.

10. To accommodate sensory and neuromuscular changes associated with aging, educational methods should be slow-paced, easily visible or audible, and include practice opportunities.

    a) To accommodate visual changes that accompany aging, color vision should be assessed. For many older adults, the yellowing of the lens with age filters out colors of short wavelengths so that patients may see gray instead of green and blue. Red, orange, and yellow are more clearly seen. Visual aids and handouts can be prepared, for example, with black lettering on yellow paper.

b) To accommodate auditory changes, speak slowly, distinctly, and augment the spoken word with visual aids. Shouting at a hearing impaired person is ineffective. Shouting accentuates vowels and masks consonants.

c) Telephone follow-up is a helpful technique with the elderly person who may have limited access to follow-up visits. If there is static over the phone lines, call again.

d) The frail elderly patient may be susceptible to sensory overload. Focus the teaching on one or two points. Use short sessions and minimize outside distractions.

C. Hyperglycemic Hyperosmolar Nonketotic Syndrome (HHNS)

1. HHNS usually is seen in the elderly and in undertreated people with NIDDM. Infection, polypharmacy, decreased thirst sensation, swallowing difficulties, and the reluctance to treat hyperglycemia in elderly people predisposes this age group to the syndrome. Nursing home residents may be particularly susceptible because of their dependence on others for medication and health decisions, and they may be less cognitively aware of their symptoms. A detailed description of HHNS can be found in Chapter XI: Hyperglycemia.

2. A small percentage of elderly people have insulin-dependent diabetes mellitus (IDDM), also called type I diabetes. C peptide measures are considered the most reliable method for determining type of diabetes.[7] In the absence of further information, an effort should be made to identify those individuals who are at risk for diabetic ketoacidosis (thin, insulin requiring) and to include urine ketone testing in their monitoring program.

D. Avoidance of Hypoglycemia

1. Although medication-induced hypoglycemia is a problem for many people with diabetes, it is particularly dangerous for elderly people. The usual early signs and symptoms may be absent, and the symptoms that are exhibited may be confused with other disease symptoms. Since hormonal counter-regulation slows with aging, recovery may be slower. Hypoglycemia may be fatal for those with a previous history of stroke or cardiac disease.

2. Inadequate food intake, decreased intestinal absorption of nutrients, and slowed metabolism of oral hypoglycemic agents compound the risks of hypoglycemia. New oral agents without hypoglycemic side effects that currently are in development will be especially beneficial to elderly people. The person who lives alone may require a "check in" system to assure early discovery if loss of consciousness occurs.

E. Long-term Complications of Diabetes

1. Amputation is twice as common in people with diabetes over age 65 than in younger people with diabetes. Neuromuscular and circulatory changes of aging are compounded by complications of diabetes. Decreased vision and sensation, as well as limited mobility, may prevent early detection of lower extremity wounds by the individual. Frequent observation of lower extremities must be planned. It may be useful for the educator to observe a patient demonstrate foot care in order to identify their specific limitations. Family, friends, and health care personnel can supplement the patient's abilities (see Chapter XXV: Lower Extremity Problems).

2. Because hypertension exacerbates other complications of diabetes, it is important to control blood pressure. Regular screening of all elderly patients for hypertension is warranted. The educator can anticipate that sodium restrictions may be

resisted by those who use heavy seasonings to compensate for decreased taste sensation. Alternate seasonings may be acceptable. Antihypertensive medications should be initiated when indicated, with close monitoring of side effects such as orthostatic hypotension and decreased cardiac output. Drug compatibilities should be examined when new medications are added.

3.   Myocardial infarction and cerebrovascular accidents are more prevalent in older people with diabetes than in those without diabetes.[8] Vascular disease may be present long before diabetes is diagnosed. Recovery and prognosis are poorer for patients with diabetes than for non-diabetic patients. Sodium restriction, exercise, weight control, lipid evaluation, blood pressure control, glucose control, and smoking cessation are appropriate interventions for the elderly when balanced with treatments for other medical conditions (see Chapter XXIV: Macrovascular Disease).

4.   Diseases of the eyes are more common with aging. Coupled with eye changes from diabetes (cataracts, glaucoma, retinopathy), elderly people with diabetes are at high risk for vision loss. Control of blood glucose, annual screening, and photocoagulation can impact vision loss, which in turn prevents vision-related self-care. Older people seek eye care less often than younger people and often have eye changes when diabetes is diagnosed. All eye diseases should be treated in order to maximize visual acuity. Functional vision for self-testing, medication administration, and foot examination should be assessed during educational sessions (see Chapter XXI: Eye Disease).

5.   Diabetic nephropathy associated with the normal changes of aging and with other causes of renal insufficiency (arteriosclerosis, hypertension, congestive heart failure, drugs, infection, cancer) can precipitate kidney failure. Since renal disease may be present at diagnosis, treatment should focus on

correcting hypertension and avoiding urinary tract infections. Low-protein diets may not be feasible if minimal protein is being consumed already. Dialysis or transplantation are options for some (see Chapter XXIII: Kidney Disease).

6. The impact of dental diseases due to aging and diabetes, and their effect on eating and nutrition, may be underestimated. Mobility or financial difficulties can result in decreased preventative care. Chronic mouth infections may be an outcome. Educators should encourage or facilitate routine oral hygiene measures and dental care (see Chapter X: Special Issues in Management).

REFERENCES

1.   Harris MI. Epidemiology of diabetes mellitus among elderly in the United States. In: Froom J, ed. Clinics in geriatric medicine. Philadelphia: Saunders Co, 1990:703-9.

2.   Perlmuter LC, Goldfinger SH, Shore AR, et al. Cognitive function in non-insulin dependent diabetes. In: Holmes, ed. Neuropsychological and behavioral aspects of diabetes. New York: Springer-Verlag, 1989.

3.   Chenitz WC, Stone JT, Salisbury SA. Clinical gerontological nursing. Philadelphia: WB Saunders, 1991.

4.   Moorley J, Kaiser F. Unique aspects of diabetes mellitus in the elderly. Clin Geriatr Med 1990;6:693-702.

5.   Graham C. Exercise in the elderly patient with diabetes. Practical Diabetol 1991;10:8-11.

6.   Halter J. Geriatric patients. In: Lebovitz HE, ed. Therapy for diabetes mellitus and related disorders. Alexandria, Va: American Diabetes Association, 1991:155-60.

7.   Madsbad S. Classification of diabetes in older adults. Diabetes Care 1990;13(suppl 2):93-95.

8.   Wilson PWF, Anderson KM, Kannel WB. Epidemiology of diabetes mellitus in the elderly. The Framingham study. Am J Med 1986; 80(suppl 5a):3-9.

KEY EDUCATIONAL CONSIDERATIONS

1. As with all learners, the elderly should be assessed and treated as individuals. However, older adults have certain learning needs that should be addressed routinely:
    a) self-care in terms of vision, mobility, mental state, functional ability, and finances;
    b) the impact of changes in weight or activity on blood glucose control;
    c) the effect of multiple medications;
    d) eating habits;
    e) the existence of concurrent illnesses;
    f) the progression of long-term effects of diabetes;
    g) undetected hypoglycemia;
    h) quality of life issues.

2. It is important to remember that the elderly patient *can* learn new things.

3. Modify the instructions based on the patient's needs, using a slower pace with simple printed/audio materials, or magnification.

4. Teaching strategies should emphasize the patient's strengths and capabilities rather than any limitations.

5. Because family support is important, include family members, a friend, or other helping person in the teaching.

6. Frequent evaluation of learning and knowledge retention should be planned because re-instruction may be necessary.

7. When negotiating proposed changes in patient behaviors, short- and long-term gains should be possible. Any changes should be viewed in the light of their effects on the patient's quality of life.

SELF-REVIEW QUESTIONS

If you are unsure of the answers to the following questions, please review the materials.

1. List four effects of aging that are similar to effects of diabetes.
2. Name an instrument that can be used to assess cognitive function.
3. What effects of aging may interfere with appropriate nutritional intake?
4. Identify one reason why hypoglycemia treatment may be inadvertently delayed by older people.
5. What are two reasons to aggressively treat diabetic eye diseases in the elderly?

CASE EXAMPLE

EP is an obese 76-year-old widow with NIDDM. She is referred to you for instruction on blood glucose monitoring. EP lives alone in a high-rise apartment in a large city. Her daughter, who is her only family, lives in a nearby suburb and has driven her to her appointment. Her doctor has become concerned that although she is taking glyburide 5 mg twice daily, her blood sugar levels as measured in his office are over 300 mg/dL (16.7 mmol/L). She states that she is not thirsty but does get up at least once nightly to urinate. Other medical problems include arthritis (which limits her mobility), cataract surgery 2 years ago, and mild congestive heart disease for which she takes digitalis.

QUESTIONS

1. What difficulties might EP have learning to do blood glucose testing?
2. What educational strategies might be helpful?
3. What long-term issues should be explored regarding future learning/management needs?

SUGGESTED SOLUTIONS

This woman is at risk for serious, short-term complications of hyperglycemia. Information is lacking about how long her diabetes has been out of control. A hemoglobin A_{1c} would help answer this question. Dehydration or subtle infections are possible. Nocturia places her at risk for falling, and given that she lives alone, help might not be available. Limited joint mobility from arthritis and limited vision increase the risk of injury. Lack of thirst, common in this age group, prevents one compensatory mechanism for her polyuria. Eliminating the polyuria is critical after you have clarified with her referring physician that her dehydration does not require hospitalization for treatment.

Because transferring the patient to insulin requires changes in self-care, you should explore other causes of elevated blood sugar, such as undetected infection, arthritis medication side effects, or possible treatment with thiazide diuretics for her congestive heart failure. Although her oral agent dose is not at the maximum level, caution is appropriate at her age to avoid toxicity secondary to age-related changes in the liver and kidneys. EP is overweight and sedentary. You suggest that she have a stress test prior to initiating aerobic exercise. EP was open to suggested flexibility exercises.

A complete nutritional assessment should be planned, with a focus on the scheduling and composition of meals. Many elderly patients who live alone do not have experience cooking for one person. EP describes frequent snacking on high-fat cheeses, especially at night. Alternative snack choices would be helpful.

Baseline information on day-to-day glucose levels will be helpful for evaluating future changes in management. Assessment of the patient's receptivity to testing, and visual and manual dexterity can be done while instructing her on a simple testing device. Her daughter should be included in instruction. Financial support for the purchase of testing strips and a meter also should be assessed.

Multiple focused, slow-paced teaching sessions should be planned, with extraneous details avoided. Several return demonstrations may be necessary.

In addition, the patient and her daughter should be made aware of the dangers of persistent hyperglycemia. They need to be told that if the above measures are not effective, insulin will be necessary. They can also be informed that additional support will be available if insulin therapy is required. Some method of daily contact between EP and her daughter should be arranged to evaluate her condition. A plan for phone contact from you should be established to evaluate her progress in learning and review the subsequent glucose results in anticipation of the need for further modifications in her management plans.

OTHER SUGGESTED READINGS

Assmann G, Schulte H. Diabetes mellitus and hypertension in the elderly: concomitant hyperlipidemia and coronary heart disease risk. Am J Cardiol 1989;63:33-37.

Baker, DE. The elderly diabetic. US Pharmacist Diabetes Management Supplement 1989:26-34.

Blunt BA, Barrett-Connor E, Wingard DC. Evaluation of fasting plasma glucose as screening test for NIDDM in older adults: Rancho Bernardo study. Diabetes Care 1991;14:989-93.

Brooks PJ, Francisco GE. Clinical aspects of type II diabetes mellitus in the elderly. J Geriatr Drug Therapy 1990;5:5-30.

Campbell RK. Diabetes mellitus in the elderly. Practical Diabetol 1987;6:10-13.

Connell CM. Psychosocial contexts of diabetes and older adulthood: reciprocal effects. Diabetes Educ 1991;17:364-71.

Davidson RA, Curanosos GJ. Should the elderly hypertensive be treated? Arch Intern Med 1987;147:1933-37.

French RL, Boen JR, Martineq AM, Bushhouse SA, Sprafka JM, Goetz FC. Population-based study of impaired glucose tolerance and type II diabetes in Wadena, Minnesota. Diabetes 1990;39:1131-37.

Funnell, MM. Role of the diabetes educator for older adults. Diabetes Care 1990;13:60-65.

Goldberg AP, Andres R, Bierman EL. Diabetes mellitus in the elderly. In: Hazard WR, Reubin A, Bierman EL, Bluss JP, eds. Principles of geriatric medicine and gerontology. New York: McGraw-Hill, 1990:739-58.

Graham C. Exercise in the elderly patient with diabetes. Practical Diabetol 1991;10:8-11.

Grobin W. A longitudinal study of impaired glucose tolerance and diabetes mellitus in the aged. J Am Geriatr Soc 1989;37:1127-34.

Hallburg JC. The teaching of aged adults. J Gerontological Nurs 1976;2:13-19.

Halter JB. Geriatric patients. In: Lebovitz HE, ed. Therapy for diabetes mellitus and related disorders. Alexandria, Va: American Diabetes Association, 1991:155-61.

Halter JB, Biby C, Duckworth WC, et al. Non-insulin-dependent diabetes mellitus in the elderly: a roundtable discussion. Kalamazoo, Mich: Upjohn, 1988:3-24.

Henry RR, Edelman SV. Advances in treatment of type II diabetes mellitus in the elderly. Geriatrics 1992;47:24-30.

Lipson LG. Diabetes in the elderly: diagnosis, pathogenesis, and therapy. Am J Med 1986;80:10-21.

Lipsky BA, Pecoraro RE, Ahroni JYH. Foot ulceration and infections in elderly diabetics. Clin Geriatr Med 1990;6:747-67.

McAvoy KH. Oral hypoglycemic agents in the management of non-insulin-dependent diabetes mellitus among the elderly. Diabetes Educ 1991;17:411-13.

Messana I, Beizer JL. Diabetes in the elderly. Practical Diabetol 1991;10:1-4.

Minaker KL. What diabetologists should know about elderly patients. Diabetes Care 1990;13:34-46.

Morley JE. Diabetes in elderly patients. Practical Diabetol 1988;7:6-10.

Morley JE, Kaiser FE. Unique aspects of diabetes mellitus in the elderly. Clin Geriatr Med 1990;6:693-701.

Mykkanen L, Markku L, Uusitupa M, Kalevi P. Prevalence of diabetes and impaired glucose tolerance in elderly subjects and their association with obesity and family history of diabetes. Diabetes Care 1990;13:1099-105.

Nettles A, ed. Guidelines for diabetic care in long-term care facilities. Minneapolis: Minneapolis-St Paul, Minn Diabetes Educators, 1992.

Peters AL, Davidson MB. Aging and diabetes. In: Alberti KGMM, DeFronzo RA, Keen H, Zimmet P, eds. International textbook of diabetes mellitus. New York: John Wiley & Sons, 1992:1103-27.

Porte D, Kahn SE. What geriatricians should know about diabetes mellitus. Diabetes Care 1990;13:47-54.

Reagan TR. Cardiac disease in the older diabetic: management considerations. Geriatrics 1989;44:91-96.

Reaven GM, Thompson LW, Nahum D, Haskins E. Relationship between hyperglycemia and cognitive function in older NIDDM patients. Diabetes Care 1990;13:16-21.

Smith DL. Patient education: tuning in to the needs of the elderly. Med Times 1986;114:27-31.

Templeton CL. Nutrition education: the older adult with diabetes. Diabetes Educ 1991;17:355-58.

The 1998 report of the joint national committee on detection, evaluation, and treatment of high blood pressure. Arch Intern Med 1988; 148:1023-38.

Tonino RP. Diabetes education: what should health care providers in long term nursing care facilities know about diabetes? Diabetes Care 1990; 13:55-59.

Wachtel TJ, Silliman RA, Lamberton P. Prognostic factors in the diabetic hyperosmolar state. J Am Geriatr Soc 1987;35:737-41.

White JR. The elderly patient with diabetes. Profile 1992;Spring:3-8.

SPECIAL POPULATIONS

XVIII. TEACHING PATIENTS WITH LOW LITERACY SKILLS

INTRODUCTION

Few would disagree that the use of printed materials for patient education is cost-effective and time-efficient. Yet, the patient's ability to read and fully understand written materials cannot be assumed or taken for granted. Diabetes educators concerned with patient adherence must ask the questions, "Are patients truly understanding what they read?" and "Can patients follow a treatment plan based on written instructions?" To answer these questions, educators must be aware that nonadherent behavior may be the result of misunderstanding or misinterpretation rather than motivational explanations. In some cases, low literacy skills are a major contributing factor. The ability to read patient education materials is particularly important for patients who have diabetes and must perform self-care behaviors. Educating patients about diet, weight control, exercise, stress management, foot care, adherence to drug therapy, and complications associated with diabetes becomes a major task for those who are unable to read and/or comprehend instructions. In addition, consequences of nonadherence related to those individuals with low literacy skills can result in unnecessary prolonged hospitalizations and/or an increased likelihood of complications that might otherwise have been prevented. Diabetes educators may choose from an array of educational strategies to work with patients who are learning impaired.

OBJECTIVES

On completion of this chapter, the learner will be able to:
- define functional literacy/illiteracy;
- identify strategies associated with determining patient understanding;
- discuss factors that contribute to reading/comprehension difficulty;
- list specific techniques that can be used to enhance readability.

A. Defining Literacy

1. Literacy implies an ability to use printed and written information in society to achieve one's goals and develop one's knowledge and potential.[1]

2. Literacy is a continuum of skills, not an all-or-none ability. It is a characteristic acquired by individuals in varying degrees. Some individuals are more literate than others, but it is not appropriate to speak of literate and illiterate persons as two distinct categories.

3. Illiteracy, the total lack of any literacy ability, is rare in the US. The problem is not that literacy skills decline to the point of illiteracy; rather, literacy demands have increased over time whereby individuals are functioning more productively in today's society. Low literacy is both chronic and common, with major consequences.[1]

4. The term "functional literacy," first used in the 1930s by the US Bureau of Census, was defined as having 3 or more years of schooling. During the 1930s it was considered appropriate that individuals completing 3 years of school could read essential printed material to function in society. Over the years, the level of education considered necessary to be functionally literate has risen steadily.[2]

5. During World War II, the Army referred to functional literacy as having attained 4 years of education. In 1947, the Census Bureau applied the term functional illiteracy to individuals with fewer than 5 years of schooling. By 1960, the US Office of Education was using 8 years of schooling as the standard.[2]

6. Evaluating literacy based upon grade equivalents alone should be done cautiously. An assumption is made that individuals who have reached a certain grade have acquired enough reading skills to function in society. Thus, the person who has

completed 8th grade is assumed to be able to function effectively in society, while the person with only 7 years of schooling is assumed to be unable to cope with the literacy demands. Setting educational attainment as a measure of functional literacy equates schooling with learning. Such an assumption is erroneous.

7. In the early 1970s, a national adult "right-to-read" movement began to assess adult literacy independent of grade levels. The challenge was to support the ability to read, write, and compute with the functional competence needed for meeting the requirements of adult living.

B. Examining the Magnitude of the Literacy Problem

1. Literacy rates in the United States vary considerably based on how one defines literacy/illiteracy. However, in 1982, US Secretary of Education Terrel Bell testified that approximately 65 million Americans were classified as functionally illiterate and unable to meet the basic requirements to function in everyday life. Educational proficiency was measured by having attained 8 years of schooling.[2,3]

2. Completing a job application, writing a letter to a friend, writing a check, reading a bus schedule, and applying for a driver's license all involve a certain degree of literacy skills.

3. Functional illiteracy is common among all races and socioeconomic strata. A larger percentage of African Americans, Native Americans, and Hispanics are marginally illiterate, however, due to a greater number of school dropouts.[2,3]

C. Methods for Measuring Literacy

1. Several methods for measuring literacy have been proposed, with no consensus (eg, educational attainment, tests of applied reading skills, comparisons of reading grade level with the reading level of common written material, investigation of job literacy requirements). Many authors indicate that a grade level equivalent should constitute the minimal standard. Grade levels have become the popular unit of measurement for literacy over time.

2. Educators need to know that reading-level estimates are replete with problems. Many individuals can read and understand material that is supposedly above their reading level. On the other hand, educators must not think that materials that are assigned an 8th-grade reading level are fully understood by all persons reading at the 8th-grade level.[2]

3. Readability formulas are used to judge patient education materials. These formulas were not popularized until the 1940s and were designed to rank the difficulty of books and other texts. Pichert & Elam[4] caution that readability formulas have flaws and have been misused.

    a) These formulas measure readability for the average reader and do not consider individual motivation and interests, all of which play a crucial role in the reading process.

    b) Readability formulas should be supplemented by other means[4] of judging the quality of patient education materials (eg, patient's background knowledge of the subject matter, patient interest and motivation, opportunity for reinforcement).

    c) In general, readability formulas evaluate sentence length and number of syllables. The most commonly used readability formulas are the SMOG,[5] Flesch,[6] Fry,[7] and Dale-Chall.[8]

        (1) The SMOG, a recently developed readability formula, is used by the US Department of Health and

Human Services, National Institutes of Health, and National Cancer Institute. The calculations depend on the total number of polysyllabic words found in a sample of 30 sentences. Based on a specific calculation, a SMOG conversion table is utilized to approximate grade levels.

(2) The Flesch Formula, developed by Rudolf Flesch in 1948, uses calculations of the average number of words per sentence, and the number of syllables per 100 words, to predict the readability level of a passage.

(3) The Fry Readability Formula selects three passages, each containing 100 words. The total number of sentences and the total number of syllables in each passage are counted and averaged. The average number of sentences and syllables per 100 words are plotted on the Fry Readability Graph, which indicates the approximate grade level.

(4) The Dale-Chall Readability Formula is based on two counts, average sentence length and percentage of unfamiliar words (those not included in the Dale List of 3000 Familiar Words).

d) The cloze procedure (test) is another method of evaluating patient comprehension. Using this procedure, a blank is substituted for every fifth word within the text. The reader is asked to fill in the blanks. One point is scored for each word that is correctly identified. The total number of correctly identified words out of 50 blanks constitutes the cloze score. Scores greater than 70% indicate the reader is able to comprehend the material independently; scores between 40% to 70% indicate that additional instruction is needed; scores less than 40% indicate the reader is unable to comprehend the material. The cloze procedure is time consuming to administer.[9]

D. Identifying Patients with Low Literacy Skills

1. Patients who have low literacy skills will go to great lengths to conceal the fact that they cannot read or write.

2. Many patients with low literacy skills have an average IQ and can speak articulately.

3. A person's comprehension skills are silent and invisible. Physical appearance is a poor indicator of skills. A roughly dressed fisherman might read at a 10th-grade reading level, while a well-dressed businessman may test at a 2nd-grade reading level.[10]

4. Patients become experts in creating defense mechanisms by manipulating a situation to avoid reading or writing.

5. Specific comments and cues that diabetes educators need to pay particular attention to include: "I forgot my eyeglasses at home." "I want my husband/wife/significant other to read this first." "Would you read it for me? My eyes are tired." "I do better if I watch you do it."

E. Ways to Determine Patient Understanding and Comprehension

1. *Paraphrasing* is the most direct and revealing method for determining patient understanding. Encourage patients to explain their condition and treatment in their own words. Paraphrasing provides ample opportunity for patients to ask about their condition. It can reveal gaps in information and misconceptions of the educational message, with a chance for immediate feedback.[11]

2. *Patient demonstration* of specific skills (eg, insulin administration, self-monitoring of blood glucose (SMBG), urine testing) provides the opportunity to correct improper techniques

quickly and answer questions about maintenance.[10,11] Food models can be used to allow the patient to plan a meal.

3. Another approach to reduce the comprehension barrier is to get *frequent feedback* from the patient. Questions such as, "Show me how you would. . .?" and "Tell me why you will. . ." are appropriate. Avoid questions like, "Do you understand. . .?" Include a variety of teaching modalities because nonreaders and poor readers are not likely to look to written materials as a primary source of information.[10,11]

F. **Teaching Patients with Low Literacy Skills**

1. Reading and listening depend upon language skills for comprehension. For those who lack vocabulary or skill conceptualizing, the ability to use written and oral information is diminished.[10] The use of illustrations and demonstration is more effective. For example, instead of reviewing a written pamphlet on foot care guidelines, demonstrate a foot exam on the patient's own foot.

2. It is important to make the distinction that a lack of comprehension skills is not a reflection of the intelligence of clients with low literacy skills.

3. Educators need to be aware of factors that contribute to reading difficulty: frequent use of polysyllabic words (vocabulary), technical terminology (concept density), and complex sentence structure.

4. Multimedia devices such as slide/tape programs or videotapes on patient education can be used. This method is less personal but provides answers/feedback in a timely manner and allows the audiotapes to be recorded in the patient's native language. An added benefit is that patients can learn in a non-threatening, private atmosphere.[10,11]

G. Methods for Reducing Literacy Demands

1. In providing patient education, the literacy demand can be reduced by utilizing the following principles based on research and experiences with individuals who are functionally illiterate.

   a) Present only essential information to meet patient needs. Think survival skills. Patients must know enough about diabetes to understand the nature and connection to treatment.

   b) Use written instructions in the sequence in which they are to be performed. Emphasize major points. Patients need relevant information to carry out appropriate behaviors. Present the most important points first. Re-emphasize points prior to conclusion and review the important points along the way.

   c) Use illustrations that show the patients' point of view.

   d) Use common words (eg, *doctor* instead of *physician*; *use* instead of *utilize*).

   e) Emphasize the desired patient action or behavior rather than underlying theory or principles.

   f) Use flip charts, food models, and homemade creative teaching tools to demonstrate a point.

   g) Paint a picture using an analogy. Try the analogy with a few patients and ask them what they think it means.

2. Use the following strategies when preparing and/or reviewing educational materials to increase the likelihood of patient comprehension.

   a) Use one- and two-syllable words (eg, *there, is, some, same, we, use, bottle, normal, contains, daily*).

   b) Write short, simple sentences. Introduce only one idea at a time in a sentence. Limit the number of new ideas on the page. Eye span should be kept to no more than 60 to 70 characters.

   c) The print should flow horizontally; print that is set in a vertical or diagonal direction is difficult to follow.

   d) State the main idea at beginning of the paragraph.

e) Use connectives sparingly (eg, *consequently, in spite of, however*).

f) Divide long stretches of narration with subtitles and captions.

g) Use the active voice to keep text less wordy and easier to read. Frequent use of the passive voice can confuse the reader.

h) Highlight important ideas.

i) Leave plenty of white space on the printed page.

j) Summarize important points in short paragraphs that are clearly labeled as "summaries." It is important to reinforce general or abstract concepts with specific, concrete examples that allow the reader to identify with the information.

k) Illustrations, photos, graphs, and cartoons, all add appeal as well as important information. For patients with low literacy skills, such visuals may be the only way to communicate desirable behavior versus non-desirable behavior. Avoid juvenile illustrations for an adult audience.

l) Write lists. Don't bury sequential information or a series of events or steps in narrative form.

m) Print size should be at least 14 point. Nobody enjoys squinting through a long page of narrative. Print style also affects both readability and motivation. Elaborate script print or ornate type (eg, italics, boldface, script) on high gloss paper are difficult to read. Underlining is more effective and easier to read than all capital letters.

REFERENCES

1.   Kirsch I, Jungeblut A. Literacy: profiles of America's young adults. Report no. 16-PL-02. Princeton, NJ: National Assessment of Educational Programs, 1986.

2.   Kaestle CF. Literacy in the United States. New Haven, Conn: Yale University Press, 1991.

3.   Kozol, J. Illiterate America. New York: Anchor Press/Doubleday and Company, Inc, 1985.

4.   Pichert JW, Elam P. Readability formulas may mislead you. Patient Educ Counseling 1985;7:181-191.

5.   McLaughlin GH. SMOG reading — a new readability formula. J Reading 1969;12:639-46.

6.   Flesch R. A new readability yardstick. J Appl Psychol 1948;32:221.

7.   Fry E. A readability formula that saves time. J Reading 1968;11:513.

8.   Powers R, Sumner W, Kearl B. A recalculation of four readability formulas. J Educ Psychol 1958;49:99-105.

9.   Taylor WS. Cloze procedure: a new test for measuring readability. Journalism Q 1953;30:415-433.

10.   Doak CC, Doak LG, Root J. Teaching patients with low literacy skills. Philadelphia: JB Lippincott Co, 1985.

11.   McCaughrin WC. Patient understanding: the key to quality patient education. Quality Rev Bull 1981;7:2-4.

12.   Haire-Joshu D, Houston C. Promoting behavior change: teaching/learning strategies. In: Haire-Joshu D, ed. Management of diabetes mellitus: perspectives of care across the life span. St. Louis: CV Mosby, 1991:565, 592.

SELF-REVIEW QUESTIONS

If you are unsure of the answers to the following questions, please review the materials.

1. Define functional literacy and illiteracy.
2. Discuss the nature and magnitude of the literacy problem.
3. What problems are associated with grade-level estimates as indicators of comprehension?
4. Identify some difficulties with using readability formulas in judging the quality of patient-education materials.
5. List the most practical means of determining patient comprehension.
6. Discuss important factors that contribute to reading difficulty.
7. List and describe strategies that diabetes educators would find helpful when preparing written instructions for patients with low literacy skills.

CASE EXAMPLE

JP is a 29-year-old male with a 2-year history of insulin-dependent diabetes mellitus (IDDM). Since his initial diagnosis of IDDM, JP has been hospitalized a number of times for ketoacidosis. During his last hospitalization, JP spoke openly about the responsibilities he had as a child. As the oldest of four children of a single, working mother, he was heavily burdened with household chores at an early age. JP never admitted he was unable to read or write, but talked about how he had trouble as a student and found it difficult to concentrate in school, often falling asleep in his chair. JP quit school in 10th grade and went to work full-time. He recently has returned to school to work toward his high-school equivalency diploma while working in a factory as a machine press operator. JP only takes his insulin when he has polyuria and polydipsia.

QUESTIONS

1. Describe the type of information that might not be readily apparent in this case study but would be appropriate for a diabetes educator to assess with regard to JP's literacy skills.
2. As a diabetes educator, identify two goals that you would like to accomplish in working with JP.

SUGGESTED SOLUTIONS

JP's childhood is one example of a home environment in which energies may have been diverted away from learning. As diabetes educators, it is important to know that young adults with low literacy skills generally have had bad experiences with formal education. They may have been labeled as having a learning disorder and may have been held back one or two grades. In general, they are reluctant to return to a formal class setting and ashamed to have others know of their limited reading and writing ability. Therefore, a learning assessment that identifies specific environmental, cultural, economic, and psychosocial factors needs to be conducted before planning diabetes education.[12]

Patients who have low self-esteem in addition to low literacy skills may have difficulty developing the confidence necessary to take actions that will improve their lives. Instead they may hold in their frustrations and rely on others to make decisions. In working with JP, the first goal should be to gain his trust. From the beginning, the educator must take the time to get to know JP and try to reduce his anxiety. The educator should be sure to recognize and emphasize his abilities, not just his problems, to focus on his strengths and to let him know that his ideas, contributions, and life experiences are just as important as the ability to read and write.

For the second goal, try to teach JP that he needs to take insulin every day. The educator can use a simple flip chart to explain that JP's pancreas does not make insulin so he must inject the insulin even when he has no symptoms. At the conclusion of the session, the educator could describe a hypothetical situation in which JP wakes up feeling great one morning and then ask, "Should you take your insulin?" If JP says no, then the educator should try again with a different teaching strategy.

OTHER SUGGESTED READINGS

Barr P. ed. Diabetes educational resources for minority and low literacy populations. Southfield, Mich: Coalition for Diabetes Education and Minority Health, 1991.

Diabetes Printed Educational Materials for People with Limited Reading Skills. National Diabetes Information Clearinghouse. June, 1991.

Falvo DR. Improving patient compliance. Quality Rev Bull 1981;7:5-8.

Farrell-Miller P, Gentry P. How effective are your patient education materials? Guidelines for developing and evaluating written educational materials. Diabetes Educ 1989;15:418-22.

Harmon D. Illiteracy: an overview. Harvard Educ Rev 1970;40:226-43.

McNeal B, Salisbury Z, Baumgardner P, Wheeler FC. Comprehension assessment of diabetes education program participants. Diabetes Care 1984;7:232-35.

Meade CD, Thornhill DG. Illiteracy in healthcare. Nurs Manage 1989;20:14-15.

SPECIAL POPULATIONS

XIX. CULTURAL SENSITIVITY IN DIABETES EDUCATION

INTRODUCTION

Minority populations in the United States are at high risk for a variety of chronic diseases and have a lower health status than the majority population.[1] Overall mortality for nonwhites is one-third greater than that for whites. Diabetes strikes particularly hard at minorities and, in the United States, the prevalence of diabetes is highest among the ethnic minorities.[2,3] The prevalence of diabetes among the nonwhite population has increased consistently and significantly since 1965. The death rate for diabetes is highest among nonwhite females, being more than twice that of white females.[1,4]

Other minority groups are also significantly affected by diabetes. The predicted incidence of non-insulin-dependent diabetes mellitus (NIDDM), also called type II diabetes, among black Americans is at least 1.6 times greater than that of white Americans.[3] The prevalence rate for diabetes among 29,000 American Indians living on reservations in the Pacific Northwest is significantly higher than the national rate. Depending on cultural area and tribe, American Indians are from 1.9 to 3.0 times more likely to get diabetes than is the general population.[5] More than 50% of Pima Indians over the age of 30 are reported to have NIDDM, and full-heritage Pimas are 1.8 times more likely to have NIDDM than are Pimas of mixed Indian-white heritage.[6] The prevalence of NIDDM among Mexican Americans and Chinese Americans is approximately twice that of white Americans.[3,7] Because of underdiagnosis and underreporting among minority populations, these estimates of the prevalence of diabetes may be low.

OBJECTIVES

Upon completion of this chapter, the learner will be able to:
- discuss the impact of diabetes on minority groups;
- identify factors associated with the development of diabetes in minority populations;
- describe components that need to be assessed to assure a culturally diverse diabetes education program;

- list the steps incorporated in the development of a culturally diverse program;
- describe the strategies for promoting minority access to diabetes care through community empowerment;
- identify strategies to assist the educator to achieve a level of sensitivity to cultural diversity;
- discuss the role of the diabetes educator as an advocate of culturally diverse diabetes education programs.

A. Etiology

1. The research to date has examined several factors as being potentially related to diabetes in minority groups. These factors include *genetics, obesity, economics, life-style factors, aging* and *continuity of care.*

   a) Genetics: Evidence of genetic tendencies for diabetes in African-American populations is substantial. Defects in insulin production and action are likely causes. Data suggesting specific versus multiple gene involvement is currently being examined.[8] Among Pima Indians, modest associations for NIDDM are found although information is not conclusive.[9]

   b) Obesity: The prevalence of obesity is generally high in African-American women specifically and in the African-American population as a whole.[10,11] Consumption of sugar, alcohol, and salt is higher among African-American populations than among other groups.[12,13] Mexican American diets are higher in fat and sodium than are the diets of those of other ethnic groups. This increased fat and sodium intake is reflected in the higher levels of blood glucose, cholesterol, and triglycerides found in Mexican Americans.[14]

   c) Economics: Socioeconomic stress is also associated with the prevalence of diabetes among minority groups. Poverty, unemployment, lack of health insurance, and limited access to medical care contribute significantly to higher rates of morbidity and mortality among minorities in the United States.[15] Socioeconomic status plays an important role in differentiating coping strategies across ethnic groups and influences various aspects of health culture. For example, middle-class families differ from lower-class families within ethnic groups because socioeconomic factors limit access to diabetes care, dietary information, and so forth.[16]

d) Life-style factors: Minority groups tend to engage in more risk-enhancing behaviors and fewer health-promotion behaviors than do whites. Blacks and Latinos engage in health habits that are associated with increased mortality; these habits include smoking, poor dietary habits, and sedentary life-style.[17] These findings are also present among American Indians. Data suggest that minority groups tend to be less knowledgeable about risk-enhancing behaviors and less aware of modifiable risk factors for chronic diseases such as diabetes.[18] Environmental determinants associated with urbanization (dietary changes, sedentary life-style, stress, etc) have resulted in increased prevalence of diabetes among numerous ethnic groups (eg, Puerto Ricans, Australian aborigines, and Polynesians). American Indian groups that have adopted a nontraditional life-style exhibit prevalence rates of diabetes that are among the highest of any group in the United States.[5,6]

e) Aging: The prevalence of diabetes in the aging population is substantial. Diabetes affects between 15% and 20% of the population over the age of 65. The majority of these individuals have NIDDM.[6] Most studies have demonstrated an increased incidence of NIDDM associated with aging.

(1) Among Pima Indians, incidence rates increase until age 44 in men and age 54 in women; after that, the incidence of NIDDM declines. This decline might be explained by disease development earlier in life.[6]

(2) A different relationship exists between aging and the prevalence of diabetes in the African-American

population. NIDDM occurs at near epidemic proportion in the African-American community. The prevalence of NIDDM among blacks is from 50% to 60% higher than among whites. The prevalence of NIDDM among elderly black women is especially alarming — one in four black women older than 55 has diabetes.[3] Furthermore, African-Americans have higher rates of complications of diabetes, including end-stage renal disease, blindness, and amputation, and they are more likely to die prematurely. Compared with elderly African-Americans without diabetes, those with diabetes are also more likely to enter a hospital or a nursing home.[12]

f)   Continuity of care: Minority groups use formal health care services less than white groups, in part because availability of services is problematic. For example, American Indians live in areas where the availability of physicians is below the national average.[17] African-Americans frequently use emergency care sources as opposed to preventive care sources. Twice as many blacks and Hispanics use hospital and emergency clinic services as do whites. Issues related to reimbursement by Medicaid and other insurers influence care-seeking decisions and may encourage acute versus preventive care visits.[19,20]

B.   Relationship of Cultural Diversity to Diabetes Education

1.   Delivery of diabetes education for minorities requires the application of comprehensive educational principles that respect the cultural differences of the specific ethnic groups.

a)   An understanding of key terminology in this area is necessary for the purpose of common communication.

b)   Some key terms and definitions are provided to encourage common communication (see Box).

2.   Ethnicity is a predictor variable in beginning to understand family health beliefs and behaviors.[16]

KEY TERMS

Cultural blindness: A set of attitudes, practices, and/or policies that adheres to the traditional philosophy of being unbiased.

Cultural competence: A set of academic and interpersonal skills that allow individuals to increase their understanding and appreciation of cultural differences and similarities within, among, and between groups.

Cultural destructiveness: A set of attitudes, practices, and/or policies that are designed to promote the superiority of the dominant culture and that purposefully attempts to eradicate the "lesser" or "inferior" culture because it is viewed as "different."

Cultural diversity: Differences in race, ethnicity, language, nationality, or religion among various groups within a community, organization, or nation.

Cultural incapacity: A set of attitudes, practices, and/or policies that, while not explicitly promoting the superiority of the dominant culture, adheres to the traditional idea of "separate but equal" treatment.

Cultural proficiency: A set of attitudes, practices, and/or policies that holds cultural differences and diversity in the highest esteem.

Cultural sensitivity: An awareness of the nuances of one's own and other cultures.

Culturally appropriate: Demonstrating both sensitivity to cultural differences and similarities and effectiveness in using cultural symbols to communicate a message.

Culturally competent: A set of attitudes, practices, and/or policies that respects, rather than merely shows receptivity to, different cultures and people.

Culturally open: Refers to attitudes, practices, and/or policies that are geared toward the learning and receptivity of new ideas and solutions to improve services rendered to one's particular target group.

Culture: The shared values, norms, traditions, customs, arts, history, folklore, and institutions of a group of people.

Ethnic: Belonging to a common group — often linked by race, nationality, and language — with a common cultural heritage.

Multicultural: Designed for or pertaining to two or more distinctive cultures.

Race: A socially defined population that is derived from distinguishable physical characteristics that are genetically transmitted.

Source: Adapted from Orlandi.[30]

a)   According to Leininger,[21] culture is a "learned and transmitted knowledge about a particular culture with its values, beliefs, rules of behavior, and lifestyle practices that guides a designated group in their thinking and actions in patterned ways." Culture influences thoughts and feelings and guides behavior. Individuals and families make different choices based on cultural forces. Information received by the learner is filtered based upon his or her own set of experiences.

b)   Application of the teaching/learning process to minority individuals requires the educator to specifically recognize the role of culture in the care decisions made by the patient. Clearly, knowledge of cultural nuances within a given population is insufficient to enable a health care provider to effectively influence choices made by clients from a different cultural experience. Thus, the educator's informed awareness, sensitivity, and incorporation of sociocultural components into the program are critical to being able to adequately address minority health care issues in diabetes.

3.   Diabetes education for minority groups should integrate and emphasize the interaction of individual, family, subcultural, and societal factors in the development of individual thought and behavior. It is important to identify and delineate the impact of multiple factors on patterns of care. This provides the means for understanding the cultural influences that affect the teaching-learning process in diabetes education. One assumption is that care-seeking choices by individuals are shaped by the interaction of individual, social group, subcultural, and societal characteristics.[22,23]

4.   The *individual* (biological/affective/cognitive level) is imbedded in a *social group*, which is imbedded in the *subculture* of the minority group which, in turn, is imbedded in the *society*, which represents the sociocultural components of the majority culture.[24] Individual thought and behavior are viewed as

developing through interaction between the individual, social group, subculture, and society at large. According to Sussman,[24] assessment using this multilevel framework is particularly appropriate for individualizing education among minority groups by providing a basis for systematic sociocultural assessment by diabetes educators (see Figure XIX.1 for a sample assessment tool). An example of a case using this framework appears at the end of this chapter.

a) Individual (biological/affective/cognitive) characteristics can affect the educational process.

(1) These include individual biology and psychology, economic resources, and attitudes and beliefs.

(a) Biological characteristics include a person's physical and psychological well-being, language and communication skills, health status, physical and emotional needs, and adaptability as well as the individual's perception and interpretation of these.

(b) Personal resources include economic resources, insurance coverage, and housing.

(c) Cognitive factors include knowledge, beliefs, attitudes, and expectations about health and diabetes care.

(2) The values reflected by the individual are also influenced by culture, as depicted in Table XIX.1. A major emphasis of this assessment is that individuals do not create their own characteristics but *reflect the layers of influence* that surround them in the form of social group, subcultural norms, and the social, political, and economic realities of the society at large.

b) Characteristics of the social group help define the individual.

(1) The immediate social group of family and friends is cross-culturally the primary source of care and support as well as the locus of many health care decisions.

FIGURE XIX.1:

Health Care Assessment Tool of Cultural Patterns of Minority Patients with Diabetes

This assessment tool is intended as a *qualitative* guide to cultural assessment of minority patients as a component of comprehensive and effective diabetes education. The diabetes educator observes, records, and rates behavior on the scale below from 1 to 4 with respect to minority or majority cultural ways. The ratings are intended to provide only a qualitative profile to guide decisions and actions. Ratings 1, 2, 3, and 4 assist in identifying *patterns* of cultural beliefs that are important factors in diabetes education.

Rating: Following each criterion, the diabetes educator documents his/her assessment of the extent to which the patient reflects patterns associated primarily with the subcultural/minority ethnic group with which the patient is primarily affiliated *versus* those patterns primarily associated with the societal or majority culture (eg, Anglo-American ethnic group).

1 = Primarily subcultural/minority patterns 2 = Moderately subcultural
3 = Moderately societal/majority patterns 4 = Mainly societal patterns

<u>Criteria</u>   <u>Rating</u>
Individual (Biological/Affective/Cognitive) Characteristics

1. Language, communication skills, and gestures (native
    or nonnative).
Specify: _____ _____

2. General environmental living context (living conditions,
    neighborhood).
Specify: _____ _____

3. Wearing apparel and physical appearance (eg, ethnic focus).
Specify: _____ _____

4   Educational values, knowledge, attitudes, or belief factors.
Specify: _____ _____

5.   Views of ways to prevent illness, maintain wellness or
     health, care for self or others.
Specify: _____ _____

6.   Food uses and nutritional values, beliefs, and taboos.
Specify: _____ _____

7.   Economic factors (cost of living, income).
Specify: _____ _____

8.   Religious or spiritual beliefs and values.
Specify: _____ _____

Characteristics of the Social Group

9.   Characteristics of kin and non-kin networks (number of
     persons in household, values, beliefs, and norms).
Specify: _____ _____

10. General social interactions and kinship ties (eg, location of
     kin, extended family contact).
Specify: _____ _____

11. Type of support received from kin (frequency of visits,
     obligations).
Specify: _____ _____

12. Family view of diabetes care (eg, knowledge, beliefs,
     attitudes, expectations of family).
Specify: _____ _____

13. Patterned daily activities.
Specify: _____ _____

Characteristics of the Subculture

14. Patterns of formal health care treatment seeking.
Specify: _____ _____

15. Folk (generic or indigenous) health care-cure values,
beliefs, and practices.
Specify: _____ _____

16. Care concepts or patterns that guide actions (what concerns
patient, support, presence, etc).
Specify: _____ _____

17. Locus of responsibilities of various age groups for health
care.
Specify: _____ _____

Characteristics of the Society

18. Political or legal influences on diabetes care.
Specify: _____ _____

19. Perception of quality, distribution, and accessibility to
health and diabetes care resources.
Specify: _____ _____

20. Unemployment rates, occupational status of neighborhood.
Specify: _____ _____

21. Geographical distribution of minority and majority groups
and characteristics of districts or neighborhoods (eg, crime
rates, housing, and transportation).
Specify: _____ _____

Source: Adapted from Leininger M. Leininger's acculturation health care assessment tool for cultural patterns in traditional and nontraditional lifeways. J Transcult Nurs 1991;2(2):40-42.

TABLE XIX.1:
Contrasting Values by Culture

Anglo-American Values	Alternative Culture Values
Personal control over the environment	Fate
Change	Tradition
Time dominates	Human interaction dominates
Human equality	Hierarchy/status
Individualism/privacy	Group welfare
Competition	Cooperation
Future orientation	Past orientation
Informality	Formality

    (a) Characteristics of the social group that help define individual behavior include the structure and networks of family, friends, neighbors and non-kin; geographic location and composition; and various resources, demands, and stressors that are present.

    (b) Also important are the characteristics of the interactions between family, friends, and individuals (such as the type of support received), and the obligations/responsibilities to the patient of family groups and friends.

    (c) Finally, the knowledge, beliefs, attitudes, values, and expectations of the individual's family and friends regarding health care in general and diabetes care in particular, and the roles played by patient and family influence a person's health care decisions.

  (2) Examination of the characteristics of kin and non-kin networks, residential proximity, and type and level of interaction can provide important information related to the structure and nature of family life and

decisions concerning diabetes care among various cultures.

    c)   Characteristics of the subculture include shared group norms of thought and behavior, values, and preferences.

        (1)   Subcultural norms influence the thought and behavior of families and individuals.

        (2)   Some subcultural components relevant to diabetes education include medical beliefs and practices, and social structure and organization.

            (a)   Relevant medical beliefs and practices include concepts of health and illness; patterns of treatment seeking and use of available diabetes resources; and attitudes about expected outcomes of diabetes, about biomedical and nonbiomedical health care providers and formal mainstream services, and about the locus of responsibility for diabetes care decisions.

            (b)   Social structure and organization norms and preferences relevant to diabetes care include family structure; household composition and flexibility; the definition and function of kin groups; roles and status of various family members; norms of interpersonal interaction; and responsibilities of various age groups.

    d)   Characteristics of the society include the health care, economic, social, and political system of the society within which the individual, as a member of a minority group, resides.

        (1)   Characteristics of the society influence subcultural norms and values, families, and individuals.

        (2)   Societal characteristics relevant to the health care of minority groups include the health care system, the economic system, and demographics.

            (a)   Aspects of the health care system that affect minorities include the distribution, cost, quality, and policies of the health and diabetes care resources.

(b) Aspects of the economic system that affect minorities include the distribution and abundance of economic resources in the society and in the minority group; the social welfare system; unemployment rates; occupational status; and educational attainment of the minority and majority groups.

(c) Demographic aspects that affect minorities include the geographical distribution of minority and majority groups, and characteristics (such as crime rates, housing, and transportation) of districts and neighborhoods.

C. Culturally Relevant Diabetes Education Programs

1. Diabetes education of minority populations relies on the delivery of culturally relevant protocols of care by culturally sensitive educators. These protocols of care acknowledge the importance of culture, assess cultural influences as they relate to diabetes management, recognize cultural differences that may affect the patient's ability to manage diabetes, and adapt programs to meet culturally unique needs (for example, the exchange lists may not include foods specific to a particular culture).

2. Conventional strategies for promoting health among minority patients have been only minimally successful. The multiple influences of sociocultural components as determinants of health behaviors suggest the need for alternative strategies of diabetes education. Diabetes education programs should assure sensitivity to various minority groups by incorporating programmatic curricula that have been adapted to reflect cultural diversity.

3. Community organization may help to mitigate environmentally induced loss of control related to social and health problems.[25]

a) Community organization approaches emphasize the use of informal networks to communicate the importance of health behavior change. A central goal of community organization is to empower both individuals and communities to increase individual and community competency.[26]

b) Through participation in health promotion activities within the community, especially those targeting diabetes education, individuals can develop a sense of control and self-confidence. For example, individuals from minority communities can be educated as peer leaders to provide diabetes nutrition information to other community members. This approach helps peer leaders to improve their own knowledge of dietary information while reinforcing appropriate dietary management behaviors among community members.

4. Key strategies must be implemented to assure culturally sensitive diabetes education programs.[17,26,27] The following strategies are recommended.

a) Conduct an assessment of the presence and types of minority groups present in the area served by the diabetes program. Recognition of the various ethnic groups that reside in the area is the first step to assuring that educational materials and curricula are culturally relevant. For example, programs that serve a large number of Asian Americans will need to assure that educational materials sensitive to the dietary preferences of that culture are represented.

b) Develop an advisory board of health professionals and/or lay persons representative of diverse cultural groups to offer advice and counsel regarding the diabetes education program. Balanced representation from ethnic groups residing in the area served by the program is needed.

(1) The committee can assist in identifying any problem associated with diabetes in the community. While the problem, as viewed by the community, may vary

from that seen by the professional, input from the advisory board can provide a basis for further educational program development.

(2) Selection of a community sponsor or lead agency, such as a social service agency, a church, or other agency respected by the community, provides a valuable resource in planning and disseminating diabetes information.[22,23,25] These agencies provide access to and a means of facilitating neighborhood ownership and decision making by involving community members through service on steering committees.

c) Work with the advisory board to evaluate existing diabetes patient education protocols, materials, and media to determine applicability and suitability to specific minority groups.[27-29] Several components of this evaluation process should be addressed.

(1) Initiate focus groups. Culturally diverse focus groups should be convened to assist with the evaluation of materials, messages and media. Focus groups should be composed of members representative of the target group.

(2) Modify measures and materials to reflect appropriate language. Assessment of the general educational level, literacy, and language preferences of the target group or community should be addressed by the focus groups. Levels of literacy should be assessed by the focus group for both the preferred language of the target group (eg, Spanish) and for the majority culture language (eg, English).

(3) Develop new patient assessment and educational materials and media as needed, tailored to the specific needs of the minority group. The need for such tools will be identified as a result of the thorough assessment. Seek the assistance of the advisory board or other ethnically diverse focus

groups in developing new materials pertinent to the target audience.

(4) Incorporate examples and pictures of culturally diverse groups in the newly developed materials and media. In addition, materials should reflect ethnic differences. For example, videos should feature people from the same ethnic groups. The use of local people or national celebrities of common ethnic origin is recommended.

(5) Integrate community values into the program, educational materials, and messages to facilitate local identification. For example, educational materials may contain photographs of landmarks (eg, churches) valued by local ethnic groups. Posters and pamphlets should be designed to reflect the ethnic diversity of the community at which they are targeted.

(6) Disseminate materials to the target groups. The advisory board and/or culturally diverse focus groups should assist in identifying communication channels pertinent to the target audience. Common ethnic variations in these channels appear in Table XIX.2.

d) Implement patient education practices and programs according to the diabetes teaching and education strategies described in Chapter I: Educational Principles and Strategies. These practices should reflect an understanding of the numerous factors that influence decision making by patients of a specific ethnic background.

e) Encourage routine follow-up and preventive care. The chronic nature of diabetes results in the need for routine preventive care visits. This is especially critical for monitoring, early diagnosis, and treatment of complications that frequently result. Various ethnic groups may hesitate to use formal health care services for a variety of reasons (eg, economic, distrust of the system, etc). In part, this may reflect the system's lack of cultural

TABLE XIX.2:
Examples of Ethnically Focused
Communication Channels

Common communication channels for specific minority groups have been specified in community-based diffusion models defined by the US Department of Health and Human Services (DHHS) (1987). These channels vary from community to community and, therefore, must be determined by a careful assessment. The following examples of variations in preferences for communication patterns are based on the experience of several health promotion projects completed in ethnically diverse communities.

American Indians
Women's clubs
Community sporting events
Grandparent-grandchild relationship
Traditional medicine men
Commodity food distribution points

Asian Americans/Pacific Islanders
Local churches
Women's groups
Businessmen's groups
Ethnic grocery stores

African Americans
Family reunions
Women's clubs
Churches and religious organizations
Workplace
Peer groups

Hispanics (Mexican Americans, Puerto Ricans, Central and South Americans)
Churches and religious organizations[*]
Gender-specific organizations[†]

[*] Religion is very important in the Hispanic culture. Disease may be seen as a punishment from God. Respect for issues of spirituality and involvement in religious organizations are important means of communicating health information.

[†] Machismo is an important phenomenon in the Hispanic community. Hispanic men typically cannot be reached through the same channels as Hispanic women.

Source: Strategies for diffusing health information to minority populations: A profile of a community based diffusion model. USDHHS, National Heart, Lung and Blood Institute, 1987.

sensitivity. Recognition and acknowledgment of these factors by the diabetes educator are important.

(1) The apparent use by ethnic group members of health care systems outside the mainstream (eg, herbalists, medicine men, and other traditional healers) should not lead diabetes educators to assume that the target population differs markedly from the majority population in its health care preference.

(2) Educators should seek to understand the patterns of use of nontraditional systems and analyze information obtained by means of these systems and resources. According to a DHHS task force report, "Recognition of existing traditional health beliefs and practices, acknowledgment of their potential effects, and attempts to work with them rather than against them or despite them is needed."[27] Sensitivity to these issues and flexibility in dealing with various ethnic groups is very important.

f) Conduct a systematic programmatic evaluation. An evaluation that addresses the effectiveness of the program's cultural competence in reaching diverse ethnic groups is needed. These findings assure the adequacy of the diabetes education interventions and direct future program planning.

(1) Cultural competence may be measured in terms of the past and present performances of an organization established to enhance the services rendered to the target population.

(2) Orlandi[30] has cited areas of needs assessment, training, staffing patterns, and prior performance that should be evaluated to determine cultural competence. By posing the following questions, evaluators can get a sense of the effectiveness of their diabetes education program.

(a) Needs assessment:

i) Has the diabetes education program done a formal needs assessment during the past

3 years pertaining to the population it intends to serve?

ii) Are data collected and kept for ethnic/racial populations?

iii) Are the collected data used for planning designed to reflect the cultural diversity of the local group?

(b) Training:

i) Has the diabetes education program engaged in any training to enhance the cultural competence of its professional staff during the past 3 years?

(c) Staffing patterns:

i) What percent of the staff is trained in cultural awareness?

ii) What percent of minority members are represented in an ethnic/racial advisory board?

iii) What percent of the minority population is represented at the administrative (or decision making) level of the diabetes education program?

(d) Prior performance patterns:

i) Is there linkage with other organizations in the community that serve the same minority groups?

ii) Does the mission statement of the organization provide for culturally competent services?

iii) What is the minority population's perception of the agency's effectiveness?

iv) Does the diabetes program distribute educational materials (eg, pamphlets or brochures) in languages that the minority population understands?

v) Does the program have an in-house ethnic/ racial researcher to add to the knowledge of culturally competent practices by conducting research?

D. Role of the Diabetes Educator

1. Diabetes education programs reflect the cultural competence of those who deliver them. Thus, the diabetes educator must strive to be culturally competent.

2. Cultural competence is a multidimensional concept involving various aspects of knowledge, attitude, and skill. These components can vary in a continuum from high to low. Table XIX.3 provides a schematic representation of a useful self-assessment tool. As an example of its use, diabetes educators who care for a significant number of Asian patients might be culturally competent in that they are knowledgeable about cultural differences related to ethnicity, and committed to the need for changes in the education program; however, these same educators may be culturally incompetent in that they are unskilled in the abilities needed to promote change. Thus, the program impact is likely to be neutral at best because the educator lacks the skills to promote cultural change. Self-awareness of this should encourage the diabetes educator to seek additional training to achieve cultural competence.

3. The diabetes educator who is committed to the development of culturally diverse programs can make a variety of contributions to assure that ethnic groups and cultural differences are respected and accounted for in diabetes education. This can be accomplished in several ways.[31]
    a) Conduct programs for other health team members that stimulate a critical understanding of the obstacles to more successful diabetes treatment outcomes based on the perceptions and experiences of members of the target minority group.
    b) Encourage the least restrictive access to diabetes education programs. Strong interagency collaboration is

TABLE XIX.3:
A Framework of Cultural Competence

	Culturally Incompetent	Culturally Sensitive	Culturally Competent
Cognitive	Oblivious	Aware	Knowledgeable
Affective	Apathetic	Sympathetic	Committed to change
Skills	Unskilled	Lacking some skills	Highly skilled
Overall Impact	Destructive	Neutral	Constructive

Source: Adapted from Orlandi.[30]

critical to such efforts. Development of case management strategies might also be effective for larger patient census.[32]

c) Develop appropriate cross-cultural communication skills.

(1) Systematic evaluation of the effectiveness of teaching methods for minority patients by professionals is an important strategy in assuring this.

(2) The use of multiple evaluation methods, including audio- and videotaping of patient sessions, might prove effective.

d) Build into diabetes health promotion efforts methods of community participation and control at all levels.

e) Promote and create environments that promote diabetes education programs as a community resource.

REFERENCES

1. Ross HS, Tseng R, Howe-Murphy R. Implications for health promotion programs among multicultural groups. J Allied Health 1986;15:318-23.

2. Pi-Sunyer FX. Obesity and diabetes in blacks. Diabetes Care 1990;13:1144-49.

3. Roseman JM. Diabetes in black americans. In: Harris MI, Hamman RF, eds. Diabetes in America. Washington, DC: US Department of Health and Human Services, 1985:chap 8.

4. Department of Health and Human Services. The prevention and treatment of complications of diabetes: a guide for primary care practitioners. Atlanta: Centers for Disease Control, Center for Chronic Disease Prevention and Health Promotion, Division of Diabetes Translation, 1991.

5. Freeman WL, Hosey GM, Diehr P, Gohdes D. Diabetes in American Indians of Washington, Oregon, and Idaho. Diabetes Care 1989;12:282-88.

6. Everhart J, Knowler WC, Bennett PH. Incidence and risk factors for non-insulin-dependent diabetes. In: Harris MI, Hamman RF, eds. Diabetes in America. Washington, DC: US Department of Health and Human Services, 1985:chap 4.

7. Fujimoto WY. Diabetes in asian americans. In: Harris MI, Hamman RF, eds. Diabetes in America. Washington, DC: US Department of Health and Human Services, 1985:chap 10.

8. Permutt MA. Genetics of NIDDM. Diabetes Care 1990;13:1150-53.

9. Harris MI. Classification and diagnostic criteria for diabetes and other categories of glucose intolerance. In: Harris MI, Hamman RF, eds.

Diabetes in America. Washington, DC: US Department of Health and Human Services, 1985:chap 2.

10. Kumanyika SK, Ewart CK. Theoretical and baseline considerations for diet and weight control of diabetes among blacks. Diabetes Care 1990;13:1154-62.

11. Kumanyika S. Obesity in black women. Epidemiol Rev 1987;9:31-50.

12. Webb H. Community health centers: providing care for urban blacks. J Natl Med Assoc 1984;76:1063-67.

13. Coreil J. Ethnicity and cancer prevention in a tri-ethnic urban community. J Natl Med Assoc 1984;76:1013-19.

14. Vega W, Sallis J, Patterson T, Rupp J, Morris J, Nader P. Predictors of dietary change in Mexican-American families participating in a health behavior change program. Am J Prev Med 1988;4:194-99.

15. Sanders-Phillips K. A model for health promotion in ethnic minority families. Wellness Lecture Series, Menlo Park, Ca: Henry J Kaiser Family Foundation, 1991.

16. Guarnaccia PJ, Pelto PJ, Schensul SL. Family health culture, ethnicity, and asthma: coping with illness. Med Anthropol 1985;(summer):203-24.

17. Heckler MM. Report of the secretary's task force on black and minority health, 1985: executive summary. Washington, DC: US Government Printing Office, 1985.

18. Phillips C, Lacey L. Cancer profiles from several high-risk Chicago communities. J Natl Med Assoc 1987;79:701-4.

19. Wan T. Use of health services by the elderly in low-income communities. Health Soc 1982;60:82-107.

20. Kotranski L, Bolick J, Halbert J. Neighborhood variations in the use of city-supported primary health care services by an elderly population. J Community Health 1987;12:231-45.

21. Leininger M. Transcultural nursing: concepts, theories, and practices. New York: John Wiley & Sons, 1978.

22. Fisher EB, Auslander WF, Sussman LK, et al. Community organization for risk reduction and chronic disease management in African-American neighborhoods. New York: Association for Advancement of Behavior Therapy, 1991.

23. Fisher EB Jr, et al. Community organization and health promotion in minority neighborhoods. Bethesda, Md: NHLBI Workshop on Health Behavior Research in Minority Populations, National Heart, Lung and Blood Institute, 1991.

24. Sussman LK. Discussion on the theoretical models of behavior and behavior change. Bethesda, Md: National Heart, Lung and Blood Institute, 1992.

25. Auslander WF, Haire-Joshu D, Houston CA, Fisher EB Jr. Community organization to reduce the risk of non-insulin-dependent diabetes among low-income African-American women. J Ethnicity Dis 1992;2:176-84.

26. Minkler M. Improving health through community organization. In: Glanz K, Lewis FM, Rimer BK, eds. Health behavior and health education. San Francisco: Jossey-Bass, 1990:257-87.

27. Report of the secretary's task force on black and minority health. Vol 3, Cancer. Washington, DC: US Department of Health and Human Services, Jan 1986.

28. Basch C. Focus group interview: an underutilized research technique for improving theory and practice in health education. Health Educ Q 1987;14:413-48.

29. National Institutes of Health. Proceedings of the NIH workshop on health behavior research in minority populations. J Ethnicity Dis 1992;2:252-305.

30. Orlandi MA. Defining cultural competence: an organizing framework. In: Orlandi MA, ed. Cultural competence for evaluators: a guide for alcohol and other drug abuse prevention practitioners working with ethnic/racial communities. Rockville, Md: Public Health Service, Office for Substance Abuse Prevention, 1992:293-99.

31. Cross TL, Bazron BJ, Dennis KW, Isaacs MR. Towards a culturally competent system of care: a monograph on effective services for minority children who are severely emotionally disturbed. Vol 1. Bethesda, Md: National Institute of Mental Health, Child and Adolescent Service System Program (CASSP), 1989.

32. Seltzer MM, Ivry J, Litchfield LC. Family members as case managers: partnership between the formal and informal support networks. Gerontologist 1987;27:722-28.

KEY EDUCATIONAL CONSIDERATIONS

1. Develop individual cultural awareness by (1) increasing cognitive knowledge of ethnic groups by reading culturally relevant materials, (2) talking with members of specific ethnic groups to familiarize oneself with beliefs and attitudes specific to the group, and (3) attending multicultural activities to increase knowledge and awareness of diverse cultures.

2. Identify cultural diversity as a goal of any diabetes education program. Work closely with the advisory board to develop an understanding of culturally diverse needs. In addition to the advisory board, identify consultants of diverse ethnicity to assist with the development and evaluation of diabetes education programs.

3. Recruit professional and lay staff from diverse ethnic groups to work as members of the diabetes education team. Conduct frequent and regular in-service training sessions that address ethnic diversity as a theme.

4. Demonstrate a high level of cultural competence in the practice of diabetes education by (1) making cultural assessment a key component of diabetes education assessments, (2) individualizing educational strategies to be pertinent to the patient's ethnic group, (3) assuring appropriate use of educational materials that are culturally relevant, and (4) evaluating diabetes education programs using criteria that incorporate an understanding of the importance of culture to state-of-the-art diabetes care.

SELF-REVIEW QUESTIONS

If you are unsure of the answers to the following questions, please review the materials.

1. Discuss the etiologic factors that influence the prevalence of diabetes in minority groups.

2. Summarize the impact of culture on diabetic patients and their families.
3. Describe the components of a sociocultural assessment that are important to diabetes education.
4. Discuss how culture influences the teaching/learning process in diabetes education.
5. What steps would you take to assure that a diabetes education program is culturally sensitive to minority patients?
6. Discuss strategies of community empowerment and their importance to diabetes education.
7. Summarize the role of the diabetes educator in assuring culturally sensitive diabetes education programs.

CASE EXAMPLE

AS is a 40-year-old black woman recently diagnosed with NIDDM. She was diagnosed during an emergency visit to the community health center for treatment of an acute asthma attack. AS is 64 inches tall and weighs 200 pounds (91 kg). A single parent with six children, she is currently employed as a clerk in a local grocery store. AS's mother and sister live with her in the same home, as do four nieces and nephews. AS's therapeutic regimen for diabetes includes dietary modifications and treatment with oral agents. Blood glucose monitoring has also been recommended. AS has been referred to the diabetes educator for education.

QUESTIONS

1. How will you systematically access the impact of culture on AS's diabetes education needs?
2. How will you tailor educational strategies to be responsive to the sociocultural needs of AS?

SUGGESTED SOLUTIONS

A sociocultural assessment of AS is basic to the development of any diabetes education program. The following assessment uses the framework of the Health Care Assessment Tool of Cultural Patterns of Minority Patients with Diabetes (depicted in Figure XIX.1) to tailor an education program that meets the specific needs of the patient.

Sociocultural Assessment

Individual characteristics: Economic resources may be strained for AS. Moreover, she has expressed the view that diabetes, much like asthma, is a condition that requires only sporadic treatment. Because she is functioning well, AS sees her diabetes as having little impact on her daily living and, therefore, as not requiring excessive financial outlay. AS is very involved with her family, which requires a great deal of her time. Economic resources are limited, and she has no health insurance. Housing is in a low-income neighborhood, with limited access to local community health centers. Cognitive knowledge and expectations about diabetes care suggest minimal understanding of diabetes or its potential severity.

Characteristics of the social group: Within her family unit, AS is a major care provider to her elderly mother as well as to her nieces and nephews. In turn, the adult members of the family are sources of emotional and financial support to AS. However, the experience of these members is that everyone in the family has "a touch of sugar" and that this should not present any major difficulties.

Characteristics of the subculture: Patterns of treatment seeking and use of available diabetes resources of the subculture within which AS resides suggest that the norm is to seek care only for acute conditions because of a basic distrust and dissatisfaction with health care provided by medical personnel. The locus of responsibility for diabetes care decisions is seen as the individual, with the family having great influence.

Characteristics of the society: A societal characteristic relevant to AS's diabetes care is the inaccessibility of routine health care because of inadequate access and unaffordability. AS resides in a low-income area with a high unemployment rate, high crime rates, and minimal access to transportation. Low occupational and educational status is common within AS's community.

Diabetes Education Priorities

Establishing a trusting relationship: A relationship of trust needs to be established between the diabetes educator, the health care team, and AS.

Distrust of the formal health care system could limit the time available for diabetes education. The need to spend time developing a trusting relationship is critical to being able to facilitate follow-up visits for AS in which comprehensive diabetes education can be delivered.

Encouraging routine visits: The behavior change required to effectively manage NIDDM takes much effort. Initial education should focus on basic diabetes information. Routine visits should be encouraged and support for behavior change consistently provided by the educator. Visits should be timed to most conveniently fit AS's schedule. Frequent contact through follow-up telephone calls, mailed information, or home visits is recommended so that AS's questions can be answered. Giving AS individual attention during visits is crucial to encouraging her continued involvement in the treatment program; it is also necessary for developing an educational assessment sensitive to the needs of the patient. The educator also needs to work with members of the health care team, such as social workers, to find adequate means of financially supporting routine diabetes care visits.

Involvement of the family: The involvement of the family is critical in diabetes care. The family can influence the extent to which AS manages her therapeutic regimen by providing instrumental support (eg, accepting dietary changes) as well as social support (eg, baby-sitting for AS's children so she can attend diabetes education appointments). The diabetes educator should teach AS that her role as primary caregiver can be used to encourage family members to engage in preventive health behaviors, which may be one way to involve the family in diabetes care. Incorporating family members in appointments whenever possible and encouraging healthy behavior by the entire family unit are strategies for involving the family in AS's diabetes education.

Identification and use of neighborhood community resources: AS's lack of access to educational information is likely. Programs offered through agencies and groups located in close proximity to AS need to be identified. Programs developed through churches, social service agencies, and local diabetes associations should be explored and identified by the educator. AS should be consistently notified about such programs and encouraged to attend.

OTHER SUGGESTED READINGS

Barr P, ed. Diabetes educational resources for minority and low literacy populations. Southfield, Mich: Coalition for Diabetes Education and Minority Health, 1991.

Bracht N, Kingsbury L. Community organization principles in health promotion. In: Bracht N, ed. Health promotion at the community level. Newbury Park, Calif: Sage, 1990:66-88.

Cottrell LS Jr. The competent community. In: Warren R, ed. New perspectives on the American community. Chicago: Rand McNally, 1977:535-45.

Fisher EB Jr. A skeptical perspective: the importance of behavior and environment. In: Holroyd KA, Creer TL, eds. Self-management of chronic disease: recent developments in health psychology and behavioral medicine. New York: Academic Press, 1986.

Gohdes DM. Diabetes in American Indians: a growing problem. Diabetes Care 1986;9:609-13.

Fruedenberg N. Shaping the future of health education: from behavior change to social change. Health Educ Monogr 1978;6:373-77.

US Department of Health and Human Services. Health behavior research in minority populations: access, design, and implementation. Bethesda, Md.: National Institutes of Health, 1992; DHHS publication no. (NIH)92-2965.

Jeffery RW. Population perspectives on the prevention and treatment of obesity in minority populations. Am J Clin Nutr 1991;53:1621S-24S.

Kumanyika SK, Obarzanek E, Stevens VJ, Hebert PR, Whelton PK. Weight-loss experience of black and white participants in NHLBI-sponsored clinical trials. Am J Clin Nutr 1991;53:1631S-38S.

Leininger M. Leininger's acculturation health care assessment tool for cultural patterns in traditional and non-traditional lifeways. J Transcult Nurs 1991;2(2):40-42.

Lieberman LS. Diabetes and obesity in elderly black Americans. In: Jackson JJ, ed. The black American elderly. New York: Springer Publishing 1989: 150-89.

Lyles M, Carter J. Myths and strengths of the black family: a historical and sociological contribution to family therapy. J Natl Med Assoc 1982;74:1119-23.

McKnight JL. Health and empowerment. Can J Public Health 1985;76:37-38.

Minkler M. Health education, health promotion and the open society: an historical perspective. Health Educ Q 1989;16(1):17-30.

Pi-Sunyer FX. Health implications of obesity. Am J Clin Nutr 1991;53:1595S-1603S.

Rothman J. Three models of community organization practice. In: Cox FM, Erlich JL, Rothman J, Tropman JE, eds. Strategies of community organizations. Itasca, Ill: Peacock, 1970:20-36.

Ruderman N, Apelian AZ, Schneider SH. Exercise in therapy and prevention of type II diabetes: implications for blacks. Diabetes Care 1990;13:1163-68.

Sievers ML, Fisher JR. Diabetes in North American Indians. In: Harris MI, Hamman RF, eds. Diabetes in America. Washington, DC: US Department of Health and Human Services, 1985:chap 11.

Sobal J, Stunkard AJ. Socioeconomic status and obesity: a review of the literature. Psychol Bull 1989;105:260-75.

Strain L. Use of health services in later life: the influence of health beliefs. Soc Sci 1991;46(3):S143-50.

Williamson DF, Kahn HS, Remington PL, Anda RF. The 10-year incidence of overweight and major weight gain in US adults. Arch Intern Med 1990;150:665-72.

SPECIAL POPULATIONS

XX.   ADAPTIVE DIABETES EDUCATION
FOR VISUALLY IMPAIRED PERSONS

INTRODUCTION

Diabetes educators interact with patients who must cope with a variety of physical challenges, including visual impairment. Some patient's visual impairment may be secondary to diabetic retinopathy, while others may have eye disorders unrelated to diabetes.

This chapter outlines the fundamental information and skills required for working with visually impaired patients with diabetes.

OBJECTIVES

Upon completion of this chapter, the learner will be able to:

- describe visual acuity and the visual field;
- state the U.S. government's legal definition of blindness;
- recognize the role of the diabetes educator to direct the visually impaired patient to the appropriate resources and/or rehabilitative services;
- describe the benefits of low vision services;
- describe three ways to adapt diabetes self-management skills for the visually impaired patient.

A. Definitions of Vision

1. Ophthalmologists employ a wide range of diagnostic modalities to describe vision. Two of the many descriptions of vision include central visual function and peripheral visual function.

    a) Central visual function can be studied, determined, and noted in many different ways. The acuity (or sharpness) of central visual function is most commonly expressed by the Snellen's fraction, which is measured by reading a Snellen's chart. The Snellen's fraction is defined as[1]:

$$\textit{Visual acuity} = \frac{\textit{distance at which the letter is read}}{\textit{distance at which it should normally be read.}}$$

Using the Snellen's chart, a person who can read letters designed to be read at 20 feet while being tested at 20 feet is said to have 20/20 visual acuity. A person who can read letters to be read at 40 feet while being tested at 20 feet is said to have 20/40 visual acuity.

b) Peripheral visual function can be determined by measuring the visual field. The visual field is usually considered to be all that is visible to one (monocular) or both (binocular) eye(s) at a given time. Traquair developed the "island of vision" analogy in which he described the visual field as an "island of vision in a sea of blindness."[2] Visual field testing results in a map of the island of vision as it exists for the patient at the time of testing. The normal visual field covers 180 degrees. A patient who has had panretinal photocoagulation and whose visual field is less than 20 degrees may misplace objects because it is difficult to scan and build a visual montage.

2. Father Thomas Carroll, a leader in visual rehabilitation in the United States, once noted that "more people are blinded by definition than by any other cause."[3] There is little national or international agreement on what visual status constitutes blindness. The categories of visual loss can be broadly divided into severe visual impairment and low vision.

a) Severe visual impairment can describe levels of visual functioning that include total visual impairment (ie, no light perception) and near total visual impairment (visual acuity of ≤20/1000 with correction or a visual field of ≤5 degrees).[4]

b) Low vision can describe a level of visual functioning that prevents a person with standard or conventional optical corrections from performing customary visual activities. Moderate low vision can include visual acuity of from 20/70 to 20/160 with correction; severe low vision (US government definition of legal blindness) can include 20/200 to 20/400 with correction or a visual field ≤20 degrees; and profound low vision can include a visual acuity of from 20/500 to 20/1000 with correction.[4]

c) Part of the confusion between the terms *blindness* and *visual impairment* stems from the "legal" definition of blindness developed by the U.S. federal government in the 1930s to classify people eligible for benefits.[5] Some "legally blind" patients can have significant useful vision or vision that can be substantially improved with devices that enhance visual performance. The American Foundation for the Blind suggests that the term *blind* be reserved for people with no usable sight at all, and the terms *visually impaired, low vision,* or *partially sighted* be used for people with some usable vision.[5] In common usage, however, the term *visually impaired* may include both totally blind and partially sighted individuals.

d) Because of the wide range of vision loss, the needs of visually impaired patients will differ and may change over time.

B. Resources and Rehabilitation

1. Diabetes educators are in a key position to direct visually impaired patients toward the resources they require, including rehabilitation, low vision services, and diabetes-specific services.

a) When vision is lost or severely diminished, routine tasks can cause the greatest frustration. Learning to pour a cup of coffee without overflowing can provide a patient with the initial self-confidence needed to take on larger tasks. Rehabilitation is essential for relearning activities of daily living such as safe mobility, household tasks, communication skills, vocational guidance, and education. In addition, rehabilitation counseling can help the patient cope with the impact of visual loss on self-image and relationships. The vocational rehabilitation agency that specializes in services for the blind and visually handicapped can direct the diabetes educator to local agencies.

b) To help a patient use remaining vision more efficiently, low vision services have been designed. Many visually impaired patients buy dime store magnifiers and are frustrated because the object or print may appear larger but not clearer. Low vision services begin with a comprehensive assessment of the patient's experience, attitude, and adjustment to vision loss. A detailed visual examination focuses on function. Acuity is tested binocularly, using the modified charts developed by the Early Treatment Diabetic Retinopathy Study (ETDRS). These charts provide simple, accurate, reproducible, determinations of visual acuity.[6] Also, patients tested with the ETDRS charts express a more positive sense of accomplishment because they see many lines of letters rather than just the "big E." The exam is followed by the prescription of low vision devices (optical lenses) and visual aids (lighting, reading stands, large print, etc).[6] The patient receives training in use of the aids and devices and is reevaluated when necessary.

c) Some diabetes educators specialize in the care and education of visually impaired patients. A list of these specialists is found in the American Association of Diabetes Educators' Membership Directory.

C. Psychosocial Aspects of Diabetes and Vision Loss

1. Visually impaired people with diabetes often report that the two conditions in combination create frustration and stressful life situations.[7] The limitations of visual loss coupled with the fear of other diabetes related complications contribute to anxiety, depression, and a sense of uncertainty about the future.

2. The diabetes educator can provide support and counseling to the visually impaired patient at any point in the patient's life. Possible strategies include active listening; recognition of both

healthy and adverse coping patterns; referral for counseling and/or rehabilitation; and participation in a support group; and education.

D. Adaptive Diabetes Education for the Visually Impaired Person

1. The goals for diabetes education do not differ for visually impaired patients, ie, they remain mutually defined and based on assessment.

2. The difference in working with those who have visual impairment lies in adapting the educational content and the delivery of the content to the special needs of the visually impaired patient.

   a) Insulin measurement

   (1) There are a variety of adaptive devices designed for accurate nonvisual measurement of insulin,[8] plus needle guides to direct the needle into the rubber stopper, and clip-on magnifiers that enlarge the numbers on the syringe. With any device that allows a dose to be drawn up to a preselected setting or measurement, the setting should be checked periodically by a sighted person.

   (2) To remove air bubbles from the syringe when filling the syringe with one type of insulin, patients are taught to pull insulin into the syringe and push it back into the insulin vial at least three times. When mixing insulins, patients are instructed to follow this procedure with the first insulin; with the second insulin, patients are taught to pull back on the plunger very slowly to avoid air bubbles.

   (3) To ensure that enough insulin is in the vial at all times, several approaches can be used. One method is to calculate how many days a vial of insulin will last and devise a way to avoid using the last 50 units of insulin in the vial. For example, if the patient takes a total of 60 units each day from a 1,000-unit

Lente vial, one vial of Lente would last 15 days (divide 950 by 60). The patient could count out the number of syringes used in 15 days and keep them in a separate place. When the last syringe is used, the patient knows to open a new vial of insulin and repeat the procedure. Patients should also be encouraged to come up with creative solutions of their own.

    (4) To avoid confusing bottles when mixing insulins, the patient can use identifying textures or color codes if applicable. Some pharmacies will mark insulin vials in Braille for Braille readers.

  b) Insulin injection

    (1) Visually impaired patients can be taught to inject themselves with insulin by using automatic needle injectors, pen injectors, needle-free jet injectors, or a conventional syringe. When using the conventional syringe without an assistive device, the visually impaired patient is taught to choose the site, pinch the skin, gently place the needle above the skin, and insert the needle into the skin. This method eliminates the usual dartlike motion so that the patient can control where the needle is injected.

    (2) Injection sites are chosen by creating a map of the area to be injected. For example, the map of the abdomen can be charted by starting from the umbilicus. One finger breadth to the right of the umbilicus under the belt line is the first injection site; two finger breadths from the umbilicus is the second injection site; and so forth. When creating the map of injection sites, a sighted person can alert the visually impaired person to varicosities, scar tissue, or other areas to be avoided. As with every patient who injects insulin, injection sites should be assessed by the educator at every opportunity.

    (3) Some of the injection devices available for purchase are not designed for use by visually impaired

persons. The needs of each patient will differ and should be continually reassessed. Some visually impaired patients are able to inject themselves but are unable to fill the syringe because of multiple health problems. Guidelines for prefilling the conventional syringe are found in Chapter VIII: Pharmacologic Therapies.

c) Blood glucose monitoring

(1) Many people with diabetes have fluctuating vision and benefit from using conventional blood glucose meters that are easily adapted with a speech module.[8] The speech module not only announces blood glucose results but annunciates the timing sequence, battery status, and other displayed messages.

(2) Assessment of the visually impaired patient's skill at using a blood glucose meter should include the following evaluations.

(a) Can the patient obtain an adequate blood sample? To obtain an adequate blood sample:

- Wash hands with soap and warm water.
- Lower arm to side to allow blood to flow to fingertips.
- Squeeze tip of finger to be used to concentrate blood at the puncture site.

(b) How does the patient know if an adequate sample has been obtained? The patient can determine wetness by touching the puncture site with another finger. To obtain an adequate sample:

- Squeeze "three" times to obtain a drop of blood (the number of squeezes will vary, depending upon the reagent used and blood flow).
- Use the Accu-Drop® device.

(c) Can the patient locate the correct area to place the blood on the reagent strip? To apply blood to the strip, the patient can use a variety of techniques:

- Place two fingers on either side of the reagent pad, then place the finger with the drop of blood between the two fingers, which will act as a guide.
- Place a finger below the reagent strip as a guide and put the finger with the blood drop above the first finger.[9]

(d) If blotting or wiping is required, can the patient remove all the blood in the allotted time? The following techniques can be used to completely remove all blood:

- When wiping, position the tissue or cotton near the fingers holding the strip and wipe the entire strip.
- When blotting, hold the reagent strip with one hand and position the other hand on the corner of the tissue used for blotting.
- The patient can periodically mail used strips to the educator for verification of technique.

(e) What system does the patient employ to ensure that the meter is clean? The speech module of certain meters can "tell" the user that the meter needs cleaning.

(f) How does the patient check the expiration date of the strips? The pharmacist can mark the vial of strips according to the patient's preference.

(g) What is the patient's system for using the control solution? Using methods similar to that for positioning blood on the reagent strip, the visually impaired patient can position the tip of the control solution above the pad of the reagent strip.

(3) Following assessment, the educator and patient may conclude that a different blood glucose meter may be better suited to the patient's needs.

d) Foot care

(1) Proper foot care for the visually impaired patient with diabetes is imperative because of the increased potential for injury and the possible inability to recognize the early signs of infection. Patients with significant renal changes must consider the additional risk factor of pedal edema. In addition to podiatric care, the visually impaired patient needs to learn a nonvisual method of foot inspection.

(2) Nonvisual foot inspection is a systematic method of feeling the outer surface of the foot. The patient is taught to divide the foot into three sections: rear, middle, and forefoot. The foot is then carefully inspected as follows:

(a) Beginning with the rear foot, move the hand slowly around the heel to feel for warmth, blisters, abrasions, or rough areas. A warm area may indicate inflammation.

(b) Then move up to the outside of the foot to the fifth toe (forefoot). Place the fingers on the bottom of the foot at the end of all the toes and slowly feel underneath the toes for openings, rough areas, or warm areas.

(c) A similar search is continued through the arch, the heel, and up the Achilles tendon to the area just above the ankle joint.

(d) Move the hand to the top of the foot and slowly move down to the ends of the toes.

(e) To check the toes, place a finger in the first space between the first and second toe. Start where the edge of the toenail begins. Squeeze each toenail. Move the finger down the inside surface of the first toe and back up the second toe. Continue the same procedure with all the toes feeling for warm areas, openings, pain and discomfort, and/or rough dry skin.[10]

  (3) Some patients are unable to reach their feet or they have neuropathic changes in their hands that affect their sense of touch. These patients require the assistance of a sighted person to visually inspect their feet. All patients are taught to feel the inside of shoes for any objects or potential irritants.

  (4) Visually impaired patients with diabetes should not cut their toenails because of the increased risk of self-inflicted injury. Regular podiatric visits are recommended.

 e) Other diabetes-related self-care activities

  (1) Adaptive devices are available to facilitate food preparation and measurement, including tactile and talking scales, timers, clocks, and adaptive kitchen utensils. Patients, with or without visual impairment, who reside alone require a nutrition assessment concerning portion sizes of foods, balancing of meals, timing of meals, and storing foods.

  (2) To assist with diabetes self-care activities, patients can be provided with large-block color comparison charts for ketone urine testing, talking weight scales, talking sphygmomanometers, talking thermometers, and devices to organize medications and facilitate the instillation of eye drops.

 f) Exercise

  (1) Exercise recommendations and precautions vary depending upon the degree of vision loss. Visual impairment alone does not prevent a patient from participating in exercise if adaptations can be made. For example, using "beeperballs" to play baseball and golf facilitates participation in these sports. People who have usable remaining vision may need to take precautions to protect their vision. The rise in systolic blood pressure that normally accompanies exercise can aggravate proliferative retinopathy by causing

pressure against weakened capillaries in the retina of patients with diabetes.[11] Patients with proliferative retinopathy or evidence of renal-retinal syndrome will require careful blood pressure monitoring and guidance from an exercise physiologist.

(2) Cardiovascular endurance may be lowered in newly visually impaired persons because of the loss of independent mobility.[12] After the patient has undergone rehabilitation, independent mobility is regained. Endurance exercise can be prescribed on the basis of a physical assessment and exercise test.

(3) There is no clear evidence that intensive physical training programs accelerate the progression of diabetic retinopathy. Resistive exercises using standard weight lifting equipment are generally not recommended (see Chapter VII: Exercise). Certain types of exercises that increase systolic blood pressure with a concomitant increase in intraocular pressure are contraindicated[12] (see Table XX.1).

TABLE XX.1: Exercise Precautions with Diabetic Retinopathy

Avoid activities that involve:

- Bending over so that the head is positioned lower than the waist.
- Valsalva type maneuvers that raise blood pressure.
- Near maximal isometric contractions.
- Vigorous bouncing (eg, high impact aerobics).
- Rapid eye-head movements (eg, contact sports or jogging).
- Extremely vigorous activity (eg, parachuting, scuba diving).

Source: Adapted with permission from Graham, Lasko-McCarthey.[12]

In educating the visually impaired patient with diabetes, the diabetes educator is challenged to use diverse skills. The diabetes educator can interpret the meaning of mysterious words, increase awareness among health professionals and industry regarding the needs of the visually impaired patient, and/or direct highly individualized diabetes education using adaptive devices. Diabetes educators continue to direct visually impaired patients to the best possible resources.

REFERENCES

1. Collins JF. Ophthalmic desk reference. New York: Raven Press, 1991:615.

2. Choplin NT. Visual field testing. In: Collins JF, ed. Ophthalmic desk reference. New York: Raven Press, 1991:617.

3. Colenbrander A. Dimensions of visual performance. Trans Am Acad Ophthalmol Otolaryngol 1977;83:332.

4. Simons K. Visual acuity and the functional definition of blindness. In: Tasman W, Jaeger EA, eds. Duane's clinical ophthalmology. Philadelphia: Lippincott, 1991;5:1-21.

5. American Foundation for the Blind. Low vision questions and answers: definitions, devices, services. New York: American Foundation for the Blind, 1987.

6. Faye EE. Low vision. In: Tasman W, Jaeger EA, eds. Duane's clinical ophthalmology. Philadelphia: Lippincott, 1991;1:1-14.

7. Caditz J. Diabetes, visual impairment, and group support: a guidebook. Santa Monica, Calif: Center for the Partially Sighted, 1988:15.

8. Petzinger RA. Diabetes aids and products for people with visual or physical impairment. Diabetes Educ 1992;18:121-38.

9. Carr RB. Blood glucose testing for the visually impaired. Diabetes Self-Manage 1986;(Summer):34-35.

10. Medford HH. Podolan daily foot care. Marysville, Calif: Podoclinic Lab, 1981:1-20.

11. Greenlee G. Exercise options for patients with retinopathy and peripheral vascular disease. Practical Diabetol 1987;6(4):9-11.

12. Graham C, Lasko-McCarthey P. Exercise options for persons with diabetic complications. Diabetes Educ 1990;16:212-20.

13. Herget MJ, Williams AS. New aids for low vision diabetics. Am J Nurs 1989;89:1319-22.

KEY EDUCATIONAL CONSIDERATIONS

1. Large print is not the only consideration when making or suggesting visual aids for patients with low vision. Enhance contrast by using bold black markers on wide-lined paper and help the patient to identify what kind of lighting is most helpful.

2. When teaching patients with total or near total visual impairment, the diabetes educator cannot use visual charts, pictures, or videotapes. Instead, try to create a mental picture using analogy, familiar objects, etc. Tactile charts can be made using raised T-shirt paint. Plastic food models can be used for teaching portion sizes. Audiotapes can be made or borrowed from the Talking Books program.

3. When teaching visually impaired patients to use a blood glucose meter or an adaptive device, organize the parts by referring to the numbers on a clockface. For example, when teaching the use of a meter, you can place the strips at 2 o'clock, the meter at 6 o'clock, the lancing device at 11 o'clock, and so forth.

4. When teaching meter use, use expired reagent strips so the visually impaired patient can practice placing the blood on the strip without wasting usable strips.

5. Let the visually impaired patient explore an adaptive aid with his or her hands before instruction. Then name the device and describe its parts and their location. Always use the same name each time you refer to a specific part. Slowly talk the patient through the entire procedure for using the device. If the process involves more than five steps, break the steps down into easy-to-remember chunks of five or fewer steps.[13]

6. Do not assume that a visually impaired person will find Braille markings useful.[13]

7. Audiotapes share a role similar to that of brochures, ie, they provide reinforcement. There is no substitute for the exchange between educator and patient.

8. Many people who have visual impairment from diabetes need an update of newer aspects of diabetes management such as syringe disposal. As with all diabetic patients, a continuing assessment of learning needs is necessary.

SELF-REVIEW QUESTIONS

If you are unsure of the answers to the following questions, please review the materials.

1. What type of vision does the Snellen's fraction describe?
2. How can a visual defect interfere with performing blood glucose monitoring?
3. What is the U.S. government's legal definition of blindness?
4. Why do visually impaired patients require reassessment of their diabetes-related skills?
5. What can a patient expect from "low vision services"?
6. Describe three strategies to assist the visually impaired person who is struggling with the demands of diabetes and visual loss.
7. Describe one technique for insulin injection used by visually impaired patients.
8. List three specific concerns when evaluating a visually impaired patient's technique in using a blood glucose meter.
9. Describe the steps in a nonvisual foot inspection.
10. What is the relationship between the rise in blood pressure during exercise and proliferative retinopathy?

CASE EXAMPLE 1

BE arrived by ambulance and was admitted to the emergency department at 10 AM. She was unconscious and her blood glucose level was 42 mg/dL (2.3 mmol/L) after an intravenous bolus of 50% dextrose was administered. At 2 PM, the diabetes educator is called for consultation. BE is alert but groggy. Her blood glucose level is 313 mg/dL (17.4 mmol/L). BE tells the diabetes educator that her fasting blood glucose level was 138 mg/dL (7.7 mmol/L) and that her usual dose of insulin is 40 units of NPH and 5 units of regular. BE, who is legally blind, realizes that in her haste she did not use her magnifier and relied on her vision to see the large N and R on the insulin vials. BE is convinced that she injected 40 units of regular insulin and 5 units of NPH. BE keeps repeating, "What would have happened if my husband wasn't home today?"

QUESTIONS

1. What would be the educational goal for BE while she is in the emergency department?
2. What other measures could be employed to insure that this error does not occur again?

SUGGESTED SOLUTIONS

Considering that BE was still not alert enough to participate in learning, the diabetes educator reviewed the discharge instructions with BE's husband and made an appointment to see BE the following day.

BE was more alert and relaxed the next day, but she confided that she insisted on her husband filling the insulin syringe that morning. BE gave detailed examples of how she has coped and adapted to her visual loss. She described her rehabilitation and brought some of her adaptive devices to the diabetes center. The diabetes educator recognized three goals for this one-time teaching session: (1) to restore BE's confidence in her ability to care for herself, (2) to brainstorm with BE regarding ways to prevent this error from happening again, and (3) to teach BE's husband the technique for administering glucagon.

By listening and using affirming statements, the diabetes educator facilitated the first goal. The diabetes educator then outlined goals 2 and 3 for BE and her husband. The diabetes educator explained to BE that many people have made a similar error. One common technique for identifying the correct vial is to put a rubber band around the regular insulin (R for rubber and regular) so that the magnified visual clue is reinforced by a tactile reminder. The diabetes educator and BE discussed other methods to clearly distinguish the insulins. BE decided that she liked the rubber band suggestion the best.

After a review of all the positive, helpful steps BE's husband took in treating BE's severe hypoglycemia, the diabetes educator taught BE's husband how and when to administer glucagon. BE's husband gave an accurate return demonstration, and he took a brochure about glucagon for reinforcement. The diabetes educator wrote a note in large print with a black felt tip pen to remind BE to have the glucagon prescription filled.

CASE EXAMPLE 2

VT is 68 years old and has been participating in the local diabetes clinic more than 7 years. Five years ago, in a hallway conference, the nurse, dietitian, and physician discussed how VT's vision had deteriorated. VT was referred to the ophthalmology clinic. The dietitian discussed some safe cooking suggestions with VT, and the nurse gently questioned VT about her insulin administration procedure. VT loved the cooking ideas but was not interested in any help with insulin administration. The nurse told VT about an array of useful gadgets to help her continue to administer an accurate dose of insulin. VT said that she'd been giving herself insulin for years now and did not need any help.

This week the nurse received a call from VT requesting information about "those insulin gadgets." "Are they expensive?" she asked. "I think I need one."

QUESTIONS

1. What does VT teach us about readiness to learn?

SUGGESTED SOLUTIONS

The diabetes team offered information to VT based on her readiness to learn. She wanted the cooking information immediately but was not open to information about the insulin devices. However, the nurse "planted the seed," and 5 years later the seed bore fruit: VT requested information.

When VT was ready for assistance and before a serious error occurred, the nurse referred VT to a local diabetes educator who specialized in working with visually impaired patients.

OTHER SUGGESTED READINGS

Barnow DH. Preparing injections: a guide for the visually impaired. Diabetes Self-Manage 1986;(Jul/Aug):30-31.

Bernbaum M, Albert SG, Brusca SR, Drimmer A, Duckro PN. Promoting diabetes self-management and independence in the visually impaired: a model clinical program. Diabetes Educ 1988;14:51-54.

Bernbaum M, Eachus G. Cooking tips for the visually impaired. Diabetes Self-Manage 1987;(Mar/Apr):38-41.

Caditz, J. Diabetes, visual impairment and group support: a guidebook. Santa Monica, Calif: Center for the Partially Sighted, 1988.

Carr RB. Blood glucose testing for the visually impaired. Diabetes Self-Manage 1986;(Summer):34-35.

Cleary ME. Aiding the person who is visually impaired from diabetes. Diabetes Educ 1985;10:12-23.

Cleary ME, Fahy C. Lighting a lamp for persons who are visually impaired. Diabetes Educ 1989;15:331-41.

Freeman PB. Finding help for a visual impairment. Diabetes Forecast 1992;(Sept):77-82.

Hoover J. The national task force on diabetes and blindness. Diabetes Educ 1988;10:27.

National Task Force on Diabetes and Vision Impairment. Help for visually impaired [Commentary]. Diabetes Educ 1988;14:482-83.

Williams AS. Adaptive diabetes education for visually impaired persons: teaching non-visual self-care. J Home Health Care Practice 1992;4:62-71.

Williams AS. Foot care for the visually impaired. Diabetes Self-Manage 1992;(Nov/Dec):46-47.

Complications

INTRODUCTION

Each chapter in this section discusses one of the long term complications of diabetes, allowing readers to focus on them individually. In reality, chronic complications usually coexist, resulting in complex management issues for patients, families, and providers. The patient with complications frequently reports: feeling betrayed by past and present providers, "nobody ever told me this could happen"; receiving confusing, competing or even conflicting advice from numerous health care providers; feeling that his or her body is "falling apart"; having difficulty maintaining the usual roles and responsibilities at home and work; experiencing frustration with the time and expense involved in seeing multiple providers and managing several chronic conditions; and blaming themselves and being blamed by family, friends, and providers for having complications.

Diabetes educators may be able to prevent some of these difficulties in their patients who do not currently have complications by:

- acknowledging gaps in scientific knowledge and limitations of treatment modalities when discussing the rationale for glycemic control and self-management;
- promoting patients' beliefs in their *capabilities* related to self-care, rather than in their total responsibility or control over long-term health;
- using the communication style of a consultant, rather than that of rescuer ("I'm an expert; I'm here to take care of you.") or parent ("These are the rules; you have to follow them, or else...!");
- being respectful and nonjudgmental when discussing regimen adherence;
- assisting patients who feel guilty about some aspect of their diabetes management to use that guilt productively and as an opportunity to reevaluate goals and problem solve.

Diabetes educators may ameliorate some of the issues faced by patients who have complications by:

- giving patients the benefit of the doubt and assuming that they did the best they could, with the resources available to them;
- recognizing and dealing with the almost inevitable feelings of guilt... acknowledging that many patients in similar situations feel guilty and face blame from others too... assisting patients and families to realize

the limitations they were operating under and turn their attention to dealing with the present situation;

- assuring frequent communication among team members so that priorities are clear to all members, especially the patient and family;
- encouraging appointment schedulers to be flexible and facilitate coordination of multiple appointments.

The next five chapters provide details of the pathogenesis, diagnosis, and treatment of chronic complications. The challenge to diabetes educators is to integrate the complications in providing comprehensive care and education to patients.

COMPLICATIONS

XXI.   DIABETIC EYE DISEASE

INTRODUCTION

Diabetes is the leading cause of new cases of blindness and visual loss among adults in the United States.[1] Although diabetic retinopathy is the most significant cause of severe visual loss, other ophthalmic sequelae of diabetes are very common and cause patients much consternation and many problems. Most of the complications are related to duration of diabetes, while others seem to be related to the level of blood glucose control. All patients with diabetes, whether insulin-dependent or non-insulin-dependent, are susceptible to the ophthalmic complications of diabetes. A clear understanding of these complications and treatment options enables diabetes educators to advise patients on prevention, diagnosis, and treatment.

OBJECTIVES

Upon completion of this chapter, the learner will be able to:
- identify patients at risk of developing diabetic retinopathy;
- describe three stages of diabetic retinopathy;
- identify current methods of treatment available for diabetic retinopathy;
- state general recommendations for ophthalmic examination of the patient with diabetes;
- list three other ophthalmic complications besides diabetic retinopathy and discuss specific treatments.

A.   Patients at Risk of Developing Diabetic Retinopathy

1.   Millions of Americans who have diabetes are unaware that diabetes is the leading cause of blindness in the United States among adults. The occurrence of diabetic retinopathy seems to be related, in part, to the duration of the disease. The earliest changes of retinopathy are seen most often after at least 5 years duration of diabetes.

2.   After 15 years duration of diabetes, 80% of all patients have developed at least some background retinopathy.

3. All patients, regardless of type of diabetes or treatment modality, (eg, insulin, diet alone, or oral hypoglycemics) are at risk of developing retinopathy.[2]

4. Patients with poorly controlled hypertension or diabetic nephropathy may have an increased risk of developing retinopathy.

B. **Classification of Diabetic Retinopathy**

1. There are three stages of diabetic retinopathy: nonproliferative, preproliferative, and proliferative.

   a) Over time, diabetes causes changes in the microvasculature of the retina (see Figure XXI.1). The capillaries become damaged and the walls of the vessels become permeable to some of the components of blood. The changes are very common and generally occur without symptoms. This stage is termed *nonproliferative retinopathy*, or *background retinopathy*, and is comprised of some or all of the following features.

      (1) Microaneurysms, or areas of weakness in vessel walls, are an early sign of retinopathy. They appear as tiny red dots in the retina. They are very common and may disappear and reappear.

      (2) Hard exudates can occur when microaneurysms leak large lipid molecules. The lipids are seen as yellowish deposits with distinct margins.

      (3) Intraretinal hemorrhages are another lesion of nonproliferative retinopathy and appear as red smudges in the retina.

   b) The lesions of *preproliferative retinopathy* represent further destruction of retinal capillaries, subsequent retinal ischemia, and development of capillary obstruction. These changes are harbingers of the more severe form of retinopathy, proliferative disease.

      (1) Venous beading is the term used to refer to a change in the appearance of retinal veins. The veins become

FIGURE XXI.1: Normal Eye

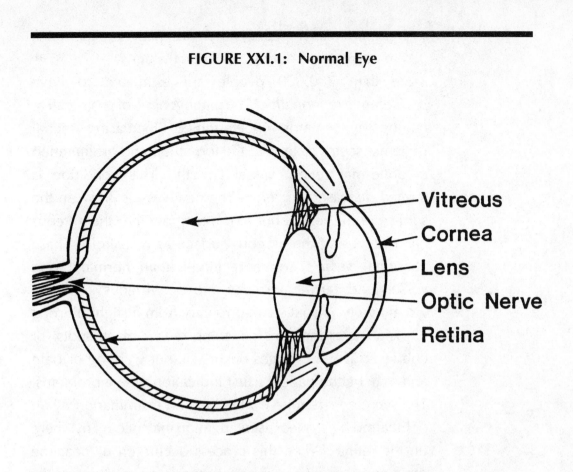

- Vitreous
- Cornea
- Lens
- Optic Nerve
- Retina

Reprinted with permission: Non-insulin-Dependent Diabetes Mellitus: a Curriculum for Patients and Health Professionals, Michigan Diabetes and Training Center, The University of Michigan, 1988.

tortuous and swollen, looping over themselves and taking on the appearance of sausages or a string of beads.

(2) Soft exudates or "cotton wool spots" are the names commonly given to areas of infarction in the nerve fiber layer of the retina. These areas in the retina are whitish and opaque with indistinct borders.

(3) Intraretinal microvascular abnormalities (IRMA) appear to be dilated capillaries or shunt vessels, and often are found near areas of capillary closure. These vessels can leak and contribute to macular edema. There generally is an increase in the size and number of intraretinal hemorrhages in

preproliferative retinopathy. Most patients experience no symptoms during this critical stage.

    c) More than 700,000 people are estimated to have *proliferative retinopathy.*[3] The pathogenesis of proliferative retinopathy remains undetermined. Increasing retinal ischemia seems to lead to the formation and proliferation of abnormal retinal vessel growth.[4] This condition is termed *neovascularization.* The new vessels grow on the surface of the retina, but also may grow into the vitreous chamber, using the vitreous surface as a scaffold. These abnormal vessels are more fragile than normal blood vessels and can hemorrhage into the vitreous, reducing visual acuity. Visual symptoms vary from a slight blurring of vision to complaints of seeing red or black spots, or cobwebs. These changes occur without warning or pain and may be the patient's first indication of eye problems. The symptoms require evaluation and examination by an ophthalmologist. Neovascularization may occur anywhere on the retina. When this process occurs on or near the optic nerve or disc, it is called *neovascularization of the disk (NVD).* A higher risk of visual loss is associated with NVD than with *neovascularization (NVE),* which occurs *elsewhere* in the retina.

2. Results of the Diabetic Retinopathy Study (DRS),[5] defined treatment of diabetic retinopathy by identifying high-risk characteristics in patients with proliferative disease who had a high risk for severe visual loss.

    a) Among these characteristics were moderate or greater NVD, or the combination of vitreous or preretinal hemorrhage with smaller NVD.

    b) Vitreous hemorrhage, the development of fibrous proliferation, retinal detachment (a separation of the retina from the choroid as the result of a hole or tear), and severe visual loss were likely outcomes of untreated, high-risk characteristics.

C. Macular Edema

1. The development of macular edema is a significant consequence of damage to retinal blood vessels. Macular edema is an important cause of moderate visual loss (a doubling of the visual angle in which 20/40 vision is reduced to 20/80) in the diabetic population, and can coexist with any of the stages of retinopathy. As many as 500,000 Americans are estimated to have this complication.

2. The *macula* is the area of the retina responsible for central vision. The macula is about the size of the head of a pin. When microaneurysms leak fluid and large lipoproteins into or near the macular area, central visual acuity may be affected. Symptoms may range from mild central blurring to 20/200 vision (legal blindness), or even worse vision.

3. Edema involving or directly threatening the center of the macula is considered to be clinically significant. This condition is best diagnosed and managed by a retinal specialist.

D. Methods of Treatment

1. The treatment of nonproliferative and preproliferative retinopathy involves blood glucose and blood pressure control plus follow up by an ophthalmologist.

2. Photocoagulation is used in the treatment of proliferative retinopathy in conjunction with blood glucose and blood pressure control.

   a) The Early Treatment Diabetic Retinopathy Study (ETDRS)[6] demonstrated that macular edema may be treated and vision stabilized with argon laser photocoagulation applied focally (eg, "spot-welding" the leaking microaneurysms). The ETDRS defined clinically significant macular edema as a stage of edema that should be strongly considered for treatment. Fluorescein angiography is an important tool in the diagnosis and treatment of macular edema because it enables identification of the leaking microaneurysms that contribute to the edema.

b) Patients who will be receiving laser treatment for macular edema should be informed that multiple treatments may be necessary and that maintaining follow-up is critical to a successful outcome. An important component of follow-up is appropriate referral to low vision services as needed.

c) The DRS[5] demonstrated that pan-retinal photocoagulation (laser treatment) is an effective treatment for patients with proliferative retinopathy and high-risk characteristics. Pan-retinal photocoagulation is the treatment of choice for patients with high-risk eyes. Initially, 1200 to 1600 burns are applied throughout the periphery of the retina in a scatter pattern, sparing the macular area. Additional photocoagulation may be required depending upon the efficacy of the initial treatment.

d) Side effects of laser treatment vary according to the type of treatment and the total amount of treatment required.

(1) About 10% of patients who are treated with pan-retinal photocoagulation experience a loss of about a line of vision, (from 20/20 to 20/25). Additionally, there may be a decrease in peripheral vision, as well as increased difficulty with dark adaptation, posing a significant problem for patients who must drive at night.

(2) Although the treatment itself usually is relatively painless, many patients find it tedious and very tiring. During treatment, the patient sees a bright, colored light flashing hundreds of times. Anxiety levels may be very high, especially before the initial treatment. Some areas of the retina are relatively sensitive and patients may find treatment in these areas somewhat uncomfortable. Most patients require nothing more than anesthetic drops, although an anesthetic injection may be given near the eye if needed.

(3) Treatment usually is done on an outpatient basis, and most patients can resume normal activities the next day. Some patients may have activity restrictions (generally with regard to weight lifting), but these recommendations are made on an individual basis.

3. Intraocular Intervention/Vitrectomy

   a) Some vitreous hemorrhages will clear on their own over time. Patients may be encouraged to sleep with the head of the bed elevated to help the hemorrhage to settle. However, when a hemorrhage does not clear after 6 or more months, or when there is a retinal detachment or risk of one, vitrectomy may be considered. An ultrasound examination can aid in determining whether a retinal detachment exists in an eye with a dense vitreous hemorrhage.

   b) Vitrectomy can aid in restoring vision in eyes that have suffered vitreous hemorrhage. Because the potential benefit must outweigh the risks involved, this procedure generally is reserved for eyes with poor vision. The surgery involves an intricate intraocular procedure to remove the hemorrhage, the vitreous, and any fibrous proliferation that may exist. Results are best when the initial surgery is successful and repeat surgeries are not necessary. This surgery is best performed by an experienced vitreo-retinal surgeon.

E. Psychosocial Issues

1. Including a social worker in the team often is beneficial as patients struggle to adapt to changes in vision and the difficulties posed by fluctuating vision. Some patients hesitate to use adaptive devices and/or continue to drive long after vision is significantly compromised. Referral to a social worker also should be made for patients with insurance or financial problems that may interfere with appropriate care.

2. The patient should be questioned carefully about activities of daily living in relation to current visual acuity. Quality of life can be enhanced greatly by a timely referral to a low vision center where there are many helpful services available for patients who have some early vision loss (see Chapter XX: Adaptive Diabetes Education for Visually Impaired Persons).

F. Recommendations for Ophthalmologic Examination

1. Because the onset of non-insulin-dependent diabetes mellitus (NIDDM), also called type II diabetes, is difficult to determine and duration is unclear, patients with NIDDM should have an ophthalmologic examination at the time of diagnosis. Persons with insulin-dependent diabetes mellitus (IDDM), also called type I diabetes, usually are seen after 5 years of duration of diabetes, but often prefer, for peace of mind, to be examined at the time of diagnosis. This approach is reasonable because many patients have fluctuations in vision at the time of initial diagnosis and treatment.

2. The ophthalmological examination schedule is best determined by the needs of the individual. However, the following is a recommended approach to this process.[7]

   a) *All patients should have a dilated fundus exam at least once per year.* This examination should include a slit lamp exam, gonioscopy (visualization of the angle of the anterior chamber to look for abnormal iris vessels), and intraocular pressure check, as well as a careful retinal exam. Fundus photography often is used to document retinal status. These photographs enable the examiner to compare retinal changes on future exams and to assess the progress of retinopathy. Fluorescein angiography may be utilized to assess the patency of the retinal vessels and to find areas of leakage that may be contributing to macular edema. Treatable lesions also may be identified.

   b) Patients without retinopathy and those with minimal background changes should be examined yearly.

c) Patients with moderate nonproliferative retinopathy or macular edema should be seen at 4- to 6-month intervals.

d) Patients with clinically significant macular edema or preproliferative retinopathy should be seen at 3- to 4-month intervals.

e) Individuals with proliferative retinopathy, but without high-risk characteristics, should be seen at 2- to 3-month intervals.

f) Laser treatment is indicated for individuals with high-risk proliferative retinopathy. These patients should be followed every 3 to 4 months after the initial treatment is completed.

g) Patients with high-risk retinopathy that is not amenable to laser treatment should be followed at 1- to 6-month intervals as indicated by the patient's condition. This schedule would include patients with dense vitreous hemorrhages waiting to clear.

h) Various concurrent medical conditions, such as pregnancy, hypertension, and renal disease, may adversely affect retinopathy and may alter the timing of laser treatment and follow-up care.

G. Other Ophthalmic Complications of Diabetes

1. *Glaucoma* is defined as an elevated intraocular pressure that has damaged the optic nerve and caused visual field loss. Normal intraocular pressure ranges from 10 to 21 mm Hg. About 5% of people with diabetes have glaucoma, compared with 2% of the nondiabetic population.

a) *Open angle glaucoma* is the most common form of glaucoma seen in people with diabetes. Aqueous humor is a fluid that normally flows out of Schlemm's canal at the angle of the anterior chamber where the cornea and the iris meet. Upon examination, this angle appears to be wide and open. For unknown reasons however, outflow is impeded and intraocular pressure rises slowly, to a moderate degree. This type of glaucoma usually is painless and the patient has no symptoms. Treatment may consist of eye drops such as timolol maleate and/or pilocarpine to enhance outflow, as well as oral agents such as acetazolamide, a carbonic-anhydrase inhibitor, to decrease production of aqueous humor. When this condition does not respond to medical measures, a surgical filtering procedure or laser trabeculoplasty may be performed.

b)   *Neo-vascular glaucoma* is a form of glaucoma specific to diabetes that is not uncommon in eyes with retinal ischemia. Abnormal vessels grow on the surface of the iris, enter the angle of the anterior chamber, and occlude the outflow of aqueous humor. This condition, rubeosis iridis, usually develops in conjunction with retinal neovascularization. Treatment usually consists of pan-retinal photocoagulation because the abnormal iris vessels tend to proliferate in response to retinal ischemia. Treatment is not uniformly successful, and some patients progress to having blind, painful eyes, necessitating either alcohol injection for pain, or enucleation.

c)   *Angle-closure glaucoma* is an acute condition that is very painful, with pressures often rising significantly above normal (40 to 60 mm Hg), secondary to angle obstruction. Patients with this condition are very ill, their eyes are red, and they may be nauseated. The associated pain usually causes patients to seek treatment, and they must be seen as soon as possible. After the pressure is lowered medically, the patient undergoes surgery to create new outflow channels. A peripheral iridectomy usually is suggested to prevent further blockage of the angle of outflow. People with diabetes are no more likely than nondiabetic individuals to suffer from this type of glaucoma.

2.   Lenticular changes affect the clarity of the lens and the focusing power of the eye. The crystalline lens of the eye is responsible for focusing at various distances. The image passes through the

lens and, with the expansion and contraction of the ciliary muscles and zonular fibers, is focused on the retina. This process is known as accommodation. With normal aging, some of the accommodative power is lost. When this happens, the individual may require reading glasses or bifocals.

a) Refractive changes may be one of the first symptoms of diabetes experienced by the patient. Patients may believe that their glasses are the wrong prescription due to eye fatigue and intermittent blurred vision.

b) Refractive changes occur because the lens of the eye swells in response to the hyperglycemic state. Some patients mistakenly believe that their vision is improving because their reading acuity improves, not realizing that distance vision is decreasing.

c) Because changes in blood glucose level can affect the refractive power of the lens, the patient should achieve a stable level of blood glucose control before being fitted for new glasses. This level of control should be maintained for 6 to 8 weeks prior to reevaluation of the glasses prescription. Patients who are instituting significant alterations in their metabolic control effort (eg, increasing frequency of insulin injections or beginning an exercise program) should be informed that these alterations may cause some refractive changes.

d) Temporary visual disturbances such as blurring, darkening, double vision, or bright flashing lights may occur at times of significant hypoglycemia. These symptoms may be due to cerebral edema.

3. *Cataracts* are opacities within the substance of the lens of the eye, not a covering or skin. The degree of opacification can vary from a few crystal-like changes in the periphery that do not interfere with vision to a total white opacification that clouds the pupil. Generally, change in visual acuity is proportional to degree of opacification. Although cataracts occur commonly in the general population, they seem to

develop at an earlier age in the person with diabetes, and may in part be initiated by hyperglycemia.

a)   *Nuclear sclerotic cataracts* have a dense nucleus that can make patients more nearsighted. As a result, patients may believe that visual acuity is improving simply because reading can be done without glasses.

b)   *Posterior subcapsular cataracts* are an opacity on the posterior surface of the lens. Patients complain of decreased acuity in bright light or when reading because pupillary constriction is forcing sight through the opacity. Patients with this kind of cataract generally prefer dim lighting.

c)   The only treatment for cataracts is surgery. Drops will not dissolve cataracts, and lasers cannot break them. However, the yttrium-aluminum garnet (YAG) laser can break up the remaining lens capsule if it should opacify after surgical lens extraction.

   (1)   Cataract surgery is done most often on an outpatient basis and usually under local anesthesia.

   (2)   Cataracts should be removed when the patient feels significantly visually handicapped, or when the retina can no longer be examined confidently.

   (3)   Previous rules about the "ripeness" of a cataract are no longer used clinically. The patient should be informed of the risks and potential benefits of the proposed surgery. A final decision should involve careful consultation with an ophthalmologist and/or retinologist.

d)   Restoring vision after cataract surgery is the goal of treatment. When the lens of the eye is removed, focusing power is lost. Patients then require correction for both distance and reading vision.

   (1)   Cataract glasses, known as aphakic glasses, are recommended for some people. They are thick and heavy, with inherent disadvantages such as a 30% magnification and a decreased visual field.

(2) Contact lenses offer restoration of peripheral vision and 10% magnification, which usually can be tolerated fairly well. However, some patients cannot comfortably wear contact lenses, or do not have the manual dexterity to manipulate the lens.

(3) Intraocular lens implant (IOL) is recommended for many patients undergoing cataract extraction. The lens usually is made of polymethacrylate and placed in the posterior chamber at the time of cataract extraction. These lenses offer a 1% to 3% size magnification, and the patient can enjoy a full visual field without having to care for the lens on a daily basis. However, there is a greater risk of inflammation and infection when a foreign body such as a lens is implanted.

4. *Ophthalmoplegias* are complications of the eye associated with neurologic changes involving the third, fourth, or sixth cranial nerves. The patient usually complains of double vision due to paresis of one of the extraocular muscles innervated by the affected cranial nerve.

a) Involvement of the third cranial nerve may cause some discomfort. The pupil usually is spared from concomitant dilation, but there is ptosis or drooping of the upper eyelid associated with paralysis of full ocular movement. The eye usually is deviated down and out. Intracranial lesions must be ruled out in any patient presenting with third nerve involvement.

b) Involvement of the sixth cranial nerve usually is indicated by an inward turning of the affected eye. Fourth nerve involvement creates vertical diplopia or double vision.

c) Most diabetic palsies resolve spontaneously within 4 to 6 months. No medical treatment is necessary, although providing support and suggesting techniques to eliminate double vision, such as fogging the lens of the glasses over the affected eye, can be helpful for the patient. Any palsy that persists beyond 6 months should be further investigated because it may be due to causes other than diabetes.

H. Reducing Modifiable Risks for Diabetic Eye Disease

1. Patients may wonder how they can protect themselves from eye diseases associated with diabetes. In answering this question, the patient's history, habits, activities of daily living, and personality must be considered. A multidisciplinary approach, including a dietitian, internist, exercise physiologist, nurse educator, and social worker, generally is beneficial to patients and their families.

2. The diabetes educator should address several key topics.
   a) Remind the patient of the importance of a regular eye exam by an ophthalmologist, including visual acuity, intraocular pressure check for glaucoma, refraction if indicated, and dilated fundus exam.
   b) Efforts to achieve normoglycemia should be intensified, if indicated.
   c) Hypertension should be controlled, if present.
   d) Patients who smoke should be encouraged to stop.
   e) The need for careful follow-up, regardless of the stage of retinopathy, should be stressed.

REFERENCES

1. National Society to Prevent Blindness. Vision problems in the US: facts and figures. 1980;Feb.

2. Patz A, Smith R. Guest editorial: the ETDRS and Diabetes 2000. Ophthalmology 1991;98:739-40.

3. Klein R, Klein BEK, Moss SE. Visual impairment in diabetes. Ophthalmology 1984;91:1-9.

4. Frank RN. On the pathogenesis of diabetic retinopathy: a 1990 update. Ophthalmology 1991;98:586-93.

5. Diabetic Retinopathy Study Research Group. Indications for photocoagulation treatment of diabetic retinopathy, DRS report no. 14. Int Ophthalmol Clin 1987;27:239-53.

6. Early Treatment Diabetic Retinopathy Study Research Group. Photocoagulation for diabetic macular edema: ETDRS report no. 1. Ophthalmology 1985:103;1796-1806.

7. American Academy of Ophthalmology Quality of Care Committee Retina Panel. Preferred practice pattern; diabetic retinopathy. San Francisco: The American Academy of Ophthalmology, 1989.

KEY EDUCATIONAL CONSIDERATIONS

1. It is important to emphasize that diabetic retinopathy often occurs without symptoms until late in the disease process. Measures designed to protect vision are best instituted early.

2. The patient must appreciate that nothing can substitute for regular dilated eye examinations by an ophthalmologist. Many patients are confused by the difference between ophthalmologists and optometrists, and need to be directed to an ophthalmologist, if possible. An ophthalmologist is a medical doctor who specializes in diseases of the eye, whereas an optometrist is a doctor of optometry whose expertise lies in the proper fitting of lenses and screening for eye disease.

3. Because many patients are not familiar with the anatomy and physiology of the human eye, explain how the eye functions using a plastic model or colorful diagrams. Comparing the eye to a camera is an excellent way to explain the functions. It may be helpful to explain retinal problems by comparing the retina to damaged film in the camera, and a cataract to a camera lens with a scratch or crack. This analogy is especially helpful for patients who have difficulty understanding why their problems cannot be corrected with stronger refractive lenses.

4. Any discussion of diabetic eye disease should include a review of visual disturbances that the patient may have experienced. Patients who have noticed visual blurring may be receptive to suggestions for improving blood glucose control, particularly if the educator relates these symptoms to the lens changes associated with hyperglycemia. Some patients may find that during periods of fluctuating blood glucose control their old eyeglasses better suit their visual needs than their current prescription.

5. A sudden loss of vision, a sudden onset of floaters, the appearance of a shade or curtain coming across the visual field, eye pain, and photophobia should be reported immediately to the ophthalmologist.

SELF-REVIEW QUESTIONS

If you are unsure of the answers to the following questions, please review the materials.

1. List two risk factors for the development of diabetic retinopathy.
2. List the major stages of diabetic retinopathy.
3. What are the current methods of treatment for each stage of retinopathy?
4. What are the symptoms of diabetic macular edema?
5. What are the recommendations for ophthalmologic examination of the diabetic patient?
6. List three ophthalmic complications related to diabetes other than retinopathy.
7. What kind of glaucoma is closely associated with diabetes? How is it treated?
8. What options are available for vision restoration after cataract extraction?

CASE EXAMPLE 1

DR is a 60-year-old male with diabetes who normally is very active in his hardware store. However, 2 months ago he became bedridden secondary to an infected great toe that has been slow to heal. He has been quite upset about the enforced bed rest and now is alarmed to find that he cannot read his supply catalogues. He states, "Great! I'll probably lose my toe, my business, and my sight!"

QUESTIONS

1. What are likely reasons for this change in reading vision?
2. Since the patient probably has had glycemic control problems during this period of infection, should the health care provider wait until control improves before referring DR to an ophthalmologist for an eye examination?

SUGGESTED SOLUTIONS

Although hyperglycemia secondary to infection and lack of activity undoubtedly have affected this patient's refractive error, it also is very possible that the patient's symptoms are secondary to clinically significant macular edema. Ask DR whether he has seen an ophthalmologist recently. If not, referral to an ophthalmologist specializing in retinal vascular disease is indicated at this time.

CASE EXAMPLE 2

MJ is a 47-year-old homemaker who does occasional freelance artwork. She is 5 ft 4 in tall and weighs 162 lb (73 kg). She is a good cook, and her specialty is a dish with Italian sausage. She was told after the birth of her last child that she might have a "touch of sugar" but she would be fine if she watched her diet. She was comfortable with a diagnosis of diabetes because she feels that she has the "good kind." Her cousin, however, has "the bad kind . . . She takes needles!" and has just begun laser treatment for diabetic retinopathy. MJ accompanied her cousin to the eye clinic for the treatment and also was examined while she was there. MJ was told that she has proliferative retinopathy with high-risk characteristics and needs to begin treatment herself. MJ was astounded. "No one ever told me this could happen. I've had my glasses changed every 2 years and my vision is good. How could I possibly need laser treatment?"

QUESTIONS

1. In addition to learning about diabetic retinopathy, what are MJ's educational needs?
2. Discuss financial issues related to the diagnosis and treatment of MJ's retinopathy.

SUGGESTED SOLUTIONS

MJ needs intervention on a multidisciplinary level. She requires intensive diet counseling and diabetes education. She will require ongoing support and guidance as she makes some lifestyle changes in exercise, diet, and in the way she views diabetes.

Proceeding in a timely fashion with pan-retinal photocoagulation may help protect against severe visual loss. However, this treatment is of long duration, requiring several visits to the retinal specialist, and also will be very expensive. MJ may have some transient or permanent disabilities as a result of the treatment. Therefore, she may require the services of a social worker to assist with potential financial problems, as well as with the associated emotional issues.

OTHER SUGGESTED READINGS

Early Treatment Diabetic Retinopathy Study Research Group: The Early Treatment Diabetic Retinopathy Study (ETDRS). Effects of aspirin treatment on diabetic retinopathy. ETDRS report no. 8. Ophthalmology 1991; 98:757-66.

Marble A, Krall J, et al. Joslin's diabetes mellitus. 12th ed. Philadelphia: Lea and Febiger, 1985.

Sunness JS. The pregnant woman's eye. Survey Ophthalmol 1988;32:219-38.

Wulsin LR, Jacobson AM, Rand LI. Psychosocial aspects of diabetic retinopathy. Diabetes Care 1987:10:367-73.

COMPLICATIONS

XXII. DIABETIC NEUROPATHY

INTRODUCTION

While neuropathies can occur as a result of AIDS, Hansen's disease, injury, metabolic disorders, alcoholism, and connective tissue diseases (eg, systemic lupus erythematosus), the primary cause of peripheral neuropathy in the Western world is diabetes.[1] As the most common long-term complication of diabetes, peripheral neuropathy is responsible for the majority of limb amputations among people with diabetes and causes a great deal of morbidity and suffering for patients who experience its devastating effects.[2] Diabetic neuropathy is thought to be the result of insulin deficiency and/or hyperglycemia.[1] Its management is directed toward early diagnosis, prudent glucose control, relief of symptoms, avoidance of secondary complications, and patient education for appropriate self-care.

In the past, patients with neuropathy were often told that pain and other symptoms of neuropathy were just something they would "have to live with." Recently, however, diabetic neuropathy has been the subject of intense research interest. There is new understanding of the classification, diagnosis, and causes of neuropathy and breakthroughs in its treatment. The purpose of this chapter is to review the pathogenesis and approaches to treatment of diabetic neuropathy as it affects the peripheral nervous system, and will include areas of current and future research.

OBJECTIVES

Upon completion of this chapter, the learner will be able to:

- define neuropathy;
- discuss the role of blood glucose control in the development and treatment of peripheral neuropathies;
- list pharmacologic and nonpharmacologic treatments for peripheral neuropathy;
- list the classifications and clinical manifestations of autonomic neuropathy;
- state the primary symptom for each of the focal neuropathies;
- list the key elements that all patients with diabetes should be taught about neuropathy.

A. Diabetic Neuropathy

1. Overview: *Diabetic neuropathy* is a descriptive term for a clinical or subclinical disorder that occurs in patients with diabetes without other causes for peripheral neuropathy.[3] It encompasses a large group of syndromes with a wide range of manifestations[1] (see Table XXII.1).

    a) Diabetic neuropathy can be defined as peripheral nerve dysfunction that occurs in people with diabetes, is of a type known to be more prevalent among people with diabetes, and cannot be attributed to any other disease.[3]

    b) Diabetic neuropathy is staged as clinical or subclinical based on signs, symptoms, and objective measures. Subclinical neuropathy can be defined only through objective measures. Clinical neuropathy is defined by symptoms, clinical signs, and objective measures.[4] Clinical neuropathy is then further divided into syndromes according to the distribution of nerve involvement and clustered under the two general headings of diffuse (multiple nerve involvement) or focal (individual nerve involvement).[2]

    c) Although each syndrome has a characteristic clinical presentation and course, multiple syndromes may overlap and coexist.[5] The majority of cases are diffuse neuropathies consisting of diabetic distal symmetric, primarily sensory polyneuropathies, and are often accompanied by diabetic autonomic neuropathy.[1]

    d) Diffuse neuropathies are generally chronic, frequently progressive, and associated with increased morbidity and mortality.[5] Focal neuropathies occur less often, are generally acute in onset, and often self-limited.[6]

2. Occurrence: Reliable prevalence estimates of diabetic neuropathy have been difficult to obtain because of the lack of standard diagnostic measures and consensus in diagnostic criteria.[7]

TABLE XXII.1: Classification and Staging of Diabetic Neuropathy

Class I. Subclinical neuropathy*
- A. Abnormal electrodiagnostic tests (EDX)
  1. Decreased nerve conduction velocity
  2. Decreased amplitude of evoked muscle or nerve action potential
- B. Abnormal quantitative sensory testing (QST)
  1. Vibratory/tactile
  2. Thermal warming/cooling
  3. Other
- C. Abnormal autonomic function tests (AFT)
  1. Diminished sinus arrhythmia (beat-to-beat heart rate variation)
  2. Diminished sudomotor function
  3. Increased pupillary latency

Class II. Clinical neuropathy
- A. Diffuse neuropathy
  1. Distal symmetric sensorimotor polyneuropathy
     - a) Primarily small-fiber neuropathy
     - b) Primarily large-fiber neuropathy
     - c) Mixed
  2. Autonomic neuropathy
     - a) Genitourinary autonomic neuropathy
       - (1) Bladder dysfunction
       - (2) Sexual dysfunction
     - b) Gastrointestinal autonomic neuropathy
       - (1) Gastric atony
       - (2) Diabetic neuropathy
     - c) Cardiovascular autonomic neuropathy
     - d) Hypoglycemic unawareness
     - e) Sudomotor dysfunction
     - f) Abnormal pupillary function
- B. Focal neuropathy
  1. Mononeuropathy
  2. Mononeuropathy multiplex
  3. Plexopathy
  4. Radiculopathy
  5. Cranial neuropathy

*   Neurological function tests are abnormal but no neurological symptoms or clinically detectable neurological deficits indicative of a diffuse or focal neuropathy are present. Class I, Subclinical neuropathy, is further subdivided into class Ia if an AFT or QST abnormality is present, class Ib if EDX or AFT and QST abnormalities are present, and class Ic if an EDX and either AFT or QST abnormalities or both are present.

Source: Adapted with permission from Greene, Sima, Pfeifer, and Albers.[1]

a) In insulin-dependent diabetes mellitus (IDDM), also called type I diabetes, the prevalence of polyneuropathy appears to parallel the duration and severity of hyperglycemia. While this is probably also true for non-insulin-dependent diabetes mellitus (NIDDM), also called type II diabetes, patients may present with symptoms and signs of neuropathy and subsequently be diagnosed with diabetes. This is most likely explained by the insidious nature of NIDDM, which may be present but undiagnosed for years, so that the duration of hyperglycemia and its relationship to neuropathy are difficult to determine.[2]

b) Estimates of the prevalence of neuropathy range from 5% to 60%, and up to 100% if patients with abnormalities of nerve conduction are included.[8] Pirart's classic study reported an 8% prevalence at the time of diagnosis (mostly in older NIDDM patients) that increased linearly to 50% after 25 years.[9] A retrospective, population-based study of NIDDM patients showed a cumulative incidence of distal symmetrical polyneuropathy of 4% after 5 years and 15% after 20 years, with a median time of 9 years from diagnosis to its development.[10] Neuropathy occurs with similar frequency in IDDM and NIDDM patients, and also in patients with various forms of acquired diabetes.[9]

c) It is generally fair to say that diabetic neuropathy is an extremely common problem that ultimately affects half of all patients with diabetes.[1] If, as has been conservatively estimated, 10% of patients with diabetes have symptoms so severe that they seek help, then 600,000 persons in the United States are affected.[7]

d) The incidence of autonomic and focal neuropathies has not been well studied.[1]

3. Pathology: The nervous system is divided into the central nervous system and the peripheral nervous system. The peripheral nervous system is made up of the autonomic nervous system (sympathetic and parasympathetic) and the sensorimotor nervous system. The autonomic nervous system controls

involuntary functions. The sensorimotor system includes the sensory nerves that send information from the skin and internal organs about how things feel, and motor nerves that send commands from the brain to the body about movement. While there may be some central nervous system involvement in diabetic neuropathies, most of the pathology occurs in the peripheral nervous system.[4]

    a)   The most common pathological lesion in distal symmetric sensorimotor polyneuropathy is loss and atrophy of longer peripheral nerve axons.[1]

    b)   Polyneuropathies occur secondarily to axonal degeneration that progresses from the distal to proximal portions of the neurons.[4] The distal portions are eventually more seriously affected.[11]

4.   Pathogenesis: While the association between diabetes and neuropathic symptoms in the legs and feet was first made by John Rollo over 200 years ago, the pathogenesis of diabetic neuropathy is still unknown.[12] Evidence suggests that insulin deficiency and its related hyperglycemia contribute to the development of diabetic neuropathy.[13] However, the degree and duration of hyperglycemia or insulin deficiency do not reliably predict its development.[4] In addition, the severity of neuropathy does not always correlate with clinical findings or symptoms.[14] As with other long-term complications of diabetes, neuropathy is thought to result from the interaction of multiple metabolic, genetic, and environmental factors.[15] Current theories are complex and beyond the scope of this chapter.

    a)   The current view is that diabetic neuropathy is a disease involving acute abnormalities in nerve fibers, followed by more chronic nerve fiber atrophy, injury, and loss. This process is complicated by microvascular dysfunction and blunted nerve fiber regeneration. All of these abnormalities can be linked to the effects of hyperglycemia on the cell constituents of peripheral nerve tissue and its supporting connective tissue and vascular elements.[16]

b) One theory of the mechanism by which these contributors produce nerve damage is based on the conversion of glucose to sorbitol by the enzyme aldose reductase and secondary abnormalities in myo-inositol, phospho-inositide, and Na, K-ATPase metabolism.[1] Unlike most other cells, insulin is not needed to transport glucose into nerve cells. Therefore, high levels of blood glucose lead to high levels of glucose within the nerve cell. Once inside the cell, glucose is reduced to sorbitol by the enzyme aldose reductase (the sorbitol pathway). The sorbitol is then oxidized to fructose by the enzyme sorbitol dehydrogenase (the polyol pathway). In diabetes, peripheral nerve glucose, sorbitol, and fructose levels are elevated. Specific aldose reductase inhibitors may improve nerve function by preventing the conversion of glucose to sorbitol.[4] The reason elevated sorbitol and glucose levels cause nerve damage is unclear, but may be related to decreased myo-inositol levels. Myo-inositol plays an important role in normal cellular function and metabolism, so that nerve function is impaired when levels are decreased. Myo-inositol molecules are very much like glucose molecules in size and shape. In the presence of hyperglycemia, the large number of glucose molecules inhibits the transport of myo-inositol into the peripheral nerves. This causes a self-reinforcing cycle of metabolic disarrangement resulting in peripheral nerve impairment.[1,4]

c) Additional theories of the pathogenesis of diabetic neuropathy are related to glycosylation of cellular proteins and microvascular disease. It has been hypothesized that glycosylation of cellular proteins may impair their function and alter cellular metabolism. The effects of microvascular disease and resulting decreased perfusion to the peripheral nerve tissue on the pathogenesis of diabetic neuropathy is unclear.[16] It is known that large blood vessel occlusive disease alone does not produce peripheral neuropathy.[1]

Focal neuropathies are thought to be caused by acute ischemic events.

5.   Diagnosis: Generally, diagnosis involves excluding other potential causes of the symptoms.

   a)   Objective measures, such as electrodiagnostic testing, or clinical signs, such as loss of Achilles tendon reflex, and decreased pinprick and vibration sensation, must be used to confirm the diagnosis.

   b)   The annual physical examination for a person with diabetes should include assessment for neuropathy through evaluation of muscle strength, deep tendon reflexes, temperature, position, and pinprick and vibration sensation.[2] Early detection of an insensitive foot and patient education can have a substantial effect on preventing injury, sepsis, ulceration, and amputation.

6.   Treatment: Treatment is generally palliative, supportive, and aimed at symptom relief.[1]

   a)   Improved control of blood glucose levels may result in a decrease in symptoms for some patients. However, symptoms may initially worsen as a result of nerve regeneration, which can be painful. Both pharmacologic and nonpharmacologic therapies may be useful for pain relief.

   b)   Recent studies of aldose reductase inhibitors show that these medications may hold promise for future treatment of neuropathies.

B.   Diffuse Neuropathies

1.   Distal symmetric sensorimotor polyneuropathy is the most widely known form of peripheral neuropathy. It primarily affects the sensory nerves,[1] and has been shown to affect 72% of patients with neuropathy.[10] Sensory deficits and symptoms begin in the distal portions of the lower extremities and move to the upper extremities, spreading in a "stocking-glove"

distribution with increasing duration and severity.[1] At its late stage, vertical bands of sensory loss in the trunk area may occur.[4] Distal symmetric sensorimotor polyneuropathy can be viewed as a disease of progressive nerve fiber loss, atrophy, and injury. In the early stages, manifestations can include deterioration of nerve function and development of subtle, sensory-motor deficits with minimal or no symptoms. Patients may present with neurological deficits found during physical examination, or with complications such as undetected trauma to an insensate foot.[9] The signs and symptoms of distal symmetric sensorimotor polyneuropathy depend on the class and stage of nerve fiber loss. Small-fiber and/or large-fiber nerves may be involved. Most cases include both large- and small-fiber damage.

a) Small-fiber neuropathy is most often associated with pain or sensory loss.

   (1) Several types of spontaneous pain may be associated with small-fiber neuropathy. Patients most often experience paresthesias (spontaneous uncomfortable sensations), dysesthesias (contact paresthesias), or pain. Pain is described as superficial and burning, shooting or stabbing, or bone-deep and aching or tearing, and is generally more severe at night.[2] The pain can become disabling in and of itself, and depression may occur as a result of unremitting pain.[1] In contrast, some patients report numb or cold extremities, and undetected trauma, particularly of the feet, is not uncommon.[2,4]

   (2) Sensory loss appears to correspond closely with the degree of nerve damage; however, pain corresponds more closely to independent processes, such as fiber regeneration or structural deformities.[17]

   (3) About 25% of all persons with diabetes have pain associated with neuropathy.[14] In acute painful neuropathy, the pain develops and then remits in less than six months. Precipitous weight loss may also occur.[2] In chronic painful neuropathy, symptoms

appear and stabilize, or disappear and are replaced by dense sensory deficits.[1]

    (4) Diminished deep tendon reflexes of the Achilles tendon and diminished temperature and pinprick sensations are often early signs of neuropathies.[4] Sensory impairment is clinically significant because it can predispose to ulceration.

    (5) Symptoms may occur in the absence of neurological deficits on physical examination.[2]

b) Large-fiber neuropathy produces diminished proprioception and vibration sensations.

    (1) Impaired balance, diminished proprioception and joint position sense, and absent or reduced vibration sensation are signs and symptoms of large fiber damage.[4]

    (2) Sensory ataxia may result in the most severe cases.

c) Motor neuropathy causes muscle weakness and atrophy of intrinsic foot muscles, leaving the pull of the long muscles unopposed.

    (1) Edema, ulceration, or structural deformities of the foot can result from motor neuropathy.

    (2) Potential deformities caused by interosseous and lumbrical muscle wasting include:

        (a) Claw toes, caused by dorsiflexion of toes at metatarsophalangeal joint and flexion at the proximal interphalangeal joint.

        (b) Hammer toes, caused by extension at metatarsophalangeal joint with flexion at the proximal interphalangeal joint.

        (c) Cock-up deformity, caused by flexion of the interphalangeal joint with extension of the metatarsophalangeal joint of the great toe.

        (d) Crowding of toes on the axis of second digit.

        (e) Loss of plantar arches.

        (f) Metatarsal head prominence, with loss of fat pad and callus formation.

        (g) Foot drop.

d) Treatment of distal symmetric sensorimotor polyneuropathy is focused around improved glycemic control; pain relief; relief from depression, which often accompanies chronic pain; and protection of the deformed foot.

(1) Nonpharmacological therapies include walking to ease leg pains; avoiding alcohol; relaxation exercises; biofeedback; hypnosis; transcutaneous electrical nerve stimulation (TENS); wearing body stockings or panty hose to keep clothes away from hypersensitive skin; brief cold water foot soaks; and referral to a pain control clinic.

(2) Pharmacological therapies include nonnarcotic analgesics, such as ibuprofen and sulindac, phenytoin (Dilantin) or carbamazepine (Tegretol) in anticonvulsive doses, and amitriptyline (Elavil) in subclinical doses either alone or in combination with fluphenazine (Prolixin). Topical capsaicin (Zostrix) has been found to be effective for some patients.[18]

(3) Lamb's-wool padding, gentle filing of callused areas, specially made shoes, and molded insoles or other orthotic devices can be used to protect deformed areas of the foot.

(4) Aldose reductase inhibitors (ARIs) (eg, Tolrestat) have been found to be effective in halting or reversing the progression of nerve damage in patients with subclinical neuropathies.[19] ARIs are available in other countries but are still under investigation in the United States.

e) Complications of distal symmetric sensorimotor polyneuropathy can be devastating to the patient. Neuropathic syndromes culminate in severe tertiary complications of sensory and motor denervation, such as insensitivity to pain, limb deformity, ulceration, neuroarthropathy, infection, and amputation, which parallel severity and proximal extension of the sensory loss.[16]

(1) Neuropathic foot ulcers often occur in areas where the fat pad is decreased and callus formation subsequently occurs as a result of weight-bearing pressure. Autonomic neuropathy further leads to decreased perspiration and a tendency for dry, cracked skin and infection. Because of diminished sensation, injuries may remain unnoticed until infection develops.

(2) Neuropathic arthropathy (Charcot's joint) can occur when motor function remains intact but sensation is impaired. The small joints of the foot (tarsals, metatarsals) are most commonly affected.[20] The foot is swollen, red, and painless in the early stages. Multiple fractures, fragmentations, and disarticulations occur in the later stages. As the patient continues to walk on the injured, insensate foot, marked deformities occur, including a flattened arch and "bag of bones" appearance.[4]

(3) Treatment for the complications of sensory polyneuropathy is aimed at removal of continued trauma, proper footwear, and patient education in appropriate foot care techniques.

2. Diabetic autonomic neuropathy (DAN) can occur with all classes of diabetes,[21] and can affect any system in the body.[22] The relationship of the occurrence of DAN and sensorimotor polyneuropathy varies, but they generally coexist. Fifty percent of patients with peripheral neuropathy will have asymptomatic DAN.[22] Because morbidity and mortality rates are closely linked with DAN, early diagnosis and treatment is of critical importance.[21] Table XXII.2 shows the most common classifications of DAN and its accompanying clinical manifestations.

a) Genitourinary involvement: Both bladder and sexual functioning may be affected.

TABLE XXII.2:
Diabetic Autonomic Neuropathies

Classification	Symptoms and Signs
Genitourinary	
Neurogenic bladder	Diminished urinary frequency Incomplete or difficult bladder emptying Frequent urinary tract infections Bladder residual volume >150 mL

Sexual dysfunction	In males:
	  Retrograde ejaculation
	  Impotence
	In females:
	  Diminished vaginal lubrication
	  Decreased frequency of orgasm

Gastrointestinal	
Gastroparesis	Early satiety Postprandial fullness Postprandial hypoglycemia
Intestinal	Nocturnal diarrhea Fecal incontinence
Cardiovascular	Postural hypotension Cardiac denervation syndrome (painless myocardial infarction, sudden death) Fixed heart rate
Impaired Insulin Counterregulation	Unawareness of hypoglycemia Brittle diabetes
Sudomotor	Areas of symmetrical anhidrosis Gustatory sweating
Pupillary	Decreased/absent responsiveness to light Decreased pupil size

Source: Adapted with permission from Cyrus, Broadstone, Pfeifer, and Greene.[21]

(1) Bladder dysfunction generally occurs in association with distal symmetric polyneuropathy and impotence (males).[2]

    (a) Afferent autonomic fibers transmit bladder fullness sensations and efferent parasympathetic fibers promote bladder contraction during micturition. Efferent sympathetic nerves maintain sphincter tone.[2] Damage can occur to all of these nerves; however, motor function usually remains intact.[22]

    (b) Symptoms of a neurogenic bladder are usually insidious and progressive. In the early stages, the sensation of the need to void may be blunted. This infrequent urination may be misinterpreted as decreased polyuria. Later, difficulty in emptying the bladder, dribbling, and overflow incontinence may occur.[21]

    (c) Bladder insensitivity must be diagnosed by a cystometrogram.[21] A postvoid urine residual volume of greater than 150 mL as determined by ultrasound or postvoid catheterization, confirms bladder dysfunction.

    (d) Untreated, neurogenic bladder often leads to urinary tract infections as a result of urinary stasis. These frequent urinary tract infections may accelerate deterioration of renal function. More than two bladder infections per year are indicative of the need for further evaluation of bladder dysfunction.[21]

    (e) Treatment involves frequent palpation for bladder fullness; urination scheduled every 2 to 4 hours during waking hours using manual suprapubic pressure (Credé's method) to ensure that the bladder is empty; vigorous antibiotic therapy for infections; and parasympathomimetic drug treatment (eg, bethanechol) to improve nerve contraction.[22]

Self-catheterization may become necessary if the nerves to the bladder are severely damaged.

(f) Patient education should stress the need for frequent, complete urination; the signs and symptoms of urinary tract infections; and the importance of early treatment for infections. Patients with bladder dysfunction should be taught Credé's method of emptying the bladder and to palpate for bladder fullness.[22]

(2) Sexual dysfunction is common. As many as 75% of men and 35% of women with diabetes experience sexual problems due to diabetic neuropathy.

(a) Male sexual dysfunction includes impotence and retrograde ejaculation.

- Retrograde ejaculation is unusual and results from damage to the efferent sympathetic nerves that normally coordinate the simultaneous closure of the internal vesicle sphincter and relaxation of the external vesicle sphincter.[2]

- Symptoms of impotence include impairment or loss of erectile ability sufficient for intercourse, despite a normal libido.[22] Organic impotence is gradual in onset (from partial to complete in 2 years), is partner nonspecific, and is characterized by lack of erections during sleep.[2] Cloudy urine following intercourse and decreased volume of ejaculate are symptomatic of retrograde ejaculation.

- Diagnosis of impotence includes ruling out other causes such as medications (eg, antihypertensives), alcohol use, hormonal deficiencies, or psychological causes.[2] The assessment process can include blood hormone levels, penile blood flow and pressure measurements, nocturnal tumescence testing (eg, Snap Gauge®), and referral to urology for further evaluation. Diabetic autonomic neuropathy is specifically associated with diminished or absent testicular pain sensation to pressure and loss of perineal sensation. The sensations are lost because of parallel loss of somatic and autonomic sacral segments two, three, and four.[22] Retrograde ejaculation is diagnosed by the presence of oligospermia, azoospermia, and sperm in postcoital urine.[2]

- Management of impotence includes counseling for the patient and his partner, vacuum devices to produce an erection, rigid or semirigid penile prostheses (surgical implants), the alpha adrenergic agonist yohimbine, or injection of papaverine or other vasoactive drugs directly into the corpus cavernosum to produce erection. Retrograde ejaculation may respond to the use of an antihistamine, desipramine, or phenylephrine.[2,22] Fertility may be possible by instructing patients to have intercourse with a full bladder or by harvesting sperm from the urine for artificial insemination.[2]

(b) Female sexual dysfunction includes difficulties in arousal, decreased vaginal lubrication during stimulation, and anorgasmia despite a normal libido.[2]

- Symptoms such as dyspareunia, decreased lubrication, and delayed or absent orgasmic response should be assessed.

- Management includes application of estrogen or lubricant vaginal creams and possible gynecology referral.

(3) Sexual difficulties not related to autonomic neuropathy include loss of libido related to depression as a result of diabetes and its complications, and the frequent occurrence of yeast and other vaginal infections in women with diabetes.[2]

(4) Patient education should include discussions of sexual function and the potential for diabetes-related problems, and the need to bring problems to the attention of health care professionals. Counseling for specific therapies should include both the patient and sexual partner.

b) Gastrointestinal involvement: Virtually all of the gastrointestinal system has autonomic innervation.[21] The parasympathetic nervous system stimulates intestinal and gastric peristalsis, dopaminergic innervation inhibits gastric peristalsis, and the sympathetic nervous system activity inhibits gastric emptying.[2]

(1) Upper gastrointestinal dysfunction may involve the esophagus, stomach, and upper small intestine.

(a) Symptoms can include heartburn, reflux, anorexia, early satiety, nausea, abdominal bloating, erratic blood glucose levels due to delayed absorption of food, and the vomiting of undigested food eaten several hours or days earlier.[2] However, delayed gastric emptying can also occur without symptoms.[22] Signs associated with gastroparesis include weight loss and gastrospasm.

(b) X-ray visualization of the upper gastrointestinal tract using a barium suspension is useful to rule out obstruction and to determine liquid-phase gastric emptying. While delayed liquid-phase emptying almost always indicates delayed solid-phase emptying, normal liquid-phase emptying does not rule out delayed solid-phase emptying. Therefore, a solid-phase gastric emptying phase study is the most specific way to diagnose delayed gastric emptying.[2]

(c) Treatment includes referral to a dietitian for a low-fat, low-fiber diet; multiple small, mostly liquid meals eaten throughout the day; and medications such as metoclopramide (Reglan) or domperidone (Motillium) taken one-half hour before all meals and snacks to increase the motility of the stomach. In the most severe stages, jejunostomy tube feedings may be necessary.

(d) While normalizing blood glucose levels may improve gastric emptying, the presence of gastroparesis complicates balancing insulin doses with food absorption. Frequent monitoring of pre- and postprandial blood glucose levels is needed to detect hypoglycemia and determine the insulin dose.

(2) Lower intestinal tract dysfunction is the result of damage to the efferent autonomic nerves. This leads to impaired motility and poor contraction of the smooth muscles to the gut, resulting in constipation.

(a) Constipation is fairly common and has been reported in up to 60% of all patients with diabetes.[2] Treatment includes increasing fiber in the diet; stool softeners; bulking agents such as psyllium (Metamucil®); judicious use of laxatives; and medications such as metoclopramide (Reglan), domperidone (Motillium), cisapride (Propulsion), or neostigmine (Prostigmin) to increase intestinal mobility.

(b) Decreased small intestinal motility may lead to an overgrowth of the normal intestinal bacteria, resulting in diarrhea. Diarrhea can also occur as a result of hypermotility without bacterial overgrowth.[21]

(c) While constipation is more common, diarrhea is usually more troublesome to patients. It may be nocturnal, intermittent with constipation, associated with fecal incontinence, and occur without cramping or pain.[21] Treatment includes antibiotics to decrease the bacterial overgrowth, if confirmed by a hydrogen breath test. Medications that may be useful to slow intestinal motility are clonidine, cholestyramine, lomotil, and somatostatin. In addition, biofeedback, relaxation, and bowel training may be helpful for some patients. Early treatment of diarrhea may help prevent the development of incontinence.[2]

(d) Patient education should include a discussion of these symptoms as they relate to diabetes; the need to inform health care professionals of symptoms to allow for early detection and treatment; and explanations of tests, test results, and any therapies initiated.

c) Cardiovascular involvement: Cardiovascular dysfunction is associated with abnormalities in heart rate control and vascular dynamics. Parasympathetic nerves slow the heart rate. Sympathetic nerves increase the speed and force of heart contractions and stimulate the vascular tree to increase the blood pressure.[2] Cardiovascular dysfunction is present in up to 40% of patients. There are two major associated syndromes.

(1) Orthostatic hypotension is defined as a drop in systolic blood pressure of more than 30 mm Hg within 2 minutes of changing from the supine to standing position. It generally occurs late in diabetes and signals advanced autonomic impairment.[22]

(a) Orthostatic hypotension can occur without symptoms but is often accompanied by dizziness, light-headedness, weakness, visual impairment, or syncope.[2]

(b) Blood pressure with the patient lying and standing, should be assessed at each visit of all patients who have diabetes.[2]

(c) Treatment includes increasing venous pressure with supportive elastic body stockings applied while still supine, wearing antigravity suits, correcting hypovolemia, increasing salt intake, and/or taking fludrocortisone to expand the plasma volume.[22] Pharmacologic therapies can include yohimbine, metaclopramide, phenylephrine, ephedrine, beta blockers, clonidine, and somatostatin analog.[2]

(d) Patient education includes proper application and use of elastic body stockings and instructing patients to rise slowly from a recumbent position.

(2) Cardiac denervation syndrome is the result of both parasympathetic and sympathetic system impairment. Initially parasympathetic tone decreases, which causes a relative increase in sympathetic tone and an increase in heart rate. Progressive impairment of sympathetic tone results in a gradual slowing of the heart. In the final stages, both parasympathetic and sympathetic tone are impaired.[2]

(a) Initially, a fixed heart rate of 100 to 120 beats per minute is common. In the later stages, the fixed heart rate will be in the range of 80 to 100 beats per minute.[2] The heart rate is unresponsive to stress, exercise, or tilting.[21]

(b) In the later stages, patients may suffer myocardial ischemia or myocardial infarction without accompanying pain. This results in delay or failure to seek treatment, thus increasing mortality rates. These patients are also at risk for cardiac arrhythmias and sudden death.[21]

(c) Cardiac denervation is assessed by checking the pulse or heart rate on ECG during deep breathing (six breaths per minute) or before and after exercise. No variation in heart rate is indicative of cardiac nerve damage.[2]

(d) Patients should be taught to avoid heavy exercise, aerobic exercise, and straining. In addition, these patients are generally not candidates for intensive insulin therapy because of the risk of hypoglycemia, which may cause a cardiac arrhythmia.[21]

d) Impaired insulin counterregulation: Maintenance of blood glucose levels during times of food deprivation and increased insulin action depends on glucagon secretion and the adrenergic nervous system.[21] The acute counterregulatory response to low blood glucose levels is an increase in the secretion of glucagon, epinephrine, growth hormone, cortisol, and glucose production by the liver.[2] Patients with autonomic neuropathy may have a defective adrenergic nervous system and defective glucagon secretion, leading to impaired recovery from hypoglycemia. These patients may further develop hypoglycemia unawareness so that the classic adrenergic warning signs of hypoglycemia do not occur.[21] Instead, when hypoglycemic, they develop neuroglycopenia, including lethargy, irritability, dullness, confusion, loss of consciousness, or seizures[2] (see Chapter XIII: Hypoglycemia).

(1) In IDDM patients, the normal glucagon response to hypoglycemia begins to deteriorate within 5 years of diagnosis. The epinephrine response declines with increasing duration of IDDM and may be lost after 15 to 30 years. Absent glucagon and epinephrine responses greatly increase the risk for severe hypoglycemia. The counterregulatory mechanism in NIDDM is largely unknown.[15]

(2) Information about hypoglycemia warning symptoms and episodes of hypoglycemia with loss of consciousness should be elicited during patient visits.

(3) More liberal glucose goals may need to be established with patients who have hypoglycemia unawareness. In general, normal glucose and glycosylated hemoglobin levels should not be goals of therapy. While improved metabolic control may reverse autonomic neuropathy, normoglycemia poses considerable risk for these patients. Long-acting insulins with only small boluses are recommended for intensive conventional therapy; boluses should not be used by patients who prefer insulin pump therapy (CSII).[22]

(4) Patient education should stress avoidance of hypoglycemia, appropriate treatment, the value of frequent blood glucose monitoring, and wearing appropriate diabetes identification. Family members should be taught signs and treatment of hypoglycemia, including glucagon administration.[2]

e) Sudomotor dysfunction: This is commonly manifested by anhidrosis in the lower extremities, with compensatory hyperhidrosis of the face and trunk.[21] Bilateral symmetrical loss of the thermoregulatory response and gustatory sweating in response to foods (cheese, spicy foods) that normally induce salivation may also occur.[22]

(1) Patients rarely think to report abnormal or diminished sweating; however, it is of importance because of the potential for heat stroke and foot ulcers. A careful history should be taken and the feet examined for dryness and fissures at each visit.[2]

(2) Propantheline hydrobromide or scopolamine patches may help to relieve gustatory sweating.[22] Dry feet should be lubricated daily.

(3) Patient education includes appropriate foot inspection and care, avoidance of offending foods, and prevention of hyperthermia and heat stroke.

f) Abnormal pupillary response: The iris is innervated by both parasympathetic and sympathetic nerve fibers. The sympathetic nerve fibers that cause the pupils to dilate are generally more severely affected.

   (1) Slow dilation of pupils in response to darkness may be observed during clinical examination.

   (2) Patients may report slow adaptation when entering a dark room.

   (3) Patient education should stress the need for caution during night driving, the importance of turning on lights when entering a dark room, and the use of night lights in darkened hallways and bathrooms to help prevent injuries.

C. Focal Neuropathies

1. The focal neuropathies generally occur acutely and unpredictably. They are not specific to diabetes and are not thought to be related to its duration. No strategies are available to prevent these neuropathies or to detect them early in their course, but this is offset by their self-limiting nature.[23] One study found that only 18% of patients with diabetic neuropathy had focal neuropathies; 12% of these patients had carpal tunnel syndrome.[10]

2. The primary symptom of focal neuropathy is acute pain. Abnormal nerve conduction that corresponds to the distribution of a single nerve, multiple peripheral nerves, the brachial or lumbosacral plexus, or nerve roots will be noted. Focal neuropathies often occur in patients with sensorimotor polyneuropathy.[2]

   a) Mononeuropathy and mononeuropathy complex: isolated neuropathies involving one or several nerves are more common among people with diabetes.[2]

      (1) Compression or entrapment of the median nerve of the wrist (carpal tunnel syndrome), ulnar nerve of the elbow, radial nerve of the upper arm leading to wrist

drop, lateral cutaneous nerve in the thigh, and the peroneal at the head of the fibula leading to foot drop are common mononeuropathies.[2]

(2) Diagnosis is based on pain, wrist or foot drop, and abnormal electrodiagnostic studies.[2]

(3) Treatment usually consists of surgical release of the nerve, physical therapy, or protection from further trauma, such as wrist splints, elbow pads, and ankle braces.

b) Plexopathy (femoral neuropathy): The sacral plexus and femoral nerves are generally affected.

(1) Pain extending from the hip to the anterior and lateral surface of the thigh is characteristic. Pain is generally worse at night, and muscle weakness and wasting are common.[4] Its occurrence is greatest among older adults.[2]

(2) Simple analgesics may be used to relieve pain. This condition generally remits spontaneously, but may recur periodically.[2]

c) Radiculopathy (intercostal neuropathy): The result of damage to the nerve root, radiculopathy is singular and unilateral, with pain localized to the chest or abdominal wall.

(1) The patient generally presents with pain or dysesthesia that is worse at night and is marked by an absence of cutaneous sensation. Profound weight loss may also occur.

(2) Simple analgesics may help to control pain that generally remits spontaneously in 6 to 24 months.[2]

d) Cranial neuropathy: The third cranial nerve is most often affected.

(1) The onset is generally abrupt, with headache, eye pain, or dysesthesias on the upper lip preceding palsy by several days. Ptosis is marked, but the pupil is generally spared from concomitant dilatation. The occurrence of cranial neuropathy is greatest among older adults.[2]

(2) An eye patch for the affected eye may help to alleviate double vision. Pain and oculomotor function will gradually improve after several weeks, with full recovery in 3 to 5 months.[2]

REFERENCES

1.   Greene DA, Sima AAF, Pfeifer MA, Albers JW. Diabetic neuropathy. Ann Rev Med 1990;41:303-17.

2.   Herman WA, Greene DA. Microvascular complications of diabetes. In: Haire-Joshu D, ed. Management of diabetes mellitus. St. Louis: CV Mosby, 1992;149-89.

3.   American Diabetes Association. Consensus statement: Diabetic neuropathy. Diabetes Care 1991;14(suppl 2):63-68.

4.   Broadstone VL, Cyrus J, Pfeifer MA, Greene DA. Diabetic peripheral neuropathy. Part I. Sensorimotor neuropathy. Diabetes Educ 1987;13:30-35.

5.   Dyck PJ, Karnes J, O'Brien PC. Diagnosis, staging, and classification of diabetic neuropathy and associations with other complications. In: Dyck PJ, Thomas PK, Asbury AK, Winegrad AI, Porte D, eds. Diabetic neuropathy. Philadelphia: WB Saunders, 1987:36-44.

6.   Asbury AK. Focal and multifocal neuropathies of diabetes. In: Dyck PJ, Thomas PK, Asbury AK, Winegrad AI, Porte D, eds. Diabetic neuropathy. Philadelphia: WB Saunders, 1987:45-55.

7.   Melton LJ, Dyck PJ, Karnes J, O'Brien PC. Epidemiology. In: Dyck PJ, Thomas PK, Asbury AK, Winegrad AI, Porte D, eds. Diabetic neuropathy. Philadelphia: WB Saunders, 1987:27-35.

8.   Harati Y. Frequently asked questions about diabetic peripheral neuropathies. Neurol Clin 1992;10:783-806.

9.   Pirart J. Diabetes mellitus and its degenerative complications: a prospective study of 4,400 patients observed between 1947 and 1973. Diabetes Care 1978;1:168-88, 252-63.

10. Palumbo PJ, Elveback LR, Whisnant JP. Neurologic complications of diabetes mellitus: transient ischemic attack, stroke, and peripheral neuropathy. Adv Neurol 1978;19:593-601.

11. Dolman CL. The morbid anatomy of diabetic neuropathy. Neurology 1963;13:135-42.

12. Rollo J. Cases of diabetes mellitus. London: C Dilly, 1978.

13. Committee on Health Care Issues, American Neurological Association. Does improved control of glycemia prevent or ameliorate diabetic neuropathy? Ann Neurol 1986;19:288-90.

14. Clements RS Jr. Diabetic neuropathy — new concepts of its etiology. Diabetes 1979;28:604-11.

15. Greene DA, Sima AAF, Albers JW, Pfeifer MA. Diabetic neuropathy. In: Rifkin H, Porte Jr D, eds. Ellenberg and Rifkin's diabetes mellitus: theory and practice. 4th ed. New York: Elsevier Science Publishing, 1990:710-55.

16. Greene DA, Sima AAF, Stevens MJ, Feldman EL, Lattimer SA. Complications: neuropathy, pathogenic considerations. Diabetes Care 1992;15:1902-25.

17. Britland ST, Young RJ, Sharma AK, Clarke BF. Association of painful and painless diabetic polyneuropathy with different patterns of nerve fiber degeneration and regeneration. Diabetes 1990;39:898-908.

18. Capsaicin Study Group. Effect of treatment with capsaicin on daily activities of patients with painful diabetic neuropathy. Diabetes Care 1992;15:159-65.

19. Giguliano D, Marfella R, Quatraro A, et al. Tolrestat for mild diabetic neuropathy. Ann Int Med 1993;118:7-11.

20.   Sinha S, Munichoodapa CS, Kozak GP. Neuro-arthropathy ('Charcot joints') in diabetes mellitus: clinical study of 101 cases. Medicine (Baltimore) 1972;51:191-210.

21.   Cyrus J, Broadstone VL, Pfeifer MA, Greene DA. Diabetic peripheral neuropathy. Part II. Autonomic neuropathies. Diabetes Educ 1987;13:111-14.

22.   Vinik AI, Holland MT, LeBeau JM, Liuzzi FJ, Stansberry KB, Colen LB. Diabetic neuropathies. Diabetes Care 1992;15:1926-75.

23.   Stevens MJ, Feldman EL, Funnell MM, Sima AAF, Greene DG. Optimal methods for detecting early neuropathy and its progression. In: Morgenstern CE, Standl E, eds. Concepts for the ideal diabetes clinic. Vol IV. Berlin: deGruyter Publications, 1993:315-32.

KEY EDUCATIONAL CONSIDERATIONS

1. The importance of foot inspection and care cannot be overemphasized for patients with peripheral neuropathy. See Chapter XXV: Lower Extremity Problems for detailed information of this content.

2. Periodically assess patients with diabetes for the presence of modifiable risk factors for peripheral neuropathy, including hyperglycemia, alcohol abuse, and smoking.

    a) Refer patients to counseling or organizations such as Alcoholics Anonymous if they identify alcohol abuse as a problem.

    b) Discuss the added risk that smoking poses and ascertain the patient's thoughts about stopping. Provide information about local smoking cessation programs. Some patients may find that nicotine patches or gum help in their attempts to stop smoking.

3. Because some manifestations of neuropathy (eg, sexual dysfunction, incontinence) may be embarrassing for the patient to discuss, a tactful assessment of these problems should be done during each visit.

4. Informing patients about the symptoms of neuropathy and encouraging them to report these to their health care professional is important and can provide the basis for group discussion. Specific information about the neuropathic symptoms that the patient is experiencing and treatment options and approaches should be provided individually.

5. This content can be difficult to teach and detailed explanations of the complexity of the nervous system are unnecessary. Present a simple concept such as, "Some nerves send information about how things feel, others tell the body to move and others control automatic body functions." Teaching should focus on what the patient needs to know such as symptoms and treatment, with pathology discussed only as needed. Visual aids can assist patient understanding.

    a) Reinforce the relationship between hyperglycemia and neuropathic pain, and discuss specific individualized options for improving blood glucose levels.

    b) Open-ended questions will often yield information about a patient's use of nontraditional therapies for pain.

c) Offer patients options for nonpharmacologic and pharmacologic treatment for pain.

d) Because most therapies to relieve neuropathic pain take time to work, prepare patients for the delay and encourage them to give therapy a fair trial before discontinuing it.

e) The depression that can accompany painful neuropathy may act as a barrier to learning. In conjunction with treatment for depression and neuropathy, focus patient teaching on what the patient can do to ease the discomfort and prevent other related problems.

f) Encourage patients with neuropathy to stay informed about new research studies and findings about the treatment of neuropathy.

6. Education about complications should be provided with sensitivity and only after the patient's readiness to hear this information has been determined. Point out the value of early detection and hope for future treatment of neuropathy.

SELF-REVIEW QUESTIONS

If you are unsure of the answers to the following questions, please review the materials.

1. What is neuropathy?
2. What are the classifications of neuropathy and their respective sub-categories?
3. What roles do aldose reductase, glucose, myo-inositol and ATPase play in the pathology of diabetic neuropathy?
4. What therapies are available for painful peripheral polyneuropathy?
5. What are the major symptoms, clinical manifestations, and treatment for autonomic neuropathy?
6. What should all patients with diabetes be taught about neuropathy?

CASE EXAMPLE

MJ is a 56-year-old black man with a 7-year history of NIDDM. His diabetes has been treated with 5.0 mg of glyburide twice a day for the past 5 years. He does not monitor his blood glucose levels at home, and his most recent glycosylated hemoglobin value was 10.6% (normal is 4% to 8%). He reports some blurred vision, but denies any other symptoms of hyperglycemia. He is 5 ft 8 in tall and weighs 198 lb (89 kg). He has been given a 1600-calorie ADA diet, but states that he is hungry all of the time when he tries to follow it. His weight has been stable at about 200 lb (90 kg) since diagnosis. MJ is married, has three grown children, and works as a carpenter. He presents today with burning and tingling sensations in his feet, impotence for the past 3 months, and occasional dizziness on standing. His wife calls you aside and tells you that she is concerned because he appears to be depressed and is withdrawing from friends and family. She is also concerned because his cigarette smoking has recently increased to two packs per day. MJ reports occasional alcohol intake on social occasions.

On physical examination, MJ has diminished bilateral vibratory and pinprick response, and dry feet. His sitting blood pressure (BP) is 148/84 mm Hg, his supine BP 136/82 mm Hg; and his standing BP, 100/76 mm Hg. His fasting blood glucose is 196 mg/dL (10.9 mmol/L). When asked, he tells you that he takes care of his feet by soaking them in hot water when he gets home from work each night.

QUESTIONS

1. What are the medical and educational concerns?
2. How would you prioritize MJ's care?

SUGGESTED SOLUTIONS

MJ's needs are complex but typical, and raise the issue of what to do first so as not to overwhelm the patient. A careful assessment of presenting symptoms and concerns help the team, including MJ and his wife, decide where to begin. After the discussion MJ is referred to a urologist for further assessment of his impotence and to a social worker for evaluation of depression.

The need for better control of blood glucose levels is discussed as a way to decrease symptoms and MJ is offered options to improve glycemic control through initiation of insulin therapy and/or meal planning. MJ is also referred to a dietitian for a meal plan that fits his lifestyle and caloric needs. If MJ elects to begin insulin therapy, the dietitian will also provide information on balancing food intake with insulin. MJ is instructed on how and when to monitor his blood glucose levels.

Basic education is also provided about neuropathy, foot care, and safety issues related to carpentry work and orthostatic hypotension. MJ's thoughts about quitting smoking are discussed, as is the impact of smoking on his circulation, neuropathy, and general health. MJ states that he would like to quit and has attempted to several times in the last year. Information is provided about methods and support available for smoking cessation.

MJ is asked to return within 2 weeks for evaluation of his symptoms and blood glucose control; reinforcement of his blood glucose monitoring technique; instruction on interpreting and acting upon blood glucose results; review of his new meal plan; and follow-up smoking cessation plans. Subsequent visits will continue to address and build on these issues as well as follow up on the treatment plan for his impotence and depression.

OTHER SUGGESTED READINGS

Albert L. Restraining pain. Diabetes Forecast 1988;41(1):39-41.

American Diabetes Association. Consensus statement: diabetic neuropathy. Diabetes Care 1991;14(suppl 2):63-68.

Barnett JL. Taking care of constipation. Diabetes Forecast 1992;45(5):25-27.

Broadstone VL, Cyrus J, Pfeifer MA, Greene DA. Diabetic peripheral neuropathy. Part I. Sensorimotor neuropathy. Diabetes Educ 1987;13:30-35.

Campbell RK, Baker DE. New drug update: Capsaicin. Diabetes Educ 1990;16:313-14, 316.

Cohen SN. Treating impotence. Diabetes Forecast 1991;44(12):54-57.

Cronin B. Nutritional concerns in gastrointestinal neuropathy. Diabetes Educ 1992;18:531-35.

Cyrus J, Broadstone VL, Pfeifer MA, Greene DA. Diabetic peripheral neuropathy. Part II: Autonomic neuropathies. Diabetes Educ 1986;13:111--15.

Fogel CI. Sexuality and diabetes: an issue for both sexes. Diabetes Spectrum 1991;4(1):13-40.

Funnell MM, McNitt PM. Autonomic neuropathy. Am J Nurs 1986; 86:266-70.

Greene DA, Sima AAF, Stevens MJ, Feldman EL, Lattimer SA. Complications: neuropathy, pathogenic considerations. Diabetes Care 1992;15:1902-25.

Graham C. Neuropathy made you stop? Diabetes Forecast 1992; 45(12):47-49.

Haire-Joshu D. Smoking, cessation and the diabetes health care team. Diabetes Educ 1991;17:54-64.

Haas LB. Chronic complications of diabetes. Nurs Clin North Am 1993;28:71-86.

Ivy J. Exercise and complications. Diabetes Forecast 1990;43(2):46-49.

Lagana DJ. Female sexuality: separating fact from fiction. Diabetes Self-Manage 1992;9(4):40-42.

Leese DL. Diabetic cranial mononeuropathies: a patient's perspective. Diabetes Educ 1988;14:527-31.

Martin FL. When the solution is a prosthesis. RN 1990;53(Mar):32-35.

Maser RE, Becker DJ, Drash AL, et al. Pittsburgh epidemiology of diabetes complications study. Diabetes Care 1992;15:525-27.

McCall AL. Impact of diabetes on the central nervous system. Diabetes 1992;41:557-70.

O'Dorisio TM, Cataland S. Gastrointestinal autonomic neuropathy. Diabetes Spectrum 1992;5(3):147-72.

Reznichek CG, Reznichek R. The problem most men won't talk about. RN 1990;53(Mar):28-32.

Schover LR. Women, sexuality and diabetes. Diabetes Forecast 1992;45(8):59-61.

Vinik AI, Holland MT, LeBeau JM, Liuzzi FJ, Stansberry KB, Colen LB. Diabetic neuropathies. Diabetes Care 1992;15:1926-75.

Vinik AI, Vinik E. The diabetes complication no one talks about. Diabetes Forecast 1992;45(7):71-74.

Wakelee-Lynch J. Relieving pain with peppers. Diabetes Forecast 1992;45(6):35-37.

Whitehead ED. Diabetes-related impotence: putting new knowledge to waste. Geriatrics 1988;43:114-20.

Wyeth-Ayerst Consensus Conference. Proceedings of a consensus development conference on standardized measures in diabetic neuropathy. Diabetes Care 1992;15:1079-1108.

COMPLICATIONS

XXIII.   KIDNEY DISEASE

INTRODUCTION

Diabetic nephropathy, the kidney disease associated with diabetes mellitus, is characterized clinically by albuminuria, hypertension, and progressive renal insufficiency.[1] Currently, diabetic nephropathy is the most common cause of new cases of end-stage renal disease (ESRD) in the United States.[2] In 1936, Kimmelstiel and Wilson,[3] after examining patients with non-insulin-dependent diabetes mellitus (NIDDM) on autopsy, termed the disease *nodular intercapillary glomerulosclerosis*. Today, *diabetic nephropathy* is the term used to describe one of the major forms of small-vessel (microvascular) disease found in diabetes. Important differences are found in the incidence and prevalence of ESRD due to diabetes among various racial groups in the United States. In insulin-dependent diabetes mellitus (IDDM), also called type I diabetes, nephropathy is more common in whites than in nonwhites. ESRD due to NIDDM, also called type II diabetes, is more prevalent among nonwhites, with the highest rates being found among American Indians, blacks and Hispanics.[4]

Caring for patients with diabetic nephropathy is challenging and requires the expertise of medicine, surgery, nursing, social services, podiatry, nutrition, and rehabilitation services. Preventing or slowing the progression of this chronic complication has received much attention recently as newer strategies have proven successful. Additionally, striving to inform and involve patients and families is critical to health promotion and treatment during all phases of kidney disease and treatments.

Interventions aimed at optimizing care and quality of life for the patient with diabetes who has renal disease include controlling blood pressure and blood glucose levels, preventing insults to the kidney, decreasing dietary protein intake and, recently, treating the symptomatic anemia of kidney disease with erythropoietin. When renal replacement therapy is required, careful consideration of individual needs must be incorporated into the decision-making process. Current options in uremia therapy include: no therapy (resulting in death), hemodialysis, peritoneal dialysis, kidney transplant, or a simultaneous kidney-pancreas transplant (for IDDM). Medical and nutrition management are incorporated into each of the modalities. No matter what the stage of renal disease or type of renal replacement therapy, both the patient and the health care team must recognize that the patient's diabetes still requires daily attention, and medical and nutritional management will be integral components of that management.

OBJECTIVES

Upon completion of this chapter, the learner will be able to:

- describe the basic functions of the kidneys;
- list the tests used to assess kidney function and to track disease progression;
- list the major stages and syndromes in diabetic nephropathy;
- describe current conservative measures to treat diabetic nephropathy;
- list current treatment options for renal replacement therapy.

A. Key Definitions

1. The *nephron* is the functioning unit of the kidneys that serves to clear the blood of waste materials and form urine. Each kidney contains about 1 million nephrons. Each nephron consists of a glomerulus leading to a long tubule in which the filtrate is concentrated and modified before it is eliminated as urine.

2. The *glomerulus* is the filtering component of the nephron. It is a tuft of capillaries in which filtration of the blood takes place. A kidney biopsy will show diabetic changes in the glomerulus in a patient with diabetic nephropathy.

3. *Glomerular filtration* initiates the production of urine with the formation of an ultrafiltrate of plasma by the glomerulus.

4. *Glomerular filtration rate (GFR)* is the amount of plasma passing through the glomerulus per minute. Normal GFR is 100 to 125 mL/min. This is a precise technique determined by measuring the renal clearance of a marker substance and is used primarily in research. GFR decreases with aging, the presence of kidney

or vascular diseases, sodium and water depletion, hemorrhage, and vigorous exercise; it increases with dietary protein intake, hyperglycemia, and pregnancy. Repeat measurements of GFR over time provide more useful information than a single value.

5. *Creatinine clearance* (CrCl) provides an estimate of GFR and is an approximate measure of kidney function. Creatinine clearance is used clinically (rather than GFR) because it is more easily determined. To calculate CrCl, a timed urine specimen and a serum or plasma sample are required. Since the clearance depends on protein intake, in the absence of renal disease, an individual's CrCl would be a reflection of his/her diet. The CrCl on a typical Western diet in an adult male is 100-120 mL/min. In women, the clearance is slightly lower, probably because women have less muscle mass, the tissue in which creatinine is formed.

6. *Blood urea nitrogen* (BUN) is the blood level of urea. Urea is the end product of protein metabolism and is formed in the liver. After synthesis, urea travels through the blood and is excreted in the urine. The normal plasma value is 8 to 20 mg/dL (2.9 to 7.1 mmol/L), varying with the quantity and quality of protein intake, state of hydration, and kidney function.

7. *Creatinine* (cr), another nitrogen compound, is formed mainly from the metabolism of muscle. The daily production rate is relatively constant in an individual. The normal plasma value is 0.5 to 1.4 mg/dL (44 to 124 µmol/L), varying with body size and gender, with men having higher levels than women. Plasma creatinine rises as kidney function deteriorates.

8. *Microalbuminuria* is an abnormal excretion of slightly increased quantities of urinary albumin. Persistent microalbuminuria (30 to 300 mg/24 h occurring in more than one 24-hour urine collection) is often the first laboratory evidence of renal

damage. An excretion rate of up to 30 mg/24 h is considered normal.

9. *Proteinuria* is the presence of protein in the urine. Excess amounts of protein are pathologic, indicating either systemic disease or intrinsic kidney disease.

10. *Nephrotic syndrome* is characterized by protein excretion >3.5 g/24 h. Typically the rate of protein excretion can rise from 4 to 30 g protein/24 h, resulting in low blood proteins and massive fluid retention, often with ascites and pleural effusion.

11. *Uremia* is a syndrome characteristic of ESRD that develops because of extreme reduction in renal function, causing urea, creatinine, and other metabolic products to accumulate in the blood. This results in anemia, osteodystrophy, neuropathy, and acidosis. Nausea, hypertension, susceptibility to infection, and generalized organ dysfunction frequently accompany this syndrome.

12. *End-stage renal disease* (ESRD) is the term used to describe advanced kidney failure. Renal replacement therapy must be employed for life to continue.

B. Description and Function of Kidneys

1. Normally, people have two kidneys located posterior to the abdominal cavity. Each kidney is the size and shape of an Idaho potato and weighs approximately 5 oz (150 g).

2. The kidneys maintain the internal environment of the body by regulating the quality of the extracellular fluid.

3. Blood flow to the kidneys is approximately 1300 mL/min and accounts for 25% of the cardiac output.

4. An excretory organ, the kidney performs metabolic and endocrine functions.
   a) The kidneys remove water, urea, creatinine, and other waste products from the blood.
   b) The kidneys form urine.
   c) The kidneys selectively maintain electrolyte (sodium, potassium) and acid-base balance.
   d) Together with the heart and endocrine system, the kidneys regulate blood pressure.
   e) The kidneys produce erythropoietin, a hormone that helps in the formation of red blood cells.

C. Diabetic Nephropathy

1. The United States Renal Data Systems (USRDS) collects information on ESRD in the United States.[5]
   a) In 1990, 195,000 persons were enrolled in ESRD programs.
   b) In 1992, 45,153 new patients initiated therapy for renal failure. Of these, 34% were diagnosed as having diabetes.

2. The incidence rate of ESRD among patients with diabetes has been increasing at a striking rate (see Figure XXIII.1).
   a) Blacks with diabetes are more than twice as likely as whites with diabetes to be treated for ESRD secondary to diabetes. This is probably due not only to the higher prevalence of diabetes among blacks, but also to differences in severity of disease and health care use between blacks and whites.
   b) Men are at particular risk for ESRD associated with IDDM.

3. Renal failure occurs in 5% to 15% of patients with NIDDM.
   a) The course of renal failure in NIDDM is more uncertain than in IDDM, in part because of the difficulty in dating the onset of NIDDM. In addition, coexisting diseases found in the older population can contribute to or cause

kidney damage, such as preexisting hypertension or systemic atherosclerosis.[6]

b)   It has been reported that patients who develop NIDDM at a later age may progress to nephropathy more rapidly than those who develop NIDDM at an earlier age, although the exact date of onset of NIDDM is often ambiguous.[7]

c)   The majority of patients with diabetes who are on dialysis in the United States have NIDDM. Although only 5% to 15% of persons with NIDDM become uremic compared with 30% to 40% of persons with IDDM, the higher prevalence of NIDDM yields an expected ratio of five uremic patients with NIDDM for every two uremic patients with IDDM.[8]

Figure XXIII.1

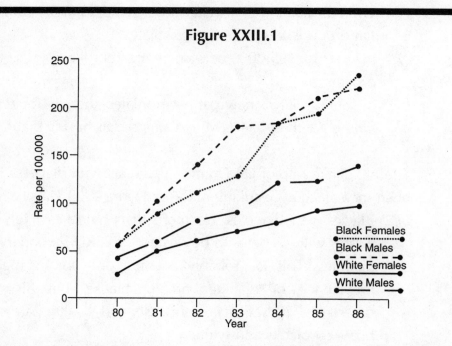

Age-standardized incidence rate of end-stage renal disease due to diabetes per 100,000 diabetic population, by race, sex, and year, United States, 1980-1986.

Reprinted from Diabetes Surveillance, 1990.

4.   Renal failure occurs in about 30% of persons with IDDM in a mean time of 20 years after diagnosis.

a) The sequence of events of diabetic nephropathy in IDDM is under debate, and research is ongoing.

b) Current theory supposes five stages of renal involvement in IDDM[9-11] (see Table XXIII.1).

  (1) *Stage I* is characterized by hyperfunction and hypertrophy.

    (a) Hyperfunction and hypertrophy are seen at diagnosis of diabetes.

    (b) Acute kidney changes include high GFR, enlarged kidneys, and hypertrophy of nephrons.

  (2) *Stage II* is "silent."

    (a) Renal hyperfunction and hypertrophy may be present without clinical or laboratory signs of disease.

    (b) Structural abnormalities are present. Two types of lesions are identifiable by a kidney biopsy: nodular glomerulosclerosis (obliteration of glomeruli segments by amorphous material first evident in the central mesangial area of the glomerulus), and diffuse glomerulosclerosis (deposition of amorphous material in all areas in the glomerulus between capillary loops). These pathologic findings have been termed the *Kimmelstiel-Wilson lesion*.

  (3) *Stage III* is incipient diabetic nephropathy.

    (a) Microalbuminuria (development to proteinuric level) may last 10 years.

    (b) Mild to moderate hypertension is present.

  (4) *Stage IV* is overt diabetic nephropathy.

    (a) Clinical disease is evidenced by the nephrotic syndrome, hypertension, renal insufficiency (declining GFR to below 25 to 30 mL/min), and azotemia.

  (5) *Stage V* is characterized by uremia, culminating in end-stage renal disease.

    (a) GFR is <15 mL/min.

TABLE XXIII.1:

Schematic Natural History Outline of Diabetic Nephropathy (IDDM)

	Stage				
	I At diagnosis, acute changes	II First Decade (≈7-13 y)	III Second Decade (≈7-25 y)	IV Third Decade (Or Last ≈8-12 y)	V ESRF (after ≈30 y)
GFR	High*	Still HF (total and single nephron)	Still HF, but declining GFR	Fall rate 12 mL/y; single-nephron-HF likely	Close to zero
UAER	High* or normal	Normal, but slightly increasing	Increasing microalbuminuria	Increasing proteinuria	Still P
BP or HT	BP usually normal	BP comparable with background population (HT seen in ≈ 5% - 10%)	BP increasing 3% per year	HT increasing 7% per year	High BP
Suggested basic changes	Metabolic and hemodynamic changes, plus hyperphagia	*Metabolic* ↑Glycemia ↑AR ↑Hormones *Hemodynamic* Normal BP but intrarenal HT likely *Diet* Usually high in protein	*Metabolic* ↑Glycemia ↑AR ↑Hormones *Hemodynamic* Systemic and Intrarenal HT *Diet* Usually high in protein	*Metabolic* ↑Glycemia ↑AR ↑Hormones *Hemodynamic* Systemic and Intrarenal HT *Diet* Usually high in protein	Nephron closure
Other concomitant abnormality	HbA$_{1c}$↑ and many metabolic changes	Possibly hyperperfusion	Retinopathy and neuropathy, lipid changes and vascular disease in general	As III, but increasing in severity	Uremia
Main structural counterparts	Hypertrophy of nephrons	Hypertrophy of nephrons, BM thickening after ≈ 2 years Mesangial expansion after ≈ 5 years	Microalbuminuria associated with more advanced ultrastructural lesions	Advancing structural lesion especially mesangial expansion and glomerular closure	Nephron closure

Abbreviations: HF, hyperfiltration; P, proteinuria; HT, hypertension; AR, aldose reductase activity; BM, basement membrane; UAER, urinary albumin excretion rate; BP, blood pressure

* Reversible.

Source: Reprinted with permission from Mogensen.[9]

(b) Patients with diabetes are clinically sicker than patients without diabetes at the same level of kidney dysfunction.

(c) Usually, patients with a serum creatinine level >5 mg/dL (>442 µmol/L) are unable to resume their normal activities because of signs and symptoms of uremia, including nausea, vomiting, lethargy, anemia, hypertension, acidosis, and fluctuating blood glucose levels. (One-fourth to one-third of injected insulin is catabolized by the kidney and, as kidney function deteriorates, exogenous insulin acts longer and in an unpredictable manner.)

5. The management and rehabilitation of these patients are further complicated by the fact that more than 95% of patients with diabetic nephropathy have some degree of retinopathy, with 50% being blind or having lost significant vision (renal-retinal syndrome).[8] Refer to Chapter XXI: Eye Disease for more information on this complication.

D. Interventions for Patients with Diabetes at Risk for Renal Disease

1. The probability that the natural history of diabetic nephropathy and the stages described will change (or have already changed) is strong because of the interventions employed for patients with diabetes in general and for those patients with early renal disease.

2. These interventions include optimizing glycemic control, controlling blood pressure, and decreasing dietary protein intake[9] (see Table XXIII.2).

   a) *Glycemic Control.* The Diabetes Control and Complications Trial (DCCT), a randomized, controlled, multicenter clinical trial, has determined that intensive

TABLE XXIII.2:

Effect of Parameters or Surrogate Endpoints in Diabetic Nephropathy

Parameter	Technical Problems	Association with Progression, Possibly to ESRF	Main Confounding Elements	Evidence of Amelioration by Intervention
Hyperfiltration or GFR measurement	Constant infusion technique required	Found by one group in retrospective analyses	Poor metabolic control	Optimized insulin treatment, somatostatin analogues; ARI, low protein diet
MA or measurement of UAE	Due to variability, multiple collections are necessary	Found in three independent studies	Marginal BP elevation noted in MA in addition to somewhat poorer control	Optimized insulin treatment, low protein diet, antihypertensive treatment (including ACE-inhibitors)
Development of BP elevation	Due to observer bias, blinded procedures or ambulatory 24-h procedures required	Not clearly documented to be independent of proteinuria	Associated with MA and proteinuria	Antihypertensive treatment almost all agents effective on BP in diabetic persons
Degree of proteinuria or development of proteinuria	Multiple collection required	Clearly associated with development of ESRF	Nondiabetic renal disease	Antihypertensive treatment (including ACE-inhibitors), low protein diet
Fall rate of GFR	Exact measurement of GFR necessary	Clearly associated with development of ESRF	Nonexact measures of GFR	Antihypertensive treatment (including ACE-inhibitors), low protein diet
Structural analysis of renal biopsies	No studies available on representativity/reproducibility	Likely, but no documentation in longitudinal studies	Predictive value not known	No data available

Abbreviations: GFR, glomerular filtration rate; MA, microalbuminuria; UAE, urinary albumin excretion; ACE, angiotensin-converting enzyme; ESRF, end-stage renal failure; ARI, aldose reductase inhibitors.

Source: Reprinted with permission from Mogensen CE. Diabetic nephropathy in IDDM patients: how to measure progression of disease and effect of treatment. J Diabetes Comp 1991;5:65-71.

insulin and dietary therapy to maintain strict glycemic control delays the onset and slows the progression of early vascular complications in patients with IDDM (including diabetic nephropathy).[12]

(1) Studies have demonstrated that IDDM patients with microalbuminuria who were treated intensively (with insulin pump therapy [CSII]) had no further progress of their nephropathy while those who were treated conventionally went on to develop clinical proteinuria.[9]

(2) Factors affecting blood glucose values vary, depending on kidney function. As renal disease progresses, blood glucose control becomes more challenging because of slower degradation of insulin, altered appetite, fluctuating nausea, restricted dietary protein intake, diuretic therapy, and emotional stress.

b) *Blood pressure control.* Treatment for hypertension must be preceded by a careful assessment of the patient.

(1) Assessment involves exploring a number of areas:

- Is the patient overweight?
- Does the patient need to be on a sodium-restricted diet?
- What is the patient's daily alcohol consumption?
- Does the patient smoke cigarettes?
- Is the patient involved in a regular exercise program?
- Is the patient taking any drug (prescribed or over-the-counter medication) known to raise the blood pressure or glucose levels?
- Does the patient have a surgically correctable form of hypertension (renovascular disease or Cushing's syndrome)?[13]

(2) Some of the drugs known to increase blood pressure include oral contraceptives, steroidal and nonsteroidal antiinflammatory agents, nasal

decongestants, appetite suppressants, and tricyclic antidepressants (see also Chapter VIII: Pharmacologic Therapies).

(3) It is important to clarify for patients that a single blood pressure reading does not constitute a diagnosis of high blood pressure but indicates that additional observation is necessary.

(4) The desired blood pressure is a standing blood pressure of approximately 120-130/70-80 mm Hg.[8]

(5) Supine hypertension and orthostatic hypotension sometimes occur in patients with autonomic neuropathy and are difficult for the patient and challenging for the practitioner. It is recommended that, in this situation, blood pressure be determined supine, immediately on standing, and after 1 minute in the upright position.

(6) To help prevent extreme orthostatic reduction in blood pressure, the blood pressure in the standing position must be considered as the therapeutic end point when evaluating treatment with hypertensive agents.[13]

(7) To establish timing and proper dosage of antihypertensive drugs, 24-hour ambulatory blood pressure recordings or at-home monitoring can be obtained. Self-monitoring of blood pressure enhances educational efforts and affords the patient and health care providers the opportunity to work together in detection, treatment, and evaluation. Reviewing patients' technique and checking blood-pressure monitoring devices regularly can help insure correct readings.

(8) Studies have demonstrated that angiotensin-converting enzyme (ACE) inhibitors given alone or with a conventional antihypertensive agent produce a reduction of urinary albumin excretion rate in early

renal disease, but long-term studies of efficacy are needed.[9]

(9) Other classes of antihypertensive agents include, but are not limited to: diuretics (hydrochlorothiazide, furosemide, metolazone), calcium channel blockers (nifedipine), sympathetic inhibitors (clonidine), and vasodilators (hydralazine).[8]

(10) Complications affecting patients with diabetes can occur when using antihypertensive agents. These complications may include worsening of lipid levels and glycemic control (because of the use of diuretics), altered symptoms of hypoglycemia (from beta-adrenergic blockers), fluid retention (from sympathetic inhibitors and vasodilators), and hyperkalemia and worsening azotemia (when using an ACE inhibitor in patients with kidney disease).[8]

c) *Decreasing Dietary Protein Intake.* The amount of protein in the diet affects renal size, structure, and function.

(1) A high protein diet has been shown to increase both renal size and GFR.

(a) Increases in GFR, termed *hyperfiltration*, occur early in diabetic renal disease.

(b) Brenner and others[14] believe that hyperfiltration increases intrarenal pressure within the glomerulus, which is instrumental to the destruction of the kidneys.

(2) Protein restriction in a rat model has reduced the degree of hyperfiltration, hence the theory that protein restriction in humans will alter the course of kidney destruction.[14]

(3) Studies in humans have demonstrated that low-protein diets can be achieved (with effort), without compromise to nutritional status and without danger to metabolic control, and they may result in positive effects on lipid profiles.

(4) The Recommended Dietary Allowance (RDA) for adults — Food and Nutrition Board (1989) — is an intake of 0.8 g protein/kg of ideal body weight (IBW) (45-65 g protein/day). Considering that the usual dietary intake of protein in US diets is 1.2 to 1.4 g/kg of body weight per day, an intake of 1.0 g/kg of IBW or the recommended 0.8 g/kg of IBW per day is in fact a decrease in protein intake for most people.[15]

(5) Low-protein diets, such as 0.67 (SEM 0.03) g/kg of IBW per day have been shown to decrease blood pressure, reduce the rate of decline in GFR, and decrease albumin excretion.[16]

(a) These preliminary results are encouraging but must be confirmed in larger prospective, controlled studies.

(b) The feasibility of achieving long-term patient adherence with such a restricted diet must be tested.[17]

(c) A reduction in daily dietary protein intake to between 0.6 and 0.8 g/kg of IBW in patients with early nephropathy has been recommended by some, but further research is needed to define diet therapy at different levels of kidney function[18] (see Table XXIII.3 for recommended daily dietary guidelines for patients with diabetes and chronic renal disease and for those receiving various forms of uremia therapy).

d) Several preventive measures are recommended for patients with diabetes who are at risk for renal disease.

(1) To avoid urinary tract infections, educate the patient about signs and symptoms; obtain cultures to detect specific organisms; repeat urine cultures after treatment with antibiotics; ascertain whether bladder dysfunction is contributory; and avoid placing an

TABLE XXIII.3:
Recommended Daily Dietary Guidelines for Diabetic Patients

(American Dietetic Association, 1981, 1987; American Diabetes Association, 1990
Kopple, 1988; Powers, 1987)

	Chronic Renal Failure Predialysis	Hemodialysis	CAPD	Post-Transplant
Protein	0.6 g/kg (50% HBV protein*)	1.0-1.2 g/kg (50% HBV protein*)	1.2-1.5 g/kg (50% HBV protein*)	0.8-1.0 g/kg
Fat	35%[†]	30%	30%	25-30%
Carbohydrate[‡]	Remainder of nonprotein calories			
Calories	35 kcal/kg unless the patient's weight is greater than 120% or the patient gains unwanted weight			Assess basal and activity needs; for weight gain add 300-500 kcal/day
Phosphorus	10 mg/kg	17 mg/kg	17 mg/kg	No restriction
Sodium	1000-3000 mg	2000 mg	3000-4000 mg	3000-4000 mg
Potassium	No restriction unless oliguric	2000-3000 mL	No restriction	No restriction
Fluid	1500-3000 mL	1000 mL	2000-3000 mL	Adequate fluid to prevent dehydration

* HBV = high biological value protein.
† With restricted protein, fat is >30% in order to meet calorie needs.
‡ Emphasis is on complex carbohydrate and fiber.

Abbreviations: CAPD, Continuous Ambulatory Peritoneal Dialysis.

Source: Reprinted with permission from Scopelite.[15]

indwelling Foley catheter (intermittent catheterization is less likely to introduce organisms).

(2) Avoid nephrotoxic drugs.

（*a*）　If such agents (eg, aminoglycosides such as gentamicin) must be used, blood levels must be monitored and the drug administered in reduced dosage to the patient with impaired renal function.

（*b*）　In addition, when possible, avoid nonsteroidal antiinflammatory drugs such as ibuprofen.

(3)　Avoid radiographic dyes.

（*a*）　If contrast media agents must be used for tests, an osmotic diuresis induced by Mannitol administered intravenously 1 hour prior to the study gives some protection.

（*b*）　Contrast media should not be administered to any person with diabetes whose serum creatinine level is >3 mg/dL (>265 μmol/L) unless the information sought is not available by any other means.

E.　Treatment Options for Uremia

1.　Providing education and information for the patient and family will enhance the chances for a positive outcome.

a)　Direct contact with other patients who are receiving different forms of uremia therapy may be valuable for education, emotional support, and instilling hope.

b)　Benefits and risks of each treatment option should be reviewed with patients and family members (see Table XXIII.4 for a comparison of options in uremia therapy).

2.　Planning for treatment should begin early, usually when the serum creatinine level reaches 3 mg/dL (265 μmol/L).

a)　Planning includes tissue typing of family members for possible kidney transplant donation, being placed on a cadaveric waiting list, and/or creating vascular access for dialysis.

TABLE XXIII.4:
Comparison of Options in Uremia Therapy
for Diabetic Patients with ESRD

	Renal Transplantation	CAPD	Home Hemodialysis
Advantages	• Permits long intervals away from treatment facility • Best rehabilitation data • "Cure" of uremia • Patient survival often >10 yr	• Avoids major surgery • Minimizes cardio-vascular "stress" (volume shifts) • Facilitates glucose control (when insulin added to dialysate) • Can be rapidly taught as a home dialysis regimen • No need for vascular access	• Avoids major surgery • NIDDM patients have survived >10 yr • rHu-EPO* may improve rehabilitation
Disadvantages	• Steroids exacerbate poor metabolic control • Cyclosporine exacerbates hypertension • Risk of infection • Inability to predict risk of diabetes in familial donors • May not be appropriate in severe cardiovascular disease or chronically infected patient • Risk of recurrent diabetic nephropathy (minimal) • Retinopathy progresses in 30% of patients	• High technique failure rate and mortality • Risk of peritonitis • Retinopathy progresses • Risk of patient burn-out because of daily repetitive nature of technique	• Requires a committed partner • "Failure-to-thrive" in about one third of patients • Mortality similar to cadaveric kidney recipients • Retinopathy progresses • Requires vascular access

* rHu-EPO = recombinant human erythropoietin.

Source: Reprinted with permission from Markell and Friedman.[6]

b) Circumstances may exist that limit the patient's choice of treatment. For example, those with vascular access problems or cardiovascular disease might not be suitable candidates for hemodialysis, or those unable to tolerate fluid in the peritoneal cavity would not be appropriate candidates for peritoneal dialysis.

3. Uremic patients have several options when deciding on treatment.

   a) If no treatment is administered, death will result — an elective decision for some patients.

      (1) The health care team and patient may need to consider this option after the patient is dialyzed and nonuremic.

      (2) Planning supportive care for the patient who wishes to forego treatment will be necessary, eg, home care, hospice care, etc.

   b) Transplantation of a healthy kidney from an appropriate donor is one solution for kidney failure.

      (1) Kidney transplantation can be performed using a kidney from a live related donor, a live unrelated donor, or a suitable cadaveric (brain dead) donor.

      (2) Once transplantation has occurred, immunosuppressive medications are required throughout the patient's life to prevent the body's rejection of the transplanted organ (see Table XXIII.5 for side effects of immunosuppression).

      (3) Patients with diabetes must take additional insulin following transplantation because the newly functioning kidney catabolizes insulin once again; posttransplant steroid therapy has a hyperglycemic effect; and the patient experiences a notable increase in appetite with subsequent weight gain.

      (4) Following transplantation, blood glucose control may be altered.

         (a) Among the factors affecting glycemic control are the degree of function of the transplanted kidney; the treatment for transplant rejection; changes in steroid dose; the patient's increased appetite and ability to consume a more liberal diet; a gain in weight; diuretic therapy; and the presence of infection (transplant patients are more susceptible to infection).

TABLE XXIII.5:
Side Effects of Immunosuppression

Prednisone

sodium (and water) retention
increased appetite
increased fat deposits
muscle wasting
increased serum cholesterol
calcium loss
sun sensitivity
increased stomach acid
night sweats
increased hair
acne
blurred vision
slowed healing
muscle weakness
hyperglycemia
susceptibility to infection
mood swings

Cyclosporine

flushing
hair growth
fine tremor
gingival hyperplasia
paresthesias
hyperkalemia
hypertension
gastrointestinal symptoms
nephrotoxicity

Sulfa drugs

liver toxicity
decreased leukocytes
allergy
sun sensitivity
gastrointestinal symptoms

Azathioprine

decreased leukocytes
liver toxicity
hair loss
allergy

Antacid drugs

diarrhea/constipation
low phosphorus
high magnesium

Antilymphocyte globin

allergy
decreased leukocytes
decreased platelets

Source: Reprinted with permission from Nettles.[20]

(b) The following are some questions to ask patients to help detect the cause of variability in blood glucose levels:

- What is your current immunosuppression regimen?

- Does that represent an increase or a decrease from your usual dose of immunosuppressive medication?

- How much weight have you gained since your transplant?
- Are you being treated for any infection?
- What antihypertensive/diuretic agents are you currently taking?
- What is your current exercise/activity schedule?

c) Patients with IDDM may consider a simultaneous kidney-pancreas transplantation.

(1) A kidney-pancreas transplantation restores both glucose metabolism and kidney function.

(2) Criteria for patient selection vary at each transplant center, but typically include: a diagnosis of insulin-dependent diabetes mellitus; evidence of secondary complications such as renal insufficiency or preproliferative retinopathy; metabolic instability; adequate financial resources/insurance coverage (insurance carriers review the patient's eligibility for payment on a case-by-case basis).

(3) Contraindications for this procedure include the presence of HIV, malignancy, psychosis, any active infection, severe neuropathies, and inoperable cardiovascular disease.

(4) Complications of this procedure include cardiac incompetence, arterial or venous thrombosis, anastomotic leaks, bleeding, and side effects of immunosuppression. Transplantation can be justified if the complications of diabetes are more dangerous than the side effects of immunosuppression.

(5) Renal transplant function is easier to measure than pancreas function.

(a) Hyperglycemia occurs late in pancreas rejection.

(b) Signs of rejection can be picked up earlier in the kidney and treatment initiated, thus providing some protection for the pancreas.

(6) Living related donors must be screened carefully because of their higher risk of developing diabetes. Brain-dead cadavers are a more common donor source.[19,20]

d) Dialysis is a process of cleansing or filtering the blood of nitrogenous wastes.

(1) The filter used for hemodialysis is a semipermeable membrane (a thin material with holes that permit the passage of small particles but keep back larger particles).

(2) During dialysis, the patient's blood passes on one side of the membrane, while dialysate (prepared dialysis solution) passes on the other side. The solution will draw fluid and particles (waste products) out of the blood.

(3) With effective dialysis treatments, the uremia can be treated and the patient returned to wellness, including a vigorous appetite.

(4) Several types of dialysis are in use:

(a) *Hemodialysis* circulates and cleanses the patient's blood outside of the body.

• The blood is withdrawn through a needle inserted in a specially prepared blood vessel, usually a synthetic graft or an arteriovenous fistula (using the patient's own blood vessels) located in the patient's forearm. The needle is attached by plastic tubing to a hemodialysis machine. A pump keeps blood moving through the dialyzer as wastes and fluid are filtered out. The cleansed blood returns to the patient through another needle in the same or an adjacent blood vessel.

• Hemodialysis can be performed in an ambulatory setting or in the patient's home. Treatments are usually given three times per week and take 3 to 6 hours to complete.

- Because the blood is not being cleansed 24 hours a day, the patient must adhere to a special diet with fluid restriction (individually prescribed).

- The use of recombinant human erythropoietin (rHu-EPO) to treat the anemia associated with renal failure has had a significant effect on rehabilitation in this population, improving quality-of-life indicators and employment status.[21]

- Patients with diabetes receiving dialytic therapy might be oliguric and therefore not experience the osmotic diuresis that typically accompanies hyperglycemia in a diabetic patient not undergoing dialysis. Satisfying the thirst that accompanies hyperglycemia might be an additional challenge for the patient when placed on a fluid-restricted diet.[15]

- Factors that can alter glucose control in the patient receiving hemodialysis treatment include: concentration of glucose in dialysate bath; appetite alteration on dialysis days and "off" days; decreased activity on dialysis days; and emotional stress.

- Examples of questions to help elicit information regarding the causes for blood glucose variability for the patient with diabetes who is receiving hemodialysis treatments include:

  - What is the pattern of glucose control on days you are having dialysis?

- What is the pattern on other days?
- When (and how much) do you eat on days you are having dialysis?
- What about other days?
- What is your hematocrit?
- What is the acceptable hematocrit range for the meter you are using?

- Sometimes a change in type of glucose meter used may be warranted to avoid measuring erroneous blood glucose values. Meter manufacturers provide specifications of hematocrit ranges for their meters (see Chapter IX: Monitoring and Management for more information).

(b) *Peritoneal dialysis* takes place inside the body by employing the body's own capillary and serosal membranes.

- Blood is filtered through the peritoneal membrane that lines the abdominal cavity. Surgery is required to place a catheter through an opening in the wall of the abdominal cavity. This opening is needed so that the dialysis solution can be instilled into the peritoneal cavity and waste products can pass from the bloodstream into the dialysis solution. The used solution is drained and replaced with a new solution on a regular basis.

- Two types of peritoneal dialysis are used today.

- Continuous ambulatory peritoneal dialysis (CAPD) is a manual method of performing peritoneal dialysis. The patient exchanges new fluid (dialysate) every 4 to 6 hours during a 24-hour period each day.

- Continuous cyclic peritoneal dialysis (CCPD) is performed with the help of a machine. The machine is responsible for the insertion and drainage of the dialysis solution.
- Patients requiring insulin can administer regular insulin directly into the dialysate before the dialysate is instilled into the peritoneal cavity. This frees the patient from subcutaneous injections.
- Regular insulin works to metabolize the dietary glucose that is consumed as well as the highly concentrated dextrose in the dialysate solution.
- Visually impaired and blind patients have been successful in performing peritoneal dialysis.
- Factors that can affect glucose regulation for patients on peritoneal dialysis include: the concentration of dialysate solution; method(s) of insulin delivery, eg, intraperitoneal, subcutaneous, or both; and infection (peritonitis).
- Examples of questions to ask to help assess the factors that may contribute to blood glucose variability include:
  - What is the dextrose concentration of the solution you are using for CAPD — 1.5%, 2.5%, or 4.25%?
  - What type(s) of insulin are you using?
  - When are you taking your insulin?
  - Where on your body are you injecting the insulin?
  - Are there any signs of infection (catheter related or peritonitis)?

F.   End-Stage Renal Disease: Psychosocial Issues

1.   Rates of depression, anxiety, and stress may be higher among dialysis patients (patients experiencing the loss of physical capacities and loss of control from the complications of diabetes) than among the general population.[22]

2.   Patients respond in a variety of ways upon hearing the diagnosis of renal disease. Some typical responses include:
   - "No one ever told me this could happen."
   - "My life is over."
   - "It's all my fault, if only I took better care of myself."
   - "It's all my doctor's fault."
   - "I feel that my body is falling apart, piece by piece."

3.   It is imperative to assess and comprehend each patient's (and family's) response to the patient's illness.
   a)   A variety of health care professionals, including mental health professionals, need to be involved in helping patients and families adjust to their losses and to a new and often complex treatment regimen.[22]
   b)   Some patients blame themselves when they develop complications of diabetes.
   c)   Educators should realize that using scare tactics ("If you don't control your blood sugar, you will go into kidney failure.") in an attempt to increase adherence to a regimen is not effective.
   d)   It is possible for complications, such as diabetic nephropathy, to develop in patients who adhere faithfully to their daily treatment regimen. It is therefore crucial that the health care team communicate this to the patient and family to help lessen the feelings of guilt and blame when the diagnosis of end-stage renal disease occurs.

4.   An effective intervention for patients with ESRD is to invite them to join a self-help group or to pair new patients with

patients who have been successfully rehabilitated as a result of one of the various renal replacement therapies.

a) Patients can learn new information, coping skills, behaviors, and positive attitudes from these "successful" patients.[22]

b) In addition, the availability of members of a self-help group in the clinic setting, ready and willing to meet new patients who face a diagnosis of renal disease, is extremely beneficial for the patients, their families, and the health care team.

REFERENCES

1. Herman HV, Hawthorne R, Hamman HK, et al. Consensus statement. Am J Kidney Dis 1989;13(1):2-6.

2. U.S. Renal Data System. USRDS 1989 annual data report. Bethesda, Md: National Institute of Diabetes and Digestive and Kidney Diseases, Aug 1989.

3. Kimmelstiel P, Wilson C. Intercapillary lesions in the glomeruli of the kidney. Am J Pathol 1936;2:83-97.

4. Rostand SG, Kirk KA, Rutsky EA, Pate BA. Racial differences in the incidence of treatment for end-stage renal disease. N Engl J Med 1982;5:172-75.

5. U.S. Renal Data System. USRDS 1993 annual data report. Bethesda, Md: National Institute of Diabetes and Digestive and Kidney Diseases, Feb 1993.

6. Markell MS, Friedman EA. Care of the diabetic patient with end-stage renal disease. Semin Nephrol 1990;10:274-86.

7. Lindblad AS, Nolph KD, Novak JW, et al. A survey of the NIH CAPD registry population with end-stage renal disease attributed to diabetic nephropathy. J Diabetes Comp 1988;2:227-32.

8. Friedman EA. Diabetic nephropathy: progress in treatment, potential for prevention. Diabetes Spectrum 1989;2:85-95.

9. Mogensen CE. Prevention and treatment of renal disease in insulin-dependent diabetes mellitus. Semin Nephrol 1990;10:260-73.

10. Hoops S. Renal and retinal complications in insulin-dependent diabetes mellitus: the art of changing the outcome. Diabetes Educ 1990;16:221-32.

11. Tuttle KR, Stein JH, DeFronzo RA. The natural history of diabetic nephropathy. Semin Nephrol 1990;10:184-93.

12. The Diabetes Control and Complications Trial Research Group. The effect of intensive treatment of diabetes on the development and progression of longterm complications in insulin-dependent diabetes mellitus. New Engl J Med 1993;329(14):977-86.

13. Working Group on Hypertension in Diabetes. Statement on hypertension in diabetes: final report. Arch Intern Med 1987;147:830-42.

14. Brenner BM, Meyer TW, Hostetter TH. Dietary protein intake and the progressive nature of renal disease. The role of hemodynamically mediated glomerular injury in the pathogenesis of progressive glomerular sclerosis in aging, renal ablation, and intrinsic renal disease. N Engl J Med 1982;307:652-59.

15. Scopelite JA. Dietary modifications: impact on diabetic nephropathy, ANNA J 1992;19:447-52.

16. Viberti G. Recent advance in the treatment of diabetic nephropathy: low-protein diet. J Diabetes Comp 1991;5:87.

17. Anderson S. Low protein diets and diabetic nephropathy. Semin Nephrol 1990;10:287-93.

18. Schafer RG. Implementation of low-protein diets for treatment of persons with early diabetic nephropathy. Diabetes Educ 1989;15:231-35.

19. Trusler LA. Simultaneous kidney-pancreas transplantation. ANNA J 1991;18:487-91.

20. Nettles AT. Pancreas transplantation: a University of Minnesota perspective. Diabetes Educ 1992;18:232-38.

21. Delano BG. Improvements in quality of life following treatment with r-HuEPO in anemic hemodialysis patients. Am J Kidney Dis 1989;14(suppl):14-18.

22. Koop J. Psychosocial correlates of diabetes and renal dysfunction. ANNA J 1992;19:432-37.

KEY EDUCATIONAL CONSIDERATIONS

Prior to any educational intervention, barriers to patient education need to be considered. The following illustrates some of the barriers and suggests possible interventions for patients with diabetes and renal disease.

1. The patient/family might be experiencing feelings of grief, anxiety, anger or rage, depression, hopelessness, guilt, and fear. These issues need to be addressed. Establishing a supportive, trusting, nonjudgmental and ongoing relationship with the patient and family is essential for them to work through these difficult and complex issues. Asking some key questions will yield useful information: What is wrong with your kidneys? Why do you think you have kidney disease? What have you heard about kidney disease or kidney treatment? What sort of things are you worried about now? What seems to help you when you are feeling down?

2. Assist in forming a supportive network of patients if one does not exist. Explain to prospective members of the group that they can have a positive impact on newly referred patients as well as help the health care team in their efforts in helping the patients. Also point out that participation in a self-help group can benefit all the members of the group. Forming a supportive group for family members/significant others is another avenue to explore.

3. Azotemia and uremia can alter the patient's ability to concentrate and think clearly. Provide concise, clear educational sessions. Create individualized handouts as the "lesson" is being given. Leave written material (large print or audiotape if necessary) after the session. Meeting with families or significant others at the same time can be helpful; it is important that all members of the "family" hear the same information.

4. There is an immense amount of new information to absorb and new health professionals to meet (perhaps in a new setting). The

patient/family often feel overwhelmed. Explain the role of each member of the team; how and when members of the health care team can be reached; and what is expected of the patient/family. Promote a comfortable environment where the patient and family can voice concerns about care if they are not satisfied.

SELF-REVIEW QUESTIONS

If you are unsure of the answers to the following questions, please review the materials.

1. What percentage of individuals with IDDM develop renal failure?
2. Why are there more patients with NIDDM than IDDM who have renal disease?
3. State three functions of the kidney.
4. Define BUN, microalbuminuria, and proteinuria.
5. List the signs and symptoms of the nephrotic syndrome.
6. Describe current interventions used to prevent or slow the progression of diabetic renal disease.
7. Describe treatment options for renal replacement therapy and their impact on diabetes management.
8. Name other factors that can harm the kidneys. How can these factors be minimized?
9. List the stages of diabetic nephropathy in IDDM.
10. Name the first clinical sign indicative of kidney involvement in a person with diabetes.

CASE EXAMPLE

GK, a 61-year-old married woman who has had NIDDM for approximately 10 years, was referred to the nephrology team. She told the examining physician, "I'm holding onto water, I get out of breath when I walk up the stairs, my sugar keeps dropping, and I don't know what's going on." Physical findings included gross edema of the lower extremities (3+); lungs clear; blood pressure reading of 196/106 mm Hg; feet dry, scaly, cold to the touch (no palpable pulses); toenails overgrown;

indentation marks on both feet from shoes and stockings. Laboratory studies disclosed the following values: proteinuria (3280 mg [3.28 g] urinary protein per 24 hr); serum albumin, 3.0 g/dL (30 g/L); glucose, 55 mg/dL (3.1 mmol/L); hematocrit 29% (normal 36-45%); and serum creatinine, 2.6 mg/dL (229.8 μmol/L). Current medical regimen includes 30 units of NPH insulin each morning and 40 mg furosemide (Lasix) daily. GK demonstrated a lack of knowledge about both diabetes management and kidney disease.

QUESTIONS

1. What are some interventions that the health care team could employ now?
2. What teaching plan would you develop for GK and how would you begin?

SUGGESTED SOLUTIONS

A priority at this first visit is to begin to establish relationships between the patient and key members of the nephrology team. Members should be introduced and each should meet individually with the patient over the next month. GK should be encouraged to become an active participant in all aspects of her care. Regular visits and telephone contact should be initiated.

GK and her family need introductory information on kidney disease: function, preventive measures, and terminology used to track kidney function (eg, *creatinine, BUN, proteinuria*). In addition, they will need support related to the patient's learning of the presence of kidney disease. Introducing GK to another patient with diabetes and kidney disease may be helpful. While renal replacement therapy is not indicated now, a brief discussion of various options may be started if the patient displays readiness.

GK's presenting complaints (and the team's management concerns) must also be addressed. Diuretic therapy is intensified by adding metolazone (10 mg twice a day) to the treatment regimen and increasing the furosemide dosage. After the extra fluid is lost, GK will be instructed to adjust the metolazone dose, guided by daily weight levels and the presence of edema. Electrolytes will be checked regularly to ascertain if an increase in dietary potassium intake or a potassium supplement is required.

Glycemic control is addressed through a decrease in insulin dose and instructing GK in blood glucose monitoring. An appropriate meter is chosen based on GK's needs and ability and after checking meter specifications for range of acceptable hematocrit values. GK is advised to monitor four times a day initially and telephone her results to the team so that further adjustments can be made if necessary. Signs and symptoms of hypoglycemia, as well as causes, treatment, and prevention are reviewed with her. At follow-up visits, her monitoring technique will be assessed and quality control checks done.

Blood pressure control must be achieved and will be facilitated by removal of extra fluid through diuretic therapy. An ACE inhibitor is prescribed. The patient is advised to obtain a blood pressure monitor and to check her blood pressure several times per day initially (prior to getting out of bed in the morning and seated at other times during the day). At a follow-up visit, the patient's technique and the machine's reliability will be verified.

Preventive measures related to foot and eye care, so critical for this high-risk patient, must be reviewed and reinforced. GK is referred to the podiatrist for care and education and to the ophthalmologist for evaluation.

Given the emotional impact of a diagnosis of kidney disease, the new medications, changes in management, and the amount of education that needs to be done, the educator arranges to speak with GK by telephone during the next week and a return visit is scheduled within the next 2 weeks.

OTHER SUGGESTED READINGS

Dullaart RPF, Beusekamp BJ, Meijer S. Van Doormaal JJ, Sluiter WJ. Long-term effects of protein-restricted diet on albuminuria and renal function in IDDM patients without clinical nephropathy and hypertension. Diabetes Care 1993;16:483-92.

Holechek MJ. Glomerular filtration and renal hemodynamics. ANNA J 1992;19:237-48.

Mann KV. Promoting adherence in hypertension: a framework for patient education. Can J Cardiol Nurs 1989;1:8-14.

Marion R, Ryan R. Nursing management of the hypertensive patient. In: Laragh JH. Hypertension: pathophysiology, diagnosis and management. New York: Raven Press, 1990.

Powers MA. Handbook of diabetes nutritional management. Rockville, Md: Aspen Publishers, 1987.

Roberto PL. Diabetic nephropathy causes, complications, and considerations. Crit Care Nurs Clin North Am 1990;2:55-66.

Thom SL, ed. Low protein diets in diabetic nephropathy. American Dietetic Association, Diabetes Practice Group. On the Cutting Edge 1991;12(4).

Voice of the Diabetic (A Support and Information Network), Diabetics Division of the National Federation of the Blind, 811 Cherry Street, Suite 309, Columbia, Mo 65201.

COMPLICATIONS

XXIV. MACROVASCULAR DISEASE

INTRODUCTION

Arteriosclerosis is a general term that describes the condition that causes blood vessel walls (both arteries and veins) to become thick, hard, and nonelastic. *Atherosclerosis* is a specific term that refers to the deposition of materials along blood vessel walls (especially arterial). *Macrovascular disease* refers to both arteriosclerotic and atherosclerotic changes in moderate- to large-sized arteries and veins. Of special importance is coronary, cerebral, and peripheral macrovascular diseases because of associated morbidity and mortality. Atherosclerosis, common in diabetes, is literally a "soft" hardening in which mounds of lipid material mixed with smooth muscle cells and calcium accumulate in the inner walls of blood vessels. These mounds, called plaques, enlarge over time. Eventually, they may completely block blood flow or cause the formation of a blood clot. These plaques may also initiate vascular spasm, which would further reduce blood flow. Plaque formations occur by several different mechanisms. For example, smooth muscle cells, which normally lie behind the inner wall, or intima, of a blood vessel, may migrate into this intima, spread across its surface, and form the base of plaque. What starts this process of migration is not known for certain. Injury to the intima may initiate this smooth muscle migration, the injury itself reflecting mechanical insult, oxygen deficiency, or lipid deposition. As the plaque forms, cholesterol becomes a major component. Calcium deposits may also cause further hardening of the plaque.

OBJECTIVES

Upon completion of this chapter, the learner will be able to:

- identify types of macrovascular disease that affect patients with diabetes mellitus;
- describe risk factors that may contribute to the morbidity and mortality of macrovascular disease in diabetes;
- describe assessment and intervention strategies that may ultimately prevent and/or minimize macrovascular disease in diabetes mellitus.

A. Types of Macrovascular Disease That Affect Patients with Diabetes

1. The three major types of macrovascular disease are: *coronary artery, cerebral vascular,* and *peripheral vascular* disease.[1]

   a) In patients with diabetes mellitus, atherosclerotic vascular disease of the coronary vessels develops at an earlier age than in the nondiabetic population, and involves coronary vessels more extensively. Also, the incidence of early-onset or midlife atherosclerotic coronary artery disease, which is much lower among the general female population than the general male population, is relatively comparable in men and women with diabetes mellitus.

   b) Patients with diabetes mellitus appear to be prone to develop cerebral vascular disease at an earlier age than persons who do not have diabetes. (The data are not quite as strong for cerebral vascular disease when compared with coronary artery disease.) Persons with diabetes also seem to be at risk for both transient ischemic attacks and thrombotic cerebral vascular accidents.

   c) Peripheral vascular disease is very common in patients with diabetes mellitus and is clinically characterized by intermittent claudication and/or lower leg and foot ulcers. In addition, other conditions such as smoking, dyslipidemia, etc, may contribute to the progression, or clinical expression of, peripheral vascular disease.

2. Complications associated with *macrovascular disease* contribute significantly to the morbidity and mortality associated with diabetes mellitus, particularly in those persons with long-standing diabetes.[1]

   a) Most clinical and epidemiological studies indicate that coronary artery disease accounts for 50% to 60% of all deaths in patients with diabetes mellitus. Persons with non-insulin-dependent diabetes mellitus (NIDDM), also called type II diabetes, are particularly at risk for coronary-associated mortality, perhaps because of age. But coronary artery disease is also the greatest cause of mortality in persons with insulin-dependent diabetes mellitus (IDDM), also called type I diabetes. In general, coronary artery disease mortality ratios in patients with diabetes are from two- to fourfold greater than in a comparable nondiabetic population. These ratios apply to both men and women with diabetes.[2,3]

(1) Patients with diabetes mellitus are not only more likely to experience an acute myocardial infarction at an earlier age than their nondiabetic counterparts but also are more likely to have complications from that myocardial infarction (eg, heart failure, arrhythmias); succumb to the initial myocardial infarction; or experience a second myocardial infarction with the passage of time.

(2) While most persons with diabetes who experience acute coronary insufficiency will display usual symptoms, eg, angina, diaphoresis, anxiety, etc, an important element of *coronary artery disease* in patients with diabetes mellitus is the so-called silent myocardial infarction. This is an entity in which patients do not manifest these typical, or indeed, any, symptoms of acute coronary ischemia. Silent myocardial infarctions occur in the general population also, but are about two to three times more common in persons with diabetes, especially if the diabetes is of long-standing duration. In some cases, these atypical symptoms (eg, indigestion, shortness of breath) may be secondary to autonomic neuropathy. Thus, in considering patient symptoms in such assessment activities as exercise prescriptions, possible atypical manifestations should be considered.

(3) There is little relationship between the duration of NIDDM and the presence of coronary events (see discussion below about Syndrome X for possible explanations). For persons with IDDM, however, the

longer diabetes is present, the more likely it is that the person will experience a coronary event.

b) Studies of *cerebral vascular disease* in patients with diabetes mellitus are limited but suggest that mortality ratios for such patients are from three to five times greater than for the nondiabetic population. There is a relationship between the level of glycemic control at admission for a stroke in persons with diabetes, and subsequent mortality. This increased likelihood of cerebral vascular death applies to both males and females.

c) Peripheral vascular disease (PVD) infrequently leads to fatal complications during the first few years after clinical expression of PVD. Thus, most epidemiologic investigations are based on nonfatal complications, symptoms, or clinical findings associated with peripheral disease (see Chapter XXV: Lower Extremity Problems for discussion of symptoms of PVD).

(1) About 50% of all nontraumatic lower extremity amputations are performed on patients with diabetes due to peripheral neuropathy and/or vascular disease. People with diabetes have a 15 times higher age-related risk for amputation than do nondiabetic individuals.[4,5]

(2) Absent peripheral pulses, due to occlusive peripheral arterial disease, are seen considerably more often in patients with NIDDM than in patients with IDDM, particularly with increasing duration of diabetes.

(3) The incidence of occlusive peripheral arterial disease is approximately four and six times higher in men and women with diabetes, respectively, than in those without diabetes. Thus, the need for preventive education about foot care is particularly important in persons with diabetes.

B. Risk Factors

1. A number of risk factors may contribute to the accelerated atherosclerotic vascular disease in patients with diabetes mellitus, including lipid abnormalities, hypertension, smoking, obesity, physical inactivity, type of diet and nutrition, blood flow dynamics and coagulation factors, hyperglycemia per se, and perhaps even the treatment of diabetes itself.[6]

   a) Elevated plasma *triglyceride* and lowered high-density lipoprotein (HDL) values are often found in patients with NIDDM. Generally, total cholesterol and LDL-cholesterol are comparable between persons with NIDDM and matched nondiabetic individuals. In persons with well-controlled IDDM, lipoprotein levels are similar to control subjects. Qualitative abnormalities in lipid components have been identified in persons with diabetes.[7]

      (1) There is controversy regarding whether elevated triglycerides are an independent risk factor for coronary artery disease, both in the general population as well as in persons with diabetes.[7,8]

      (2) Plasma triglyceride levels correlate positively with blood glucose and glycosylated hemoglobin levels. In both IDDM and NIDDM patients, improved metabolic control results in lowered triglyceride levels and some degree of reciprocal increase in HDL levels.

      (3) The impact of plasma *cholesterol* levels on the subsequent development of cardiovascular disease is probably similar in individuals with or without diabetes. Thus, if an elevated *cholesterol* level doubles the chance of a myocardial infarction in a nondiabetic individual, a similar cholesterol level will likely have a comparable effect in a patient with diabetes mellitus.[6] Persons with diabetes seem to start from a higher baseline regarding mortality in the absence of any other risk factor (eg, cholesterol), probably as a result of diabetes per se.

b) Plasma *fibrinogen* levels are increased in diabetes, and this elevation is strongly associated with diabetic macrovascular disease.[3] Indeed, recent epidemiologic studies in the general population have identified an elevated plasma fibrinogen level as a potent risk factor for future cardiovascular morbidity and mortality. Fibrinogen levels are raised by both cigarette smoking and hyperglycemia, underscoring the importance of smoking cessation and glycemic control in the possible prevention of coronary disease.

(1) In both IDDM and NIDDM, the correlation between hyperglycemia and high-density lipoprotein (HDL) levels is poor. This suggests that the relationship between HDL levels and diabetic atherosclerotic disease is complex, ie, achieving glycemic control, by itself, will not necessarily increase HDL levels.

(2) Effective and safe ways to increase HDL levels need to be identified, as low HDL levels are a powerful and independent predictor of subsequent vascular events.[6]

c) Hypertension is approximately twice as common in patients with diabetes mellitus. Hypertension is an independent risk for cardiovascular disease in patients with diabetes as in the general population. In IDDM, there is a correlation between duration of diabetes, the presence of renal dysfunction, and the development of hypertension. In persons with NIDDM, the pathogenesis of hypertension may be associated with Syndrome X. Syndrome X represents at least four elements commonly seen together in clinical practice — hyperglycemia, hyperlipidemia, hypertension, and central obesity[9,10] A central role of insulin resistance and subsequent hyperinsulinemia and hypertension, even prior to the onset of hyperglycemia, is proposed. An "atherosclerotic environment" may thus exist for years before the onset of hyperglycemia. This would explain the lack of a time relationship between the onset of hyperglycemia and hypertension in persons with NIDDM.[11,12]

d) Persons with diabetes smoke tobacco, on average, with the same frequency as the general population. Unfortunately, younger people with diabetes smoke *more* often than their nondiabetic peers.[13] In any case, for patients with diabetes, smoking appears to have an independent additive impact on the risk for subsequent development of cardiovascular disease. Whether the mechanisms of the effects of smoking on vascular function in persons with diabetes are due to cigarette toxins per se, or mediated through lowered HDL or elevated fibrinogen levels is not clear.

e) The majority of patients with either impaired glucose tolerance or NIDDM are obese. The independent contribution of obesity to atherosclerotic vascular disease in these patients has not yet been established, perhaps because these same individuals also often have dyslipidemia and/or hypertension.

f) Little direct information is presently available on the relationship between physical activity and the risk for development of atherosclerotic vascular disease in patients with diabetes mellitus. However, a well-planned cardiovascular exercise program, with careful cardiovascular assessment prior to exercise, is a prudent adjunct to therapy for hyperglycemia, and may even prevent the onset of NIDDM in those at risk for this condition.[14]

g) Because blood coagulation factors are important in the formation and dissolution of arterial thrombi, they may contribute to both acute and chronic atherosclerotic lesions. A number of platelet and clotting-factor abnormalities have been reported in patients with diabetes. Importantly, platelet behavior tends to improve with better metabolic control.

h) In the past, attention has been directed to a possible role of therapeutic agents used to treat diabetes mellitus and associated conditions in the pathogenesis of macrovascular disease.

(1) While the University Group Diabetes Program (UGDP) suggested an increased risk of cardiovascular complications in diabetic patients treated with an oral hypoglycemic drug, subsequent overall experience with sulfonylureas does not support this association.

(2) In nondiabetic subjects, hyperinsulinemia is associated with increased risk for coronary artery disease. Whether this represents a variant of Syndrome X is not clear at present. Some clinical studies of patients with NIDDM suggest that high plasma insulin levels may also be associated with atherosclerotic vascular disease. Additional studies are needed to establish whether a relationship exists between hyperinsulinemia and atherosclerotic vascular disease.[15]

(3) In the treatment of hypertension, concern has been expressed that side effects from certain antihypertensive agents (eg, diuretics, beta-blockers), may attenuate if not reverse the benefits of blood-pressure-lowering medications.[16,17] These studies indicate the need for careful selection of blood pressure medication in persons with diabetes.

i) Because hyperglycemia is the hallmark of diabetes mellitus, the possible contribution of chronically elevated levels of blood glucose to the development of atherosclerotic vascular disease must be considered.

(1) With hyperglycemia, sorbitol accumulates in the intima, causing this layer to enlarge. This may contribute to atherosclerotic plaque formation.

(2) In an environment of hyperglycemia, protein glycosylation within the artery wall may contribute to atherosclerotic vascular disease by altering the normal protein function within the intima.

(3) Red blood cell deformability and oxygen release are reduced when diabetes is poorly controlled, interfering with tissue oxygen delivery and affecting blood flow.

2. While a number of risk factors may account for excessive macrovascular disease in diabetes mellitus, their exact individual role is unclear. It is likely that each risk factor for macrovascular disease contributes to the overall prevalence of coronary, cerebral, and peripheral vascular disease.

   a) The strength of the relationship between the presence of the three major risk factors — elevated plasma cholesterol level, high blood pressure, and smoking — and the development of atherosclerotic vascular disease is probably the same in patients with diabetes mellitus as in comparable individuals without diabetes.

   b) Studies indicate, however, that only a relatively modest proportion of the excess atherosclerotic vascular disease seen in diabetes can be explained by the levels of the general risk factors for vascular disease, ie, smoking, dyslipidemia, and hypertension. The major component of excess atherosclerotic vascular disease in patients with diabetes is probably due to the effects of hyperglycemia per se through the substantial number of mechanisms briefly discussed above. It is important to note that some of these perturbations can be improved by better glycemic control. In addition, interventional strategies directed at stopping smoking and treating dyslipidemia and hypertension may further attenuate the tendency for macrovascular disease.

C. Assessment of Atherosclerotic Vascular Disease

1. The medical history should focus on coronary (eg, angina, dyspnea, etc); cerebral (eg, dizziness, transient weakness, etc); and peripheral (claudication, foot ulcers, etc) symptoms; and

the presence of risk factors such as smoking status, family history, history of cholesterol or blood pressure problems, etc.

2. The physical assessment should include blood pressure (at least two measurements either lying or sitting), the presence of vascular bruits, and the status of the feet.

3. Laboratory assessment should include glycemic control measures and a lipid profile (HDL, cholesterol, LDL, triglyceride).

4. Lifestyle/behavioral assessment should focus on dietary and exercise/activity habits, coping mechanisms, relevant knowledge, beliefs, attitude and skills.

D. Intervention Strategies

1. Because macrovascular disease accounts for such significant morbidity and mortality in patients with diabetes mellitus, therapeutic measures to reduce atherosclerotic risk are imperative.

2. Intervention goals for patients with diabetes mellitus include aggressive treatment of hypertension, cessation of cigarette smoking, treatment of hyperlipidemia, and optimal control of hyperglycemia — all designed to slow the development of atherosclerotic disease.

3. Underlying each of these strategies, nutrition efforts are essential. Caloric restriction in overweight patients, restriction of cholesterol and saturated fat intake, and use of soluble fibers are some of the important elements (see Chapter VI regarding nutritional therapy, Chapter VII for exercise therapy, and Chapter VIII for a discussion of pharmacologic treatment of hyperglycemia).

4. *Hypertension.* There are several generally accepted principles regarding hypertension in persons with diabetes.

   a) Pharmacological treatment is likely to be initiated in persons with diabetes who have only modest elevations of blood pressure compared with the general population.

   b) The selection of initial antihypertensive agents will differ from that of the nondiabetic patient because of the presence of diabetes. Thus, angiotensin-converting enzyme (ACE) inhibitors or calcium channel blockers are often selected as initial therapy. In contrast, if thiazide diuretics or beta blockers are selected, they would be used very cautiously and at the lowest possible dose.

   c) Serious efforts would be made to achieve good control of blood pressure, with frequent reassessment and change in medication should acceptable blood pressures not be achieved.[6,16,17]

5. *Smoking.* It is important that smoking status be routinely assessed in all patients. Materials and other resources, including availability of smoking cessation programs, should be made known to persons with diabetes who smoke. Generally, if members of the health care team indicate seriousness about smoking cessation and display persistence in establishing efforts to help the individual with diabetes to stop smoking, efforts will be rewarded.

6. *Dyslipidemia.* In approaching persons with diabetes and dyslipidemia, the following sequence of interventions should be considered:

   a) Nutrition and exercise are prime considerations. Focus should be on caloric restriction for individuals needing to lose weight, limitations in total and saturated fat, cholesterol restriction (see Chapter VI: Nutrition) and increased physical activity (see Chapter VII: Exercise).

   b) Optimization of glycemic control should be achieved if possible, prior to or at least concordant with any pharmacological therapy for dyslipidemia.

c) Pharmacological treatment includes several classes of lipid-lowering agents for treatment of dyslipidemia. Several of these agents have been carefully studied regarding metabolic effects as well as prevention of adverse macrovascular outcomes. Persons with diabetes, however, have either been excluded from these studies or participate in inadequate numbers to make firm judgments about specific agents. Thus, recommendations are by inference.[7] Bile acid binding resins (eg, cholestyramine) are effective but difficult to use over long periods and may increase triglyceride levels. Fibric acid derivatives (eg, gemfibrozil) do not alter diabetes control, and seem effective in controlling dyslipidemia. Their full effect may require 3 to 6 months to achieve, however. HMG-CoA reductase inhibitors (eg, lovastatin) block cholesterol synthesis and seem to be associated with a favorable lipid profile in persons with diabetes. They can be quite expensive, and long term safety studies need to be completed. Nicotinic acid is inexpensive and effective but is associated with side effects (eg, flushing) and often with worsening of glycemic control in NIDDM. Antioxident agents that may prevent LDL oxidation still await results of ongoing coronary prevention trials. Finally, while estrogen replacement is quite logical, especially given the loss of "gender protection" from atherosclerosis in diabetic women, there is still some concern about the effect of estrogens on triglyceride levels. Clearly, there are a number of therapeutic pharmacological agents; selection of the most appropriate medication must be based on individual patient characteristics.

REFERENCES

1.   Vinicor F. Features of macrovascular disease of diabetes. In: Haire-Joshu D, ed. Management of diabetes mellitus: perspectives of care across the life span. St Louis: Mosby-Year Book Inc, 1992:190-214.

2.   Kannel WB. Coronary heart disease risk factors: Framingham study update. Hosp Pract 1990;25:119-127.

3.   Kannel WB, D'Agostino RB, Wilson PW, Belanger AJ, Gagnon DR. Diabetes, fibrinogen and risk of cardiovascular disease, the Framingham experience. Am Heart J 1990;120:672-676.

4.   Pecoraro R, Reiber G, Burgess E. Pathways to diabetic limb amputation: basis for prevention. Diabetes Care 1990;13:513-521.

5.   Reiber G, Pecoraro R, and Koepsell T. Risk factors for amputation in patients with diabetes mellitus: a case-controlled study. Ann Intern Med 1992;117:97-105.

6.   American Diabetes Association. Role of cardiovascular risk factors in prevention and treatment of macrovascular disease in diabetes: consensus statement. Diabetes Care, 1989;12:573-79.

7.   American Diabetes Association. Detection and management of lipid disorders in diabetes. Diabetes Care 1993;16:828-834.

8.   Criqui M, Heiss G, Cohn R, et al. Plasma triglyceride level and mortality from coronary heart disease. N Engl J Med 1993;328:1220-25.

9.   Reaven G. Role of insulin resistance in human disease. Diabetes 1988;37:1595-1607.

10. Kaplan N. The deadly quartet: upper body obesity, glucose intolerance, hypertriglycerides, and hypertension. Arch of Intern Med 1989;149:1514-20.

11. Haffner S, Stern MD, Hazuda HP, Mitchell BD, Patterson, JK. Cardiovascular risk factors in confirmed pre-diabetic individuals: Does the clock for coronary heart disease start ticking before the onset of clinical diabetes? JAMA 1990;263:2893-98.

12. Saudek, C. When does diabetes start? JAMA 1990;263:2934.

13. Ford E, Newman J. Smoking and diabetes mellitus: findings from the 1988 behavioral risk factor surveillance system. Diabetes Care 1991;14:871-74.

14. Helmrich S, Ragland D, Lewng R, Paffenbarger R. Physical activity and reduced occurrence of non-insulin-dependent diabetes mellitus. N Engl J Med 1991;325:147-52.

15. Stout R. Insulin and atheroma: 20-year perspective. Diabetes Care, 1990;13:631-54.

16. Kaplan N, Rosenstock J, Raskin P. A differing view of treatment of hypertension in patients with diabetes mellitus. Arch Intern Med 1989;147:1160-62.

17. Christlieb A. Treatment selection considerations for the hypertensive diabetic patient. Arch Intern Med 1990;150:1167-74.

KEY EDUCATIONAL CONSIDERATIONS

1. Explain to the patient the importance of macrovascular disease in diabetes — the increased susceptibility of patients with diabetes, the synergistic effect of risk factors, which risks are modifiable, and the manifestations of macrovascular disease in diabetes. Use videotape if possible as a visual reinforcement of the concepts presented.

2. Inform the patient and family that the health care team will follow the status of lipid and blood pressure control in addition to blood glucose control. Orient the patient to normal and elevated levels of lipids and blood pressure.

3. A diet low in fat should be encouraged from the onset of diabetes, with special emphasis on low saturated fat and high soluble fiber.

4. Resources (programs and materials) related to the modification of cardiovascular risk factors should be explored and information provided to patients as appropriate.

5. Adding nutritional and/or pharmacological therapy for hyperlipidemia or hypertension bring an additional element of complexity to an already challenging treatment program. Thus, health professionals need to apply greater effort and resources in dealing with these patients. Priorities need to be clear to all team members, especially the patient and family.

6. Use labels of empty food containers to teach label reading for food content.

7. In a group class, use menus from local fast-food and fine dining restaurants to reinforce low-fat choices when eating out.

8. Create visual aids that will reinforce the fat content of commonly used regional foods such as sausage, biscuits and gravy, or lasagna.

SELF-REVIEW QUESTIONS

If you are unsure of the answers to the following questions, please review the materials.

1. Define *macrovascular disease* and distinguish it from microvascular complications of diabetes mellitus.
2. How do macrovascular complications contribute to morbidity and mortality in patients with diabetes mellitus?
3. What factors may contribute to accelerated macrovascular disease in patients with diabetes mellitus?
4. How would you assess the presence of these risk factors in your patients with diabetes?
5. What interventional programs should be initiated to minimize the development of macrovascular disease in patients with diabetes mellitus?

CASE EXAMPLE

RS, a 46-year-old black woman, mother of three teenagers, and with a 13-year history of NIDDM, is seen in your clinic for the first time. She has been treated with insulin (24 units of NPH insulin in the morning; 8 units of NPH insulin before supper), but has followed "no particular" meal plan or exercise program. She tests her blood glucose level periodically, when she feels "bad," and she has come to the clinic to be evaluated for shortness of breath and headaches. Both symptoms have been present for about 2 months but have been increasing in severity over the past 2 weeks. RS has not been routinely followed in any health facility over the past 4 years; she occasionally visits an emergency room for care.

Initial questioning reveals that RS doesn't adjust her insulin but does take her "shots" each day. She had a random blood glucose reading of 283 mg/dL (15.7 mmol/L) last week. She urinates frequently and has never had a "low blood sugar reaction" (she does know what this means). She had been told during a past emergency room visit that she had "some high blood pressure," but she wasn't put on medication and has not had her blood pressure checked in about 2 years. She has smoked cigarettes for 18 years. She is unaware of any cholesterol, heart, or kidney problems.

Physical assessment reveals a blood pressure of 195/108 mm Hg, background diabetic retinopathy, bilateral rales, a heart gallop, 2+ edema, left ventricular hypertrophy by ECG, proteinuria and glucosuria, and a random capillary glucose level of 268 mg/dL (14.9 mmol/L).

QUESTIONS

1. Discuss general approaches to complex cases such as this one.
2. What should be done now?
3. Outline an educational plan for RS.

SUGGESTED SOLUTIONS

The fact that RS has not been receiving regular evaluation and care is disturbing. That she is now coming to the clinic, when this has not been her pattern over the past 4 years, should make one particularly sensitive to her presenting complaints.

Because of the complexity of the case and the fact that RS is new to your clinic, you must obtain a lot of information during this first visit. Such information is essential to the development of an appropriate treatment plan. In addition, depending on the way this information is collected, the "process" of interacting with the patient can help establish rapport so that the chances of her returning are enhanced.

Concerns are: her diabetes has not been regularly evaluated and her glucose control seems inadequate; she has both microvascular (eye) and likely macrovascular (heart) problems, the latter associated with hypertension and tobacco use; and she may have lipid problems (although we don't know this yet). This is a lot to deal with.

Some initial attention to her glycemic and blood pressure status is essential. While it might seem reasonable to bring RS into the hospital to initiate treatment, she indicates that she must return home to care for her family, she also notes that she has only very basic health insurance. Thus, in addition to altering her dietary intake and insulin programs to begin to improve her blood glucose control, and starting her on antihypertensive medication for her hypertension and other her major complaints, it is necessary to establish some mechanisms for follow-up at home before her scheduled return visit.

The educator should be concerned with establishing rapport, addressing RS's concerns, and not overwhelming her with too much information at this first visit. A thorough assessment of her diabetes knowledge, skills, self-care, and attitudes is indicated, as well as her socioeconomic situation and the status of cardiovascular risk factors. Because attention to her blood pressure and blood glucose control is indicated, the teaching plan should include assessing her monitoring technique, ability (including financial) and willingness to do more frequent blood glucose monitoring. If she is able to test her blood glucose levels reliably and more frequently, then a plan should be developed to determine when to test and how to use the results to improve glycemic control. A plan for telephone follow-up may be useful.

OTHER SUGGESTED READINGS

American Diabetes Association. Detection and management of lipid disorders in diabetes. Diabetes Care 1993;16:828-34.

American Diabetes Association. Role of cardiovascular risk factors in prevention and treatment of macrovascular disease in diabetes: consensus statement. Diabetes Care 1989;12:573-79.

Colwell J, Lopes-Virella M. A review of the development of large vessel disease in diabetes mellitus:the genesis of atherosclerosis in diabetes mellitus. Am J Med 1988;85:113-18.

Jarrett R. Cardiovascular disease and hypertension in diabetes mellitus. Diabetes Metab Rev 1989;5:547-58.

Jarrett R. Type II (non-insulin-dependent) diabetes mellitus and coronary heart disease — chicken, egg, or neither? Diabetologia, 1984;26:99-102.

Pyorala K, Laasko M, Uusitupa M. Diabetes and atherosclerosis: an epidemiologic view. Diabetes Metab Rev 1987;3:463-524.

Sabo CE, Michael SR. Drug therapy for the hypertensive diabetic patient: implications for the diabetes educator. Diabetes Educ 1989;15:378-79.

COMPLICATIONS

XXV.   LOWER EXTREMITY PROBLEMS

INTRODUCTION

Multiple causes usually interact to necessitate each lower extremity amputation in people with diabetes. Minor trauma, skin ulceration, faulty wound healing, infection and gangrene are present in a majority of patients who undergo amputation[1].

Each year, more than 50,000 lower extremity amputations are performed on Americans with diabetes. The risk of lower extremity amputation in blacks with diabetes is 1.5 to 2 times higher than the corresponding risk in whites with diabetes, and the risk among men is 1.5 to 2 times higher than among women with diabetes.[2] It is estimated that only about 50% of patients who undergo amputation will survive 3 years.[3] Half of the patients who have had an amputation for gangrene face problems with their other leg within 18 to 36 months. Thus efforts to protect the second foot must be the paramount objective for both patient and health care providers.[4-6]

OBJECTIVES

Upon completion of this chapter, the learner will be able to:
- describe four symptoms of angiopathy;
- identify the effects of neuropathy on the autonomic, sensory, and motor functions of the foot;
- recognize the role of infection as a cause of amputation;
- list three major considerations in foot care;
- identify two factors that contribute to saving the diabetic foot;
- list four guidelines for teaching foot care to patients.

A. Angiopathy

1. Macroangiopathy denies oxygen and nutrients to the tissues and, in the presence of infection, the delivery of antibiotics.[4] This atherosclerotic process can attack all the arteries of the lower extremity. However, in persons with diabetes, the vessels involved are those found primarily below the knee. The toes may show vascular insufficiency, yet the dorsalis pedis or posterior tibialis pulses may be palpable.

2. Microthrombi, secondary to infection, create ischemic changes, decreasing nutrition of the tissues, and paving the way for necrosis and gangrene. The ischemia predisposes to atrophy of subcutaneous tissue, blisters, fissures, heat insensitivity, susceptibility to fungi, and a tendency to infection at injury sites and pressure points, such as corns and calluses.

3. Symptoms include intermittent claudication, cold feet, nocturnal pain, and rest pain. Nocturnal and rest pain are relieved by dependency of the extremity. Signs of vascular insufficiency are absent pulses, blanching on elevation of the feet with delayed venous filling after putting the feet down, and dependent rubor. Atrophy of subcutaneous fatty tissue, shiny skin, hairless feet and toes, and thickened nails with frequent fungus infections and gangrene are other signs of angiopathy.

B. Neuropathy

1. Neuropathy destroys the diabetic foot through loss of sensory-motor or autonomic nerve function.

2. Sensory loss is the cause of the majority of diabetic foot problems. In the neuropathic foot, pain is not a reliable early signal of problems, and the risk of major foot lesions is increased without this protection. Progressive loss of sensation may allow prolonged painless trauma. Mechanical, thermal, or chemical traumas set the stage for amputation.

    a) Common causes of mechanical trauma include ingrown toenails, ill-fitting shoes, wrinkled stockings, foreign objects in shoes, unprotected feet, and inappropriate care of nails, corns, and calluses. These create the potential for injury and infection, which may go untreated if not noticed.

    b) Thermal injuries often result from hot foot soaks, hot water bottles, or heating pads and can cause severe burns to the insensitive and vascularly compromised foot.[7]

c) Chemical trauma results when caustic substances such as over-the-counter corn and callus removers come in contact with fragile tissue and destroy it.[5]

3. Autonomic involvement prevents perspiration, leading to dryness, cracks, and fissures, making the broken skin easy prey to infection.

4. Motor neuropathy causes muscle atrophy leading to new pressure points and callus formation as well as changes in gait.
   a) Not uncommonly, ulceration of the callused pressure points occurs and vascular disease prevents healing of the lesions. Infection can result in gangrene and amputation.
   b) Examination may disclose deformities of toes and metatarsals and evidence of pressure.

5. Charcot's joint is a classic example of foot deformity probably caused by diabetic neuropathy. In the acute stage, the foot is warm, swollen, reddened, and somewhat painful. Because of relative insensitivity, patients continue to walk, creating stress fractures in addition to dissolution and fragmentation of the distal ends of the metatarsals and frequent involvement of the tarsometatarsal joint. Aggressive treatment in the acute stage focuses on avoiding weight bearing, frequently with the aid of a contact cast. Without aggressive treatment, the foot ultimately develops a "rocker bottom" configuration, which may result in ulceration of the plantar surface in the arch region.

6. Signs and symptoms of neuropathy are paresthesia, hyperesthesia, hypoesthesia, radicular pain, loss of deep-tendon reflexes, loss of vibratory and position sense, anhidrosis, and heavy callus formation over pressure points. Infection that complicates trophic ulcers, changes in foot shape due to muscle atrophy and bone/joint changes, and radiographic signs of demineralization, osteolysis, and Charcot's joint may also be suggestive of neuropathy[4] (see Chapter XXII: Diabetic Neuropathy).

7. A simple and fast test to identify feet that are vulnerable to trauma and need protection has been described by Coleman and Brand.[8,9] The ability to perceive touch is evaluated using the Semmes Weinstein monofilaments. These fibers come in three thicknesses, 1-g fiber (SW 4.17 rating), 10-g fiber (SW 5.07 rating), and 75-g fiber (SW 6.10 rating). The monofilament is placed against the skin and pressure applied until the filament buckles. The monofilament is usually applied to different areas of the bottom of the foot. The patient should be able to detect the presence of the monofilament when it buckles and identify the area being touched. The 5.07 thickness monofilament is equal to 10-g of linear pressure and determines the presence or absence of protective sensation, thus identifying the foot in need of special protection and care.

C. Infection as a Cause of Amputation

1. Infection in the diabetic foot can lead to gangrene and amputation and, on occasion, patient death.

2. Traditionally, diabetic foot infections are characterized according to the primary tissues involved — ie, skin and subcutaneous tissue, fascia, muscle, bone — and whether or not they are associated with dry or wet gangrene.

3. Dry gangrene is caused primarily by ischemia; wet gangrene is associated with an underlying process of infection and deep-tissue necrosis.

4. Signs of infection include fever, erythema, warmth, discharge with ulceration, leukocytosis and, frequently, increased blood glucose levels.

5. Infection is more significant in the patient with diabetes because hyperglycemia interferes with leukocyte function. Atherosclerosis prevents leukocyte transport and impairs delivery of parenteral antibiotic therapy.[4]

6. A culture of the infected area will routinely reveal a mix of aerobic bacteria, usually staphylococci and streptococci, and Gram-negative organisms (eg, *Escherichia coli*), plus anaerobes, especially *Bacteroides fragilis*. Culturing for both aerobic and anaerobic bacteria is mandatory to determine treatment.[4]

7. After obtaining appropriate cultures, antibiotics should be administered orally or parenterally, depending on medical judgment. Patients who have infections should be hospitalized and given parenteral antibiotics. Broad spectrum antibiotics are started at once. When culture reports return, antibiotic coverage is adjusted.[10] The foot must not bear weight, and radical surgical debridement should be instituted. Hot compresses or soaks must be avoided at all times because they increase metabolic demands in a foot deprived of arterial blood supply and also increase the possibility of burns in a numb foot.[7]

8. Microthrombi develop as a result of infection, decreased blood flow, and increased platelet aggregation, leading to gangrene and necrosis.

D. Foot Care Guidelines for Patients

1. Measures should be instituted to prevent injury and infection.

   a) Fissures are caused by dry skin, especially around the heels. They can be prevented by regular application of moisturizers or creams after bathing (no moisturizers should be used between the toes) and avoidance of prolonged foot soaks. Maceration between the toes caused by perspiration or inadequate drying after bathing can also lead to cracks. This can be prevented by adequate, gentle drying after bathing and insertion of lamb's wool between the toes.

   b) Blisters result from friction from shoes or wrinkled socks, foreign objects in shoes, and exposure to heat, cold, or chemical irritants. New shoes should be objectively evaluated for proper fit.

c)   Toenail problems are often the result of incorrect cutting. Toenails should be cut slightly curved, to the contour of the toe. Ingrown toenails cause injury to the nail groove and can result in infection. An emery board is the safest tool for filing nails. Elderly patients or patients with decreased vision, neuropathy, or ischemia should routinely see a podiatrist or have a family member cut and inspect their toenails.

d)   Trauma to the foot may be caused by improperly fitting shoes, injury to an unprotected foot, "bathroom surgery," or foreign objects in the shoe. Trauma can be prevented by wearing protective footwear, purchasing shoes that fit properly, checking the insides of shoes before putting them on each time, and not walking barefoot. Sport injuries can be minimized through the use of proper footwear.

e)   Corns and calluses are a physiologic response of the skin to irritation where bony prominences come in contact with shoes or the floor. Patients should be discouraged from trimming calluses or using chemicals (over the counter foot care products) to remove corns. This will help prevent problems. Regular attention to corns and calluses by a podiatrist is recommended. Infection and osteomyelitis may develop under the corn or callus.

f)   First aid measures include cleaning the skin opening, and using an antimicrobial that does not color the skin and mask the redness of infection.

g)   Circulation can be compromised by sitting with legs crossed or wearing tight garments such as support hose, tight knee-high stockings or garters.

2.   Early detection and treatment of problems are essential and can be promoted by a careful daily inspection of the feet.

a)   Patients should be encouraged to link foot inspection with a compatible daily routine, such as bathing.

    b) Patients should inspect the top, bottom, and sides of each foot and between each toe, using a hand or magnifying mirror if needed.

    c) Patients should be instructed to look for redness, swelling, cuts, blisters, calluses, dryness, cracks, corns, and any change in appearance from their last inspection.

    d) Even "small" problems should be considered potential ulcers, and medical care should be sought within 48 hours if improvement is not noticeable.

    e) A podiatrist should be seen regularly for care, assessment and evaluation.

E.   Saving the Diabetic Foot

1.   Six major approaches are necessary to save the feet of the person with diabetes.[4]

    a) Prevent foot problems through patient education in foot care.

    b) Reduce modifiable risk factors (ie, tobacco use, hypertension, hyperglycemia, hyperlipidemia, and obesity).

    c) Recognize the existence and degree of peripheral vascular disease and neuropathy (ie, identify high-risk patients).

    d) Improve circulation whenever possible.

    e) Manage foot ulcers with aggressive, multifaceted treatment, including no weight bearing.

    f) Use a multidisciplinary team in the treatment of complicated problems.

2.   The best tools to save the diabetic foot are patient education in foot care, special shoes when indicated, and regular evaluation that begins with the simple request, "Please remove your shoes and stockings."

REFERENCES

1.   Pecoraro RE, Reiber GE, Burgess EM. Pathways to diabetic limb amputation: basis for prevention. Diabetes Care 1990;13:513-21.

2.   Geiss LS (ed). Diabetes surveillance, 1991. Atlanta: US Dept of Health and Human Services, 1992:27-9.

3.   Bild DE, Selby JV, Sinnock P, Browner WS, Braveman P, Showstack JA. Lower-extremity amputation in people with diabetes: epidemiology and prevention. Diabetes Care 1989;12:24-31.

4.   Levin ME. Pathophysiology of diabetic foot lesions. In: Davidson JK, ed. Clinical diabetes mellitus: a problem oriented approach. 2nd ed. New York: Thieme, 1991:504-20.

5.   Hobgood E. Conservative therapy of foot abnormalities, infections, and vascular insufficiency. In: Davidson JK, ed. Clinical diabetes mellitus: a problem oriented approach. 2nd ed. New York: Thieme, 1991:521-30.

6.   Kilo C. Vascular complications of diabetes. Cardiovasc Res Rep 1987; (June):19-23.

7.   Lippmann HI. The foot of the diabetic. In: Grodoff BM, Bleicher SJ, eds. Diabetes mellitus and obesity. Baltimore, Md: Williams & Wilkins, 1982:712-34.

8.   Coleman WC, Brand PW. The diabetic foot. In: Davidson JK, ed. Clinical diabetes mellitus: a problem oriented approach. 2nd ed. New York: Thieme 1991:496-503.

9.   Brand PW, Coleman WC. The diabetic foot. In: Rifkin H, Porte Jr, D, eds. Ellenberg and Rifkin's diabetes mellitus: theory and practice. 4th ed. New York: Elsevier, 1990:792-811.

10. American Diabetes Association. Position statement. Foot care in patients with diabetes mellitus. Diabetes Care, 1991;14:18-9.

KEY EDUCATIONAL CONSIDERATIONS

1. Encourage patients to remove their shoes and socks at every physician visit, even if they are not asked to.

2. Reinforce that pain is not a reliable indicator of problems and that loss of sensation is gradual. An injury may not be noticed right away or may be deemed less serious than it is because it doesn't hurt. Poor circulation can delay or prevent healing of injuries.

3. If patients have some neuropathy or angiopathy, the educator should examine their feet, pointing out signs of diminished sensation or circulation. ("I see your hair growth stops at mid calf, that indicates some decreased blood supply to the area below.") This helps patients learn what to look for.

4. Encourage institution of two habits: daily foot inspection and feeling the inside of shoes each time before putting them on. Assist patients in planning how to incorporate new behaviors into existing routines.

5. This content area presents excellent opportunities to use case examples as a teaching aid. Patients are often surprised that very large foreign objects in shoes can go undetected. However, in doing this, the educator must use sensitivity and not turn to "scare tactics."

6. Because the objectives of foot care instruction are related to the acquisition of skills (inspection and care), appropriate teaching methods include explanation, demonstration and return demonstration, and assistance with incorporating new skills into practice. Frequent reinforcement in the form of foot inspections by health professionals, coupled with feedback on the condition of the feet and appropriateness and fit of shoes sends a strong message.

SELF-REVIEW QUESTIONS

If you are unsure of the answers to the following questions, please review the materials.

1. Define the role of vascular disease and its contribution to diabetic foot lesions.
2. What are four signs and symptoms of vascular disease in the diabetic foot?
3. Identify and explain the origin of most diabetic foot problems.
4. List two signs and symptoms of autonomic, sensory, and motor neuropathy in the diabetic foot.
5. Describe the effect of hyperglycemia on the body's response to infection and the role this process plays in problems of the diabetic foot.
6. What are three major components to consider in foot care?
7. Name three approaches that may "save" the diabetic foot.
8. List four important guidelines to teach patients about foot care.

CASE EXAMPLE

SV is a 40-year-old smoker, with an 18-year history of insulin-dependent diabetes mellitus (IDDM). She has been taking two injections of insulin for years, and has evidence of background retinopathy, mild hypertension, and microalbuminuria. At her clinic visit, you notice that she is wearing very high heeled shoes and ask her to remove her shoes and stockings for a foot exam. She replies, "I don't have any problems with my feet!" After explaining why you want to examine her feet, you do so, and note some decrease in sensation, thick calluses on pressure points and very short nails, with an ingrown toenail on the left great toe.

QUESTIONS

1. How would you explain your rationale for being concerned about SV's feet?
2. Outline your foot care teaching plan for SV.

SUGGESTED SOLUTIONS

SV is at risk for foot problems because of her long-standing diabetes, hypertension, tobacco use, existence of other chronic complications of diabetes, diminished sensation, and foot care practices.

Explanation is needed of these factors that put her at risk for foot problems. Referral to a podiatrist is indicated for evaluation and care of her calluses and ingrown toenail. Techniques for foot inspection and care (including trimming/filing of nails) should be demonstrated and practiced. Appropriate footwear should be discussed. Reduction of other modifiable risk factors may be addressed now or at a follow-up visit, as appropriate, including smoking cessation and improvements in glycemic and blood pressure control. SV, now identified as being at risk for foot problems, should have a foot exam at each visit, with positive reinforcement for good self-care habits and encouragement to adopt other necessary practices.

OTHER SUGGESTED READINGS

Christensen MH, Ehrlich M, Fellows E, Funnell M, Tarolli J. Diabetes foot care: a complete guide to professional education. Ann Arbor: University of Michigan, 1989.

Donovan J, Rowbothom JL. Foot lesions in diabetic patients: cause, prevention and treatment. In Marble A, Krall LP, Bradley RF, Christlieb AR, Soeldner JS, eds. Joslin's diabetes mellitus. 12th ed. Philadelphia: Lea & Febiger, 1985;732-36.

Fylling CP, ed. Wound healing: an update. Diabetes Spectrum 1992;5:328-59.

Guthrie DW, Guthrie RA. Nursing management of diabetes mellitus. 3rd ed. New York: Springer Publishing Co, 1991:156-62.

Guthrie DW, Guthrie, RA. The diabetes source book. Los Angeles: Lowell House, 1990:71-74.

Scheffler NM. Foot care. Diabetes in the News 1989 Feb.

Research

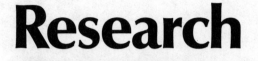

RESEARCH

XXVI.   RESEARCH: CONTINUING EDUCATION

Portions of this chapter have been published in the Research Core Course Training Manual of the Advanced Studies Institute for Diabetes Educators, American Association of Diabetes Educators.

INTRODUCTION

One may wonder why the topic of research is embodied in a book of core knowledge in diabetes education. As a health care professional engaged in direct patient care and teaching, you may not perceive research to be relevant or pertinent to your job; or you may feel that your lack of research knowledge/skill precludes you from conducting research; or you may find there is insufficient time to engage in research, considering all the other dimensions of your job and the demands made on your time by colleagues, administration, and patients. Besides, isn't research something done by those folks in academia in some foreign language called statistics?

This chapter is designed to focus your attention on the fact that knowledge of the research process is a core requirement for diabetes educators. All health care professionals are participants in research at one level or another. In reality, research is the foundation of clinical practice and patient care in diabetes education. Conversely, clinical practice serves as a critical foundation for research. Within the scope of this chapter, various aspects of the research process will be discussed to facilitate (1) critical reading of research papers; (2) evaluation of the appropriateness of applying research findings to your clinical practice setting; and (3) use of resources for applying research to practice.

OBJECTIVES

Upon completion of this chapter, the learner will be able to:
- define research in terms of a problem-solving process;
- describe methods in which diabetes educators participate in research;
- distinguish the two basic approaches to scientific inquiry;
- describe the purpose and aims of research;
- describe selected aspects of the process of critically reading research papers.

A. Defining Research

1. In the most general sense, research is the scientific approach to solving a problem.[1] Clinical practitioners are faced with problems every day. For example, what is the best approach to teaching diabetes self-care to a patient with low-literacy skills? What is the most practical means of validating the efficacy of diabetes education to warrant third-party reimbursement? How does one document patient teaching in accordance with quality assurance guidelines?

2. Such questions represent just a sample of the problems clinicians face in the course of providing diabetes education services. Obtaining answers to these questions, and any others relevant to your particular practice setting, involves a process of, first, assessing and identifying a problem; second, designing a plan to solve the problem; third, implementing the plan; and, fourth evaluating the outcome(s) of the plan. You likely engage in this four-step process several times during the course of any given day. This process of problem solving is often called the *scientific method*.

3. Most times, in the hectic pace of your job, this process is more likely informal. For example, you may have encountered the situation where a patient who attended a teaching session on the use of a glucose meter was unable to demonstrate proper use of the meter. You probably sat back to assess the situation while thinking, "We've got a problem here." Hence, you have undertaken step 1 of the process — assessing and identifying the problem. You try to think of ways to present the information again to the patient so that critical knowledge can be imparted. In doing so, you have reached step 2 — designing a plan to solve the problem. You now say to the patient, "OK, let's go through just the first three steps of the procedure." You have now moved to step 3 — implementing the plan. After going through the first three steps of the procedure with the patient, you again ask the patient to return a demonstration of

his or her skill. You listen and watch the patient. As the patient demonstrates, you judge the person's ability to properly execute the first three steps in the use of the glucose meter. By doing this, you have performed step 4 — evaluating the outcome(s) of the planned approach you have selected to teach the patient how to use a glucose meter.

4. The scenario described is an informal version of the research process. As health care professionals, we are all involved in research. We can understand and appreciate research as a problem-solving process through which we come to know something about the effects of our interventions. Knowledge is the most important product of research, whether formal or informal.[2] In the patient scenario above, you derived some knowledge of the patient's ability to use a glucose meter.

5. The remaining sections of this chapter will focus on explaining facets of the formal research process and your role as a participant in this process.

B. Research Involvement by Health Care Professionals

1. Health care professionals facilitate research conducted by others. Providing a researcher access to subjects is an example of this kind of involvement. You may allow a researcher to use your clinic/hospital for data collection, or you may serve as a subject by completing a survey received in the mail. Many research programs rely on the availability of subjects from a wide range of health care facilities. Regardless of the means by which you facilitate another's research, this basic level of involvement is extremely important. Researchers may have the means by which to design a research study, statistically analyze data, and evaluate and interpret study outcomes but lack access to subjects on which to conduct their study. You may not have the research proposal, but you have the subjects or are the subject of study.

2. Health care professionals use the research process in routine problem solving. Both formally and informally, health care professionals use the research process to solve clinical problems. An example would be the use of the research problem-solving process to find out why fewer people are attending your classes. Use of the research process (as a problem-solving approach) provides a framework for the identification, development, and evaluation of a plan to solve a clinical problem.

3. Health care professionals incorporate research findings into their clinical practices. At this level of involvement, health care professionals can critically read published research and apply the outcomes of formal research studies to clinical practice. For example, a diabetes educator might modify a patient-teaching program to include a stress-reduction topic because findings suggest a significant, positive correlation between stress and blood glucose levels. Other examples might be the use of a valid and reliable test evaluated by others to assess patient knowledge before and after a teaching intervention, or reliance on research studies demonstrating the effectiveness of a product you may wish to use in practice.

4. Health care professionals conduct formal research. This refers to the actual implementation of a formal research study. Your role in the conduct of research may range from coordinator of a clinical trial to principal/coinvestigator of a funded research study.

C. **Approaches to Scientific Study**

1. There are two basic types of scientific research — quantitative and qualitative.
   a) Quantitative studies that reflect the "scientific and empirical" research process represent much of the published research in diabetes. In this type of research, specific rules, guidelines, and methods determine the

means by which the research process is formulated and structured.[3] Research in the basic sciences, for example, reflects the quantitative approach to scientific study.

  b) Qualitative research involves the nonnumerical interpretation of observations for the purpose of discovering important underlying dimensions and patterns of relationships.[4,5] In qualitative research, the researcher seeks to capture and describe the "lived experience" of diabetes. The data are critically analyzed for emerging themes or patterns of thought, affect, or behavior. Such knowledge may serve as the foundation for new theory so that, for example, diabetes self-care behavior in elderly people may be better understood. Ethnography, phenomenology, historical studies, case studies, and grounded theory are examples of qualitative research.

2. The qualitative approach to research offers a dimension to patient education research that the quantitative scientific process may not capture. An increasing number of studies in the behavioral and psychological sciences include qualitative findings applicable to the study of diabetes self-care. A wide range of funded research programs in nursing, for example, reflect qualitative studies or a combination of qualitative-quantitative approaches to inquiry. The reader is directed to the suggested readings at the end of this chapter for sources that explain this approach to scientific inquiry.

D. Purpose and Aims of Research

1. Scientific research is designed to discover new knowledge, expand existing knowledge, or validate existing knowledge.[6]

  a) Knowledge is the most significant outcome of research. Improving, expanding, or validating our knowledge about diabetes education and management greatly enhances our ability to provide service and care to patients.

  b) The following example shows how research can discover new knowledge. Many studies in diabetes education have attempted to examine any given number of factors hypothesized to influence patient teaching and learning. However, little research has explored diabetes education among minority groups. We do know about factors that may influence patient teaching and learning among nonminority populations. To positively affect minority care, research must discover new knowledge relevant to specific ethnic groups.

2. The scientific research process contributes to our knowledge by describing, explaining, predicting, or controlling phenomena.[1]

   a) *Description*: A research study may simply describe a phenomenon or event in diabetes education. The use of the word *simply* is not to be taken lightly, for descriptive research can result in powerful contributions to diabetes education. For example, a study may yield data that describe the process by which elderly patients learn to use a glucose meter. Knowledge of this process can be integrated into teaching protocols so that elderly patients may benefit from specific teaching interventions. By describing the learning process for older adults, we may come to know how their learning processes differ from those of adolescents. Research aimed at describing phenomena or events may yield knowledge that can greatly affect the expenditure of time, money, energy, and resources in today's age of skyrocketing health care costs.

   b) *Explanation*: We know that elderly people differ in their ability to learn the use of a glucose meter. Why does this occur? By exploring key variables, research can offer insight into this difference and explain why some elderly people are better able to learn than others.

   c) *Prediction*: The power of research becomes more evident when the findings of a study yield predictive knowledge. Suppose a researcher wants to find any significant factors that may predict whether an older person will learn the correct use of a glucose meter. After collecting and analyzing the data, the researcher finds that a patient's educational level and socioeconomic status are significant predictors of patient learning outcomes. Assuming that the study design and implementation were appropriate and sound, this means that the higher a patient's level of education and socioeconomic status, the greater the likelihood of a successful learning outcome.

d) *Control*: Research can yield knowledge regarding factors that control phenomena or events. Suppose you had knowledge of one or more factors that, when controlled, could affect patient learning outcomes. Continuing with the example of elderly people learning to use a glucose meter, the clinical practitioner is not able to influence the ability of elderly patients to learn to use a glucose meter by changing their socioeconomic status. However, the educator may be able to improve outcomes by applying the results of a study that demonstrated that controlling the format and length of lecture presentation may influence patient outcomes.

E. The Research Process

1. This chapter is not intended to discuss all of the components in design and implementation of research. Many texts cover the basic fundamental descriptions, and others describe experimental designs and statistical analysis techniques. (A sampling of these texts is included in the suggested readings.) Instead, this chapter focuses on selected aspects of the research process — specifically, on those related to quantitative studies. Figure XXVI.1 presents an outline of the entire research process for your review.

2. The purpose of this discussion is twofold: (1) to illustrate selected aspects of the research process, and (2) to critically analyze these aspects as they are presented in research literature. This approach is designed to increase the application of research to practice.

FIGURE XXVI.1: The Process of Research

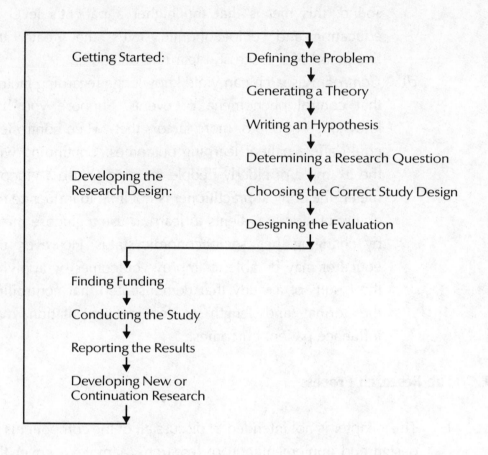

Getting Started:

Defining the Problem

↓

Generating a Theory

↓

Writing an Hypothesis

↓

Determining a Research Question

↓

Developing the
Research Design:

Choosing the Correct Study Design

↓

Designing the Evaluation

Finding Funding

↓

Conducting the Study

↓

Reporting the Results

↓

Developing New or
Continuation Research

Reprinted with permission: Aspen Publishers, Inc. from Handbook of Diabetes Nutritional Management, 1987.

a)   *Research Problem*: The research problem selected for exploration in any research study had its origins "somewhere."[7] In diabetes education, many research problems are identified within the practice setting in which clinicians function every day. Other research problems emerge from literature reviews. For example, gaps in knowledge become evident when you cannot find any published information on a particular problem you face in clinical practice, or when the published research does not apply to your patient population.

(1) Regardless of the source, the problem under investigation should be clearly stated in a research paper. The feasibility of studying the problem and the relevance of the problem to diabetes education should be evident in the research problem statement. The problem statement, in a nutshell, serves to justify the undertaking of a research study. When reading a research paper, ask yourself, Why was this study done? The paper should give you the answer, and that answer represents the research problem.

(2) The research problem statement typically leads directly to the purpose of the study. A specific purpose may not be explicitly stated. There should, however, be some indication of the reason(s) why the problem is worth exploring. Consider the following example:

Research problem statement: Elderly people with non-insulin-dependent diabetes mellitus (NIDDM) appear to have more difficulty learning correct use of a glucose meter than do younger adults. No published studies explore the effectiveness of small group lecture as a means of teaching blood glucose monitoring to older adults. The purpose of this study is to measure the benefits of small group instruction in teaching older adults the skill of blood glucose monitoring.

(3) The purpose of the study, in other words, is to test a method of teaching applied to a specific population. This simplified example represents how the research problem and the purpose of the study are related.

b) *Theoretical Framework*: Often published studies abbreviate the explanation of the theory guiding a study or exclude it because of space limitations. Instead, the theory is inferred from the review of the literature. It would be beneficial for research studies to explain/describe the theoretical framework that supports a line of study.

(1) When study outcomes are obtained, authors attempt to "make sense" of the findings within the larger scope of diabetes practice or diabetes education. Keep in mind that theory guides research.[8] Results obtained from research should be placed back in the context of the theory used to guide formal inquiry. Doing so greatly contributes to our knowledge base regarding the efficacy of our practice. When you read a research paper, part of your critical appraisal is based on whether you agree with the theory guiding the research study. Furthermore, do you agree with the manner in which the author has placed the context of the study within the stated theoretical framework?

In the research problem described above, findings from the exploratory study can best be understood if one knows the educational theory or principles that led the researcher to hypothesize that a small group lecture would be a viable approach to teaching older adults how to use a glucose meter. If this study was your idea and you had to justify its implementation to a colleague, part of that justification would include the efficacy of teaching strategies among older adults. Knowledge regarding those teaching strategies is derived from educational, teaching, and/or learning theory.

c) *Review of Literature*: A review of the pertinent literature serves several purposes.

(1) Published research represents one of the primary ways in which health care professionals stay informed about relevant research findings.

(2) Research literature is also a primary source of research problems.[3] In the last section of most research papers, where researchers discuss their findings, the authors often state what areas of research are still needed to better understand a phenomenon.

(3) The literature review included in research studies serves to justify the study. Authors should cite both supportive and opposing literature as well as the strengths and weaknesses of previous research studies. Sometimes different research studies on the same topic yield discrepant outcomes. Authors should discuss possible reasons for these discrepancies and state why their study provides a more viable means of addressing the research problem.

(4) The literature review should be organized and comprehensive, citing current references (past 3 to 5 years) related to the specific problem statement. Relevant classic studies may also be included. For example:

If a colleague asks, "Well, what is known about this problem? What does the literature suggest about effective teaching strategies for older adults?" you will be prepared to respond to your colleague because you have undertaken a review of the literature that lends support for the study.

(5) Literature reviews can be extremely time consuming, especially for the one who has to actually obtain the articles from the library. Reference librarians are equipped to conduct computerized literature searches based on key words, terms, or phrases, which they can help the researcher identify. Even if you are not actually conducting a research study, you may wish to review research papers of interest

or relevant to your practice setting.[8] The reference librarian is your best source of such information.

d) *Research Questions and Hypotheses*: In a research paper, the research questions and hypotheses are usually presented following the purpose statement. Research questions and hypotheses should clearly state and reflect the essence of a study.

(1) Research questions are statements of the characteristics, actions, or events to be studied and how they relate to each other.[1,6,9]

(2) Hypotheses are statements of the researcher's predictions of the answers to the research questions.[1,6,9] There should be no surprises in this section of a research paper.

Continuing the example of elderly people learning to use a glucose meter, in a descriptive study the research question might read: Does small group lecture significantly improve the skill of using a glucose meter among older adults with diabetes?

Suppose you encounter the following question: Does small group lecture significantly increase psychological stress among elderly people learning to use a glucose meter? You should be critical of this question because psychological stress has nothing to do with the research problem, purpose statement, education/learning theory, or review of literature described up to this point. Remember, the purpose of the study is to explore the efficacy of small group lecture, not psychological stress.

(3) When conducting research, questions and hypotheses should be drawn up before the study is initiated as they will guide the study design. They will also dictate the methodology and subsequent analysis of data.

e) *Study Design*: The structural blueprint of a research study is its design. The design involves a plan, structure, and strategy.[10-12]

(1) The design used in a research study should be consistent with, and appropriate for, the research problem under study. Many authors of research papers will explicitly state the research design used in their study. For example, "This study employed a one-group pretest/posttest. . .," or ". . .survey research methods were used. . .," or "a one-group repeated measures design was used."

(2) Before the actual implementation of a research study, a pilot test may be conducted to determine if the design of the study is practical and feasible for use.

(3) If a research design is not explicitly stated and you do not feel comfortable critiquing this aspect of a research paper, let intuition guide you. Go back to the stated research problem, purpose statement, and research questions and hypotheses. Does the study design appear to consistently address the problem? Does it help achieve the purpose of conducting the research? Does the design appear to offer a means of answering the research questions or testing the hypotheses?

(4) Numerous experimental and nonexperimental research designs within the domain of quantitative research are available for use in diabetes education. A review of the literature should provide information about how others have studied the same or similar topics. You are also encouraged to explore resources listed in the suggested readings at the end of this chapter.

(5) For any investigator, the evaluation and selection of an appropriate research design entails a sophisticated knowledge of the scientific method. Many health care professionals rely on consultants to assist them in planning a research study.

In the proposed research study of the effectiveness of small group lecture on helping elderly patients learn how to use a glucose meter, you may want to consult a researcher to help you design the study.

(6) Good sources of possible consultants are colleges and universities. Academicians are typically involved in research as an integral part of their job. Research consultants can also be found within hospital-based settings, as more hospitals are employing doctorally prepared researchers.

f) *Sample Group:* This is one of the most important aspects of a research study, particularly in the behavioral, educational, and social sciences, because research in these fields involves the use of a sample group from which data regarding the variables of interest are gathered.

(1) Sample groups are used for very practical reasons. For example:

It is not possible to gather and analyze data on every elderly person in this country. (All elderly people in the country represent the *target population*, that is, the population to which the outcomes of a study should apply.[1]) *Instead, a researcher would use a sample of elderly people, which ideally is representative of all elderly people in the country. A sample group is obtained from an accessible population of older adults, such as all older adults who attend your outpatient diabetes clinic. Supposedly these older adults from your outpatient clinic are representative of all elderly people with diabetes in the country. But are they? Probably not. Therefore, the ability of researchers to apply the findings of their study to the target population is threatened.*

(2) The ability to apply the findings of a study beyond the sample group used to obtain data is referred to as generalizability or *external validity*.[13] External validity means that researchers would like the results of their studies to be valid outside of (ie, external to) the sample group.

  (a) Many factors may threaten the external validity of a study including random versus nonrandom sampling, sampling bias, and convenience sampling.

  (b) The size of the sample group used in a research study is also very important. Generally, the larger the size of the sample group, the greater the chance of obtaining a more representative sample of the target population.[13]

(3) Measures can be incorporated into a study to enhance the representativeness of a sample group to its target population. In a research paper, these measures will usually be stated.

In your hypothetical study of elderly patients learning to use glucose meters, what sample of patients would be available for your use, considering your practice setting? How many patients would you study? (You would obtain a better representation of your patient population if you studied 100 patients rather than just 5.)

(4) Why are the concepts of sample group and external validity so important to you as a practitioner? Because, when reading a research paper that appears to yield significant results that could impact the quality or nature of care you provide your patients, you must consider whether your patients resemble those used in the research study. If your patients are different, the findings of the research study may not apply to your patients, or to your practice setting.

One example of weak external validity can be found in the cardiovascular-related studies that excluded women from participation. The findings from these studies can not be applied to both genders. This is not to say that the research was not significant, it was merely limited in its external validity by gender. Limiting research to an all-white population is another example of weak external validity of research. The results of such research are valid for the population studied. However, care should be used in applying the results to minority or other populations. Studies with questionable external validity may be excellent examples of studies to be replicated.

(5) Sampling is extremely important not only in designing a research study but in critically appraising it. To use research findings in practice requires an understanding of the strengths and limitations of study design and sampling procedures.[14]

g) *Evaluation and Instrumentation*: This aspect of research involves the means and measures used to obtain or gather data regarding the variables of study.[15,16]

Continuing the example of elderly people learning to use a glucose meter, what "instrument" would you propose to use to measure the learning — that is, the change in skill of the elderly patients after they have completed the small group lecture? Whatever the instrument, does it measure what it purports to measure? In other words, is it valid? In this case, you would like the instrument to measure skill in use of a glucose meter in elderly people with diabetes. You do not want an instrument that measures psychological stress in elderly patients. Psychological stress is not the primary variable of study — skill regarding use of a glucose meter is the variable of interest.

(1)   Any instrument, measuring tool, or device must be *valid*. Examples of instruments include attitude scales, diabetes knowledge tests, and biomedical devices. If an instrument to measure a variable is not available, an instrument may need to be developed. This tool should be tested in a pilot study to determine its validity.

(2)   *Reliability* of a measuring tool is also important. Reliability refers to the ability of an instrument to measure the variables of the research study each time the instrument is employed.[15] If you were to conduct the study of elderly patients learning to use a glucose meter and wished to assess their skill before and after a teaching session, you would administer the tool to measure their skill both times. Each time the tool is used, it must measure the variables under study. If the tool does not, then the instrument is not reliable.

(3)   As a general rule, a valid instrument will tend to be reliable. However, it is possible to have an instrument with good reliability but poor validity. For example, if you administer an instrument that does not measure glucose meter skill but measures psychological stress associated with self-monitoring of blood glucose levels, the instrument would be considered reliable but with poor validity. In other words, the tool measured psychological stress (good reliability) but did not measure the variable of interest — skill in use of a glucose meter.

(4)   A note of caution regarding instrumentation, especially in the educational and behavioral sciences. The establishment of validity and reliability of instruments, such as those that measure diabetes patient knowledge, is highly related to the sample/population in which the psychometric properties of the instrument were established.[15] If you administered a glucose meter skill test to elderly

patients using an instrument that was designed to measure meter skill in adolescents, the validity and reliability of the instrument may not be applicable with older adults unless tested with the elderly.

(5) This caveat also applies to the use of patient knowledge tests in various ethnic populations when the validity and reliability of the knowledge test was never established (ie, that particular ethnic group was never sampled). Language or cultural differences could change the validity and reliability of an instrument.

(6) One of the greatest areas of need in diabetes education research is the establishment of valid and reliable instruments to measure patient knowledge, behavioral practices, and other self-care skills. The research literature is replete with studies that include "diabetes patient knowledge" as a variable of study. However, a recent meta-analysis of diabetes education research conducted over a 30-year period revealed that the single most flawed methodological research problem associated with this line of study was the use of patient knowledge tests with no indices of the establishment of psychometric properties of validity and reliability.[17] With diabetes education based on providing patients with the self-care and problem-solving skills required to manage and control diabetes, a good deal of research attention is drawn to the need for more valid and reliable instruments.

F. Statistical Analysis of Data

1. Upon completion of data collection, researchers will statistically analyze the information obtained from subjects primarily to determine if the results of a study are *significant*.

    a) Statistical analysis of data involves a more sophisticated level of research knowledge. Typically, researchers employ a statistical consultant to assist them in the design and interpretation of statistical tests used to answer research questions or test research hypotheses.

b) When critically reading a research paper, let intuition guide you in this section of a reported study. Ask yourself if the statistical outcomes were consistent with the purpose of the study. Did the methods of data analysis answer the research questions or test the hypotheses? If the outcomes of a particular research study are of interest to you, you may want to obtain the help of a statistician in interpreting the analysis.

2. *Level of significance* is a statistical term used in research reports. Level of significance refers to the probability that a result, outcome, or finding occurs as a function of chance.[13] A .05 level of significance is most often used. What does this mean? Let's say that your study regarding the use of small group lecture yields "significant" outcomes regarding increased skill in accurate use of a glucose meter, with findings at the .05 level. In other words, there are 5 chances out of 100 that you would not find a real increase in skill or put another way, in 95 of the 100 times you conducted this study, you would find a true/real increase in older adults' skill in the use of a glucose meter. This same principle applies to other levels of significance. For example, the .01 level means that in 99 times out of 100, findings of a study are true; in 1 time out of 100, the results of the study would occur by chance alone.

3. The P value is another important factor in statistical tests. The P value represents the "probability" value associated with the study outcome.[18] If the P value is *less than* the level of significance, the findings of the study are statistically significant. Example: the level of skill regarding the use of a glucose meter increased 10 points among elderly people who participated in small group lecture versus elderly people who did not. The difference in skill between the two groups was associated with a P value equal to .0319. This value is less than .05, therefore

the difference between the groups is statistically significant. If the P value equals .0732, this value is greater than .05 and, therefore, not statistically significant.

G. Discussion of Research Results

1. Published research reports conclude with a discussion of the results of the study. Researchers will summarize the outcomes of their study and discuss the implications of their findings as they relate to clinical practice or knowledge of therapy or science.

    a) The discussion section of a research report should include how the current study relates to what is known about the topic of study from previous research studies conducted in the same area.

    b) Authors will typically include information about the "limitations" of their study — ie, areas of research design or methods of implementation that may have accounted for study outcomes. For example, outcomes of your study of glucose meter skill in elderly people may have resulted from the use of subjects who had previously attended a class on self-monitoring with a glucose meter versus subjects who had no prior training.

2. Limitations of a study can serve as fertile ground for the identification of research problems. If a study reports a methodological limitation, you may wish to propose conducting a study with a stronger methodological approach.

H. Increasing Your Research Role in Diabetes Education

1. The above discussion of selected aspects of the research process provides a sample of the breadth and scope of conducting or evaluating research. Additional elements in this process require their respective due attention to detail.

2.   Various methods can be used to facilitate the role of research in your diabetes education practice.

   a)   *Critically read research journals.* Professional publications serve as the primary means by which research is disseminated. In diabetes, *The Diabetes Educator* and *Diabetes Care* are examples of such publications. *The Diabetes Educator* includes a section on pertinent and relevant research abstracted for concise and succinct review. By consistently reading research papers, you increase your knowledge of research problems under study as well as those requiring further study; you learn about research methodology and design used to explore phenomena or events; you discover research outcomes that may be relevant to your practice; and you become aware of individuals actively engaged in conducting research in your area of interest.

   b)   *Attend professional meetings.* Regularly attend the local and annual meetings of specialty organizations. Professional conferences update knowledge relevant to diabetes education practice. Much of the information shared by speakers is research based whether it is specifically acknowledged as such or not. Furthermore, professional conferences may offer research seminars in which active researchers present their findings for discussion. If so, then you have a unique opportunity to ask questions about any facet of the research process used by the researcher.

   c)   *Attend journal club presentations.* Journal clubs are designed for the purpose of critically appraising one or more research-based publications. Try to attend these consistently even if the topics presented are not within the scope of your interest or practice. Journal clubs are helpful because research is critically appraised, including the means of identifying and assessing the research problem, the research methods/design, the statistical analysis techniques, and the implications for practice. Participating in these clubs increases your exposure to the research process, thereby increasing your knowledge. If a journal club is not available in your area, consider starting one. Choosing a topic relevant to a current practice issue often increases involvement in the journal club.

d) *Continue your formal education.* Higher, or advanced, education is structured to increase the knowledge and skill of the student in theory and research. If you do not have an advanced degree such as a master's or doctorate, consider auditing a research course at a local university or college. Courses may be available to you as a "nondegree" student as well. Varying levels of research knowledge and skill are embodied in higher degree courses; one of these courses may be helpful to you in the translation of research to practice.

e) *Attend patient grand rounds.* Grand rounds typically represent a "case study" in which virtually all dimensions of the research problem-solving process are evident. Presenters identify a patient's medical problem, along with assessment data supporting their diagnosis; discuss clinical approaches to address the problem; describe the implementation of the plan of care; and discuss the outcomes of care. Furthermore, clinical outcomes are discussed from a research perspective. Outcomes are considered on the basis of what is "known" about the phenomenon, thereby often requiring a discussion of previous research in the clinical field. Patient grand rounds are a common feature in medicine. Any discipline or disciplines working together can initiate patient grand rounds to discuss any phenomenon related to a particular professional field.

f) *Collaboration and consultation.* Research is never undertaken by just one person. Even people considered to be the most advanced researchers involve a number of collaborators and consultants in their research programs. Consultants are used for various reasons.

(1) They have expertise in a certain facet of research methodology.

(2) They have expertise in cultural/ethnic dimensions affecting patient care.

(3) They have expertise in selected theoretical approaches to the study of research variables.

(4) They have knowledge of selected statistical approaches.

(a) Many individuals hold expert knowledge in any given domain of the research process. Find out who these experts are and seek their assistance. If your level of interest is to interpret research findings from a particular study because of possible clinical significance to your patient population, contact someone at a local college or university for assistance.

I. Summary

1. Research is, fundamentally, a problem-solving process using a scientific approach — a process that we, as clinical practitioners, engage in many times during the course of our day. Knowledge of the research process is a core requirement for diabetes educators. The problem-solving approach provides us with "knowledge" regarding the efficacy of teaching interventions. Knowledge serves as the most important outcome derived from use of the problem-solving approach. So, too, is the role of knowledge as the outcome of formal research.

2. The formal research process represents systematic, careful examination of phenomena or events that are postulated to be associated with any given facet of diabetes patient care. The implementation of formal research aims to increase and expand our knowledge of diabetes and educational interventions. Research findings provide knowledge in the form of descriptions and explanations that help us better understand our methods of educational practice and the outcomes of our teaching interventions. As diabetes health care professionals, we are all involved in the research process. This involvement

ranges from facilitating another's research program, to conducting an independent research study, to critically appraising the research literature. By enhancing our knowledge of research, we increase our appreciation of its role in the provision of quality and effective patient care.

3. Research is the foundation of diabetes care. Our role as health care professionals is to maximize the contributions of research to practice by implementing our knowledge of the ways and means to improve patient care in settings where patients receive care.

REFERENCES

1.   Polit DF, Hungler BP. Nursing research: principles and methods. Philadelphia: Lippincott, 1991.

2.   Keeves JP. Knowledge diffusion in education. In: Keeves JP, ed. Educational research methodology and measurement: an international handbook. New York: Pergamon Press, 1988:211-19.

3.   Mateo MA, Kirchoff KT. Conducting and using nursing research in the clinical setting. Baltimore: Williams & Wilkins, 1991.

4.   Morse JM. Qualitative nursing research: a contemporary dialogue. Rockville, Md: Aspen Systems Corp, 1989.

5.   Lincoln YS, Guba EG. Naturalistic inquiry. Beverly Hills, Calif: Sage Publications, 1985.

6.   Ary D, Jacobs LC, Razavich A. Introduction to research in education. New York: Holt, Rinehart & Winston, 1990.

7.   Wheeler ML, Fineberg N. An introduction to research. In: Powers MA, ed. Handbook of diabetes nutritional management. Rockville, Md: Aspen Publishers, 1987:433-37.

8.   Strauch K, Linton R, Cohen C. Library research guide to nursing. Ann Arbor, Mich: Pierian Press, 1989.

9.   Nieswiadomy RM. Foundations of nursing research. Norwalk, Conn: Appleton & Lange, 1993.

10.   Kazdin AE. Methodological issues and strategies in clinical research. Washington, DC: American Psychological Association, 1992.

11.   Rubinson L, Neutens JJ. Research techniques for the health sciences. New York: Macmillan, 1987.

12. Aronson E, Ellsworth PC, Carlsmith JM, Gonzales MH. Methods of research in social psychology. New York: McGraw-Hill, 1990.

13. LoBiondo-Wood G, Haber J. Nursing research: methods, critical appraisal, and utilization. St. Louis: CV Mosby, 1990.

14. Meinert CL. A critical eye: the science of reading clinical research papers. Diabetes Spectrum 1988;1:13-15.

15. Waltz CF, Strickland OL, Lenz ER. Measurement in nursing research. Philadelphia: FA Davis, 1991.

16. Digman MB. Measurement and evaluation of health education. Springfield, Ill: Charles C Thomas, 1989.

17. Brown SA. Quality of reporting in diabetes patient education research: 1954-1986. Res Nurs Health 1990;13:53-62.

18. Schott S. Statistics for health professionals. Philadelphia: WB Saunders, 1990.

SELF-REVIEW QUESTIONS

If you are unsure of the answers to the following questions, please review the materials.

1.   List two ways that diabetes educators participate in research.
2.   Define two basic types of scientific research.
3.   State the three purposes of research.
4.   Describe two aspects of the research process that can be applied to critical appraisal of a research study.
5.   List two ways to build a research-based practice.

OTHER SUGGESTED READINGS

Digman MB. Measurement and evaluation of health education. Springfield, Ill: Charles C Thomas, 1989.

Kelly LJ. Dimensions of professional nursing. 6th ed. New York: Pergamon Press, 1991.

Monson ER. Research: successful approaches. Chicago: American Dietetic Association, 1992.

Pasovac ER, Corey RG. Program evaluation: methods and case studies. Englewoods Cliffs, NJ: Simon & Schuster, 1992.

Strauch K, Linton R, Cohen C. Library research guide to nursing. Ann Arbor, Mich: Pierian Press, 1989.

Waltz CF, Strickland OL, Lenz ER. Measurement in nursing research. 2nd ed. Philadelphia: FA Davis Co, 1991.

Wylie-Rosett J, Wheeler M, Krueger K, Halford B. Opportunities for research-oriented dietitians. J Am Diet Assoc, 1990;90:1531-34.

INDEX